Artificial Intelligence in Clinical
Medical Imaging

Artificial Intelligence in Clinical Medical Imaging

Editor

Daniele Giansanti

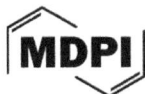

Basel • Beijing • Wuhan • Barcelona • Belgrade • Novi Sad • Cluj • Manchester

Editor
Daniele Giansanti
Centro nazionale per le
tecnologie innovative in
sanità pubblica
ISS
Rome
Italy

Editorial Office
MDPI
St. Alban-Anlage 66
4052 Basel, Switzerland

This is a reprint of articles from the Special Issue published online in the open access journal *Diagnostics* (ISSN 2075-4418) (available at: www.mdpi.com/journal/diagnostics/special_issues/3FXN9682V0).

For citation purposes, cite each article independently as indicated on the article page online and as indicated below:

Lastname, A.A.; Lastname, B.B. Article Title. *Journal Name* **Year**, *Volume Number*, Page Range.

ISBN 978-3-7258-0876-2 (Hbk)
ISBN 978-3-7258-0875-5 (PDF)
doi.org/10.3390/books978-3-7258-0875-5

© 2024 by the authors. Articles in this book are Open Access and distributed under the Creative Commons Attribution (CC BY) license. The book as a whole is distributed by MDPI under the terms and conditions of the Creative Commons Attribution-NonCommercial-NoDerivs (CC BY-NC-ND) license.

Contents

About the Editor vii

Preface ix

Daniele Giansanti
Joint Expedition: Exploring Clinical Medical Imaging and Artificial Intelligence as a Team Integration
Reprinted from: *Diagnostics* **2024**, *14*, 584, doi:10.3390/diagnostics14060584 1

Antonia Pirrera and Daniele Giansanti
Human–Machine Collaboration in Diagnostics: Exploring the Synergy in Clinical Imaging with Artificial Intelligence
Reprinted from: *Diagnostics* **2023**, *13*, 2162, doi:10.3390/diagnostics13132162 8

Clerimar Paulo Bragança, José Manuel Torres, Luciano Oliveira Macedo and Christophe Pinto de Almeida Soares
Advancements in Glaucoma Diagnosis: The Role of AI in Medical Imaging
Reprinted from: *Diagnostics* **2024**, *14*, 530, doi:10.3390/diagnostics14050530 12

Pao-Chun Lin, Wei-Shan Chang, Kai-Yuan Hsiao, Hon-Man Liu, Ben-Chang Shia, Ming-Chih Chen, et al.
Development of a Machine Learning Algorithm to Correlate Lumbar Disc Height on X-rays with Disc Bulging or Herniation
Reprinted from: *Diagnostics* **2024**, *14*, 134, doi:10.3390/diagnostics14020134 26

Shu Wu, Hang Yu, Cuiping Li, Rencheng Zheng, Xueqin Xia, Chengyan Wang and He Wang
A Coarse-to-Fine Fusion Network for Small Liver Tumor Detection and Segmentation: A Real-World Study
Reprinted from: *Diagnostics* **2023**, *13*, 2504, doi:10.3390/diagnostics13152504 40

Daniele Giansanti
AI-Enabled Fusion of Medical Imaging, Behavioral Analysis and Other Systems for Enhanced Autism Spectrum Disorder. Comment on Jönemo, J.; Abramian, D.; Eklund, A. Evaluation of Augmentation Methods in Classifying Autism Spectrum Disorders from fMRI Data with 3D Convolutional Neural Networks. *Diagnostics* 2023, 13, 2773
Reprinted from: *Diagnostics* **2023**, *13*, 3545, doi:10.3390/diagnostics13233545 52

Daniele Giansanti
An Umbrella Review of the Fusion of fMRI and AI in Autism
Reprinted from: *Diagnostics* **2023**, *13*, 3552, doi:10.3390/diagnostics13233552 55

Marijana Stanojević Pirković, Ognjen Pavić, Filip Filipović, Igor Saveljić, Tijana Geroski, Themis Exarchos and Nenad Filipović
Fractional Flow Reserve-Based Patient Risk Classification
Reprinted from: *Diagnostics* **2023**, *13*, 3349, doi:10.3390/diagnostics13213349 84

P. Kiran Rao, Subarna Chatterjee, M. Janardhan, K. Nagaraju, Surbhi Bhatia Khan, Ahlam Almusharraf and Abdullah I. Alharbe
Optimizing Inference Distribution for Efficient Kidney Tumor Segmentation Using a UNet-PWP Deep-Learning Model with XAI on CT Scan Images
Reprinted from: *Diagnostics* **2023**, *13*, 3244, doi:10.3390/diagnostics13203244 99

Ashwini B., Manjit Kaur, Dilbag Singh, Satyabrata Roy and Mohammed Amoon
Efficient Skip Connections-Based Residual Network (ESRNet) for Brain Tumor Classification
Reprinted from: *Diagnostics* **2023**, *13*, 3234, doi:10.3390/diagnostics13203234 . . . . **116**

Yi-You Chen, Po-Nien Yu, Yung-Chi Lai, Te-Chun Hsieh and Da-Chuan Cheng
Bone Metastases Lesion Segmentation on Breast Cancer Bone Scan Images with Negative Sample Training
Reprinted from: *Diagnostics* **2023**, *13*, 3042, doi:10.3390/diagnostics13193042 . . . . **134**

Hui Wu, Jing Zhao, Jiehui Li, Yan Zeng, Weiwei Wu, Zhuhuang Zhou, et al.
One-Stage Detection without Segmentation for Multi-Type Coronary Lesions in Angiography Images Using Deep Learning
Reprinted from: *Diagnostics* **2023**, *13*, 3011, doi:10.3390/diagnostics13183011 . . . . **153**

Johan Jönemo, David Abramian and Anders Eklund
Evaluation of Augmentation Methods in Classifying Autism Spectrum Disorders from fMRI Data with 3D Convolutional Neural Networks
Reprinted from: *Diagnostics* **2023**, *13*, 2773, doi:10.3390/diagnostics13172773 . . . . **170**

Usharani Bhimavarapu, Nalini Chintalapudi and Gopi Battineni
Automatic Detection and Classification of Diabetic Retinopathy Using the Improved Pooling Function in the Convolution Neural Network
Reprinted from: *Diagnostics* **2023**, *13*, 2606, doi:10.3390/diagnostics13152606 . . . . **180**

About the Editor

Daniele Giansanti

Dr. Giansanti received an MD in Electronic Engineering at Sapienza University, Rome, in 1991; a PHD in Telecommunications and Microelectronics Engineering at Tor Vergata University, Rome, in 1997; an Academic Specialization in Cognitive Psychology and Neural Networks at Sapienza University, Rome, in 1997; and a Specialization in Medical Physics at Sapienza University, Rome, in 2005.

Dr. Giansanti was in charge of the Design of VLSI Asics for DSP in the Civil Field (1991–1997) during his MD and PHD, and he served as a CAE-CAD-CAM System Manager and Design Engineer in the project of electronic systems (Boards and VLSI) for the Warfare at Elettronica spa (1992–2000), one of the leaders in the military field.

More importantly, he also conducts varied research at ISS (the Italian NIH) (2000–today) in the following fields: (1) biomedical engineering and medical physics with the development of wearable and portable devices (three national patents); (2) telemedicine and e-health: technology assessment and the integration of new systems in the field of telerehabilitation, domiciliary monitoring, digital pathology, and digital radiology; (3) Mhealth: recent interest in the integration of smartphones and tablet technology in health care with particular interest in the opportunities and the relevant problems of risks, abuse, and regulation; (4) the acceptance of, and consensus in, the use of robots for assistance and rehabilitation; (5) challenges in, and the acceptance of, the use of artificial intelligence in digital radiology and digital pathology; and (6) cybersecurity in the health domain.

Dr. Giansanti is a Professor at Sapienza and Catholic University in Rome and a tutor of theses. He is a Board Editor and reviewer for several journals. He has 171 publications indexed on Scopus and numerous scientific contributions, such as monographies, chapters, congress papers, and Special Issues.

Preface

The rapid evolution of clinical medical imaging in recent years has been nothing short of extraordinary, driven largely by the integration of artificial intelligence (AI) techniques. This convergence of technology and medicine holds immense promise, poised to revolutionize clinical practices by offering more accurate, efficient, and personalized diagnoses and treatments than ever before.

We find ourselves amidst a revolutionary metamorphosis in the landscape of clinical imaging, with every sector feeling the profound impact of AI integration. The infusion of AI in this field of the health domain signifies not merely a surface-level enhancement, but a fundamental reshaping of its technological fabric.

In the midst of these transformative developments, it is paramount to recognize the dual focus required, i.e., not only on the driving force of scientific and technological innovation instigated by AI, but also on the intricate process of seamlessly embedding AI into the broader health domain. This integration is not just a matter of technological advancement but a strategic imperative aimed at optimizing healthcare practices, enhancing diagnostic accuracy, streamlining workflows, and ultimately elevating the abilities of clinical imaging to unprecedented heights within the dynamic landscape of modern medical science.

In response to these considerations, we introduced a Special Issue, entitled "Artificial Intelligence in Clinical Medical Imaging", now presented in a reprint. This initiative aims to comprehensively outline ongoing developments, share established experiences, explore prospects, and highlight persisting challenges in this dynamic field. The Special Issue represents a significant milestone, featuring 14 contributions, each offering unique insights and perspectives.

These contributions, categorized into editorials, full scientific articles, reviews, and commentaries, collectively reflect the breadth and depth of AI's impact on clinical medical imaging. From foundational concepts to cutting-edge applications, each contribution contributes to our understanding and advancement in this critical area of healthcare.

We extend our sincere gratitude to all contributors for their invaluable insights and efforts which have made this Special Issue possible. It is our hope that the knowledge shared within these pages will inspire further innovation, collaboration, and ultimately improved patient care.

My sincere thanks goes to Dennis Zhu, who provided exceptional support in every phase of the creation of this collection.

Daniele Giansanti
Editor

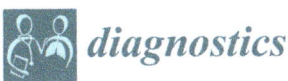

Editorial

Joint Expedition: Exploring Clinical Medical Imaging and Artificial Intelligence as a Team Integration

Daniele Giansanti

Centro Nazionale Tecnologie Innovative in Sanità Pubblica, Istituto Superiore di Sanità, Via Regina Elena 299, 00161 Roma, Italy; daniele.giansanti@iss.it

Citation: Giansanti, D. Joint Expedition: Exploring Clinical Medical Imaging and Artificial Intelligence as a Team Integration. *Diagnostics* 2024, 14, 584. https://doi.org/10.3390/diagnostics14060584

Received: 29 February 2024
Accepted: 8 March 2024
Published: 10 March 2024

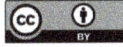

Copyright: © 2024 by the author. Licensee MDPI, Basel, Switzerland. This article is an open access article distributed under the terms and conditions of the Creative Commons Attribution (CC BY) license (https://creativecommons.org/licenses/by/4.0/).

1. The Joint Expedition Exploring Clinical Medical Imaging and Artificial Intelligence

The field of clinical medical imaging has seen remarkable advancements in recent years, particularly with the introduction of artificial intelligence (AI) techniques. AI has the potential to revolutionize clinical medical imaging by enabling more accurate, efficient, and personalized diagnoses and treatments.

The landscape of clinical imaging is currently undergoing a revolutionary metamorphosis (contribution 1), with every sector impacted by the integration of artificial intelligence (AI). This paradigm shift is not confined to one specific domain but spans the diverse realms of medical imaging, encompassing imaging diagnostics for organs and functionality [1,2], the dynamic field of digital pathology (encompassing both cytology and digital histology) [3,4], the intricacies of digital dermatology [5,6], and various other niches within the expansive field of clinical imaging.

The infusion of AI into these sectors is not merely a superficial addition but a fundamental reshaping of their technological fabric. The integration processes, fuelled by advancements in AI technologies, experienced a noteworthy acceleration, with the upheavals brought about by the COVID-19 pandemic further propelling this momentum [7,8].

In the face of these transformative developments, it becomes increasingly crucial to direct attention not only towards the driving force of scientific and technological innovation instigated by AI but also towards the intricate process of embedding AI seamlessly into the broader health domain. This integration is pivotal not just for the sake of technological advancement but as a strategic imperative to optimize healthcare practices, enhance diagnostic accuracy, streamline workflows, and ultimately elevate the capabilities of clinical imaging to new heights within the dynamic landscape of modern medical science.

In light of these considerations, we introduced a Special Issue entitled Artificial Intelligence in Clinical Medical Imaging: https://www.mdpi.com/journal/diagnostics/special_issues/3FXN9682V0, accessed on 29 February 2024.

The objective was to comprehensively outline the ongoing developments, share established experiences, explore prospects, and highlight persisting challenges in this dynamic field.

The Special Issue successfully achieved a significant milestone, featuring 13 contributions (Co)s (excluding this editorial) (Co. 1–Co. 13).

The published papers, according to the selected categories, encompass 1 introductory editorial (Co. 1), 10 full scientific articles (Co. 2–Co. 11), 1 review (Co. 12), and 1 comment (Co. 13).

2. Conclusive Discoveries: A Closer Look at the Contributions

2.1. An Overview of the Contributions

Below, we present a concise overview encapsulating the key points and insights from the contributions featured in the special issue. This summary aims to provide a brief yet comprehensive glimpse into the diverse and impactful content published within this specialized collection.

2.1.1. Pirrera, A. et al. (Co. 1): Exploring the Synergy in Clinical Imaging with Artificial Intelligence

The Editorial by Pirrera and Giansanti (Co. 1) introduced the aims of the SI and reflected on the progress and status of the introduction of AI into clinical medical artificial intelligence. The focus was on assessing the current state and briefly exploring both the evolution and the recent trends. The editorial introduced the need for an initiative Special Issue and suggested fields and directions for exploration.

The 12 contributions (Co. 2–13) covered various topics of interest to the SI. Below are detailed the focus and a brief excerpt of the content.

2.1.2. Lin, P.-C. et al. (Co. 2): Machine Learning for Lumbar Disc Height Correlation on X-rays

The study focuses on lumbar disc bulging or herniation (LDBH), a major cause of spinal issues necessitating surgery. Due to limited access to MRI, lumbar X-rays are explored for diagnostic support. Analyzing 458 patients, machine learning methods identify key predictors, with L4-5 posterior disc height, age, and L1-2 anterior disc height emerging as crucial factors. A decision tree algorithm is proposed as a valuable tool for clinical decision-making by surgeons. The study underscores the importance of machine learning-based decision tools, particularly highlighting the role of L1-2-disc height in the context of LDBH. Future research aims to develop a comprehensive decision-support model.

2.1.3. Stanojević Pirković, M. et al. (Co. 3): Fractional Flow Reserve-Based Patient Risk Classification

The study addresses the global impact of cardiovascular diseases (CVDs), emphasizing the significance of preventing and detecting risks, particularly focusing on acute myocardial infarction (AMI) responsible for 3 million deaths annually. The research aims to develop a technique using fractional flow reserve (FFR) measurements for patient evaluation and predicting the risk of death. A random forest machine learning model is employed, achieving a 76.21% prediction accuracy, with mean accuracies ranging from 74.1% to 83.6% across different test sample sizes. Additionally, a numerical approach involving the 3D reconstruction of coronary arteries for stenosis monitoring is implemented, showing promising results even with limited data. The study suggests that future improvements can be achieved by incorporating additional data, enabling the exploration of different machine learning algorithms.

2.1.4. Rao, P.K. et al. (Co. 4): Efficient Kidney Tumor Segmentation with UNet-PWP Deep-Learning Model on CT Scan Images

This study addresses the complexity of early detection in kidney tumors, introducing the UNet-PWP architecture tailored for efficient segmentation. Notably, adaptive partitioning breaks down the UNet architecture into smaller submodels, optimizing computational resources. The model incorporates pre-trained weights, boosting its capacity for intricate tasks, and employs weight pruning for further efficiency without compromising performance. The evaluation against the DeepLab V3+ model on the "KiTs 19, 21, and 23" kidney tumor dataset demonstrates the UNet-PWP model's outstanding 97.01% accuracy on both training and test datasets, outperforming the DeepLab V3+ model. To enhance interpretability, the study fuses attention and Grad-CAM XAI methods, providing valuable insights into decision-making and critical regions of interest. This interpretability is crucial for healthcare professionals to trust and understand the model's reasoning, making the UNet-PWP architecture a promising advancement in kidney tumor segmentation.

2.1.5. Kaur, M. et al. (Co. 5): ESRNet for Efficient Brain Tumor Classification

This paper introduces an Efficient Skip Connections-Based Residual Network (ESRNet) to address challenges in brain tumor classification using deep learning. ESRNet utilizes ResNet with skip connections to overcome limitations like vanishing gradient issues. It employs multiple stages with increasing residual blocks for enhanced feature learning and pattern recognition. The architecture ensures smooth gradient flow during training, preventing information loss. ESRNet integrates downsampling techniques and batch normalization for robust performance. Experimental results demonstrate ESRNet's superior accuracy, sensitivity, specificity, F-score, and Kappa statistics, with median values of 99.62%, 99.68%, 99.89%, 99.47%, and 99.42%, respectively. The proposed ESRNet showcases exceptional efficiency in brain tumor classification, offering potential advancements in clinical diagnosis and treatment planning.

2.1.6. Chen, Y.-Y. et al. (Co. 6): Bone Metastases Segmentation on Breast Cancer Bone Scans

This study focuses on employing deep learning for the automatic detection and quantification of bone metastases in bone scan images, providing clinical assistance in diagnosis. Using an internal dataset of breast and prostate cancer patients, the study adopts the Double U-Net model with modifications for multi-class segmentation. Techniques like Otsu thresholding, negative mining, background pre-processing, and transfer learning are employed to enhance model performance. Through 10-fold cross-validation, the best model achieves a precision of 69.96%, a sensitivity of 63.55%, and an F1-score of 66.60%. Compared to the baseline model, this represents improvements of 8.40%, 0.56%, and 4.33%, respectively. The developed system holds the potential for providing pre-diagnostic reports to aid physicians in final decisions and calculating the bone scan index (BSI) when combined with bone skeleton segmentation.

2.1.7. Wu, H. et al. (Co. 7): One-Stage Detection for Multi-Type Coronary Lesions with Deep Learning

This study introduces a rare approach using a one-stage model, YOLOv5, for the automatic detection of coronary lesions without segmentation. Enrolling 200 patients with significant coronary issues, the images were categorized into two views. YOLOv5 demonstrated precision, recall, mAP@0.1, and mAP@0.5 at the image level, with values ranging from 0.66 to 0.73. At the patient level, the model exhibited precision, recall, and F1 scores, ranging from 0.64 to 0.65 and 0.91 to 0.94. YOLOv5 performed best for Chronic Total Occlusion (CTO) and Local Stenosis (LS) lesions. The study concludes that YOLOv5 is feasible for automatic coronary lesion detection, particularly for LS and CTO types.

2.1.8. Jönemo, J. et al. (Co. 8): Augmentation Methods for Autism Classification with 3D CNN

This study explores the application of deep learning to resting-state functional MRI data for classifying subjects as healthy or having autism spectrum disorder. Notably, the focus is on investigating the impact of various 3D augmentation techniques on test accuracy. Using derivatives from 1112 subjects in the ABIDE dataset, a 3D Convolutional Neural Network (CNN) is trained. The findings reveal that while augmentation is employed, it only leads to minor improvements in test accuracy. This highlights the limited impact of 3D augmentation in enhancing classification performance in the context of neuroimaging data.

2.1.9. Bhimavarapu, U. et al. (Co. 9): Automatic Diabetic Retinopathy Detection with CNN

This study focuses on the diagnosis of Diabetic Retinopathy (DR), a diabetes-associated eye disease with the potential for blindness. Employing deep learning for automatic DR diagnosis from fundus images, the study introduces an enhanced Convolutional Neural Network (CNN) model. The improved model incorporates a novel pooling function within the ResNet-50 architecture, aiming to increase diagnostic accuracy while reducing computational complexity and processing time. Trained and tested on APTOS and Kaggle datasets, the proposed model achieves impressive accuracies of 98.32% and 98.71%, respectively. The comparative analysis highlights the superior performance of the proposed model in DR diagnosis when compared to state-of-the-art approaches with retinal fundus images.

2.1.10. Wu, S. et al. (Co. 10): Coarse-to-Fine Fusion Network for Small Liver Tumor Detection

This paper presents a novel approach for liver tumor semantic segmentation in medical image analysis, focusing on small tumors across various sizes. The proposed method integrates a detection module and a CSR (convolution-SE-residual) module, featuring a convolution block, an SE module, and a residual module for fine segmentation. Evaluating a private liver MRI dataset with 3605 tumors, including 3273 smaller than 3.0 cm, the method outperforms single-stage end-to-end networks and fusion networks, demonstrating superiority over 3D UNet and nnU-Net. In testing on 44 images, the proposed method achieves an average Dice similarity coefficient (DSC) and recall of 86.9% and 86.7%, respectively, surpassing comparison methods. Notably, for small objects (<10 mm), the proposed approach sets a state-of-the-art performance with a Dice score of 85.3% and a malignancy detection rate of 87.5%.

2.1.11. Bragança, C.P. et al. (Co. 11): Advancements in AI for Glaucoma Diagnosis

This article delves into the increasing role of artificial intelligence (AI) algorithms in digital image processing and the automated diagnosis of glaucoma, a significant eye disease. It provides an overview of glaucoma types, traditional diagnostic methods, and the global epidemiology of the disease. The focus is on how AI algorithms can potentially aid in early glaucoma diagnosis through population screening. The related work section explores key studies and methodologies utilizing AI for the automatic classification of glaucoma from digital fundus images. It also highlights the main databases with labeled glaucoma images available for training machine learning algorithms.

2.1.12. Giansanti, D. (Co. 12): Umbrella Review of fMRI and AI Fusion in Autism

This study conducts an umbrella review analyzing emerging themes in the integration of Functional Magnetic Resonance Imaging (fMRI) and artificial intelligence (AI) in autism diagnosis. Utilizing a structured process, it reviews 20 systematic reviews, emphasizing the significance of technological integration, especially fMRI and AI. The study acknowledges the potential in this field while recognizing challenges and limitations. It notes a growing emphasis on AI research but highlights the need for attention to healthcare process integration, including regulation, acceptance, informed consent, and data security. The study suggests focusing on health domain integration for routine implementation of these applications, pointing out the promising yet unexplored area of integration into personalized medicine (PM) in autism research.

2.1.13. Giansanti, D. (Co. 13): AI-Enabled Fusion for Enhanced Autism Spectrum Disorder Diagnosis

The proposal is a comment on contribution 8. It underscores the substantial enhancement achieved in the realms of diagnosis and classification through the incorporation of 3D augmentation. This augmentation, when synergistically combined with artificial intelligence (AI) and Functional Magnetic Resonance Imaging (fMRI), presents a formidable approach. The integration of these technologies not only elevates the accuracy and efficacy of diagnostic processes but also holds the potential to unravel more nuanced insights into the intricacies of the data, thereby further refining our understanding and application of advanced medical imaging techniques.

2.2. Conclusive Global Reflection

All the works have made noteworthy contributions to the field of clinical medical imaging, particularly at the intersection with AI. These contributions provide valuable insights and innovative approaches, enhancing our understanding of how AI can improve medical imaging processes. The integration of artificial intelligence highlighted in these studies has practical implications for advancing diagnostic accuracy, efficiency, and overall capabilities in the realm of clinical medical imaging, signifying a significant step forward in this domain.

3. Common Message, Key Emerging Themes, and Suggestions for a Broader Investigation

3.1. Common Messages

Twelve distinct contributions (Co. 2–13) weave through the intricate field of medical research focused on the integration of clinical medical imaging with AI. These studies, spanning diverse medical domains, collectively leverage several AI approaches, making an important contribution to the landscape of medical diagnostics.

Commencing with lumbar disc exploration (Co. 2), the ensemble progresses into the cardiovascular sector (Co. 3), where a novel technique employing fractional flow reserve measurements proves adept at predicting patient risks. Kidney tumor detection takes a prominent role in Co. 4, introducing an architecture optimizing computational resources with impressive accuracy. In the cerebral domain of brain tumor classification (Co. 5), ESRNet showcases notable accuracy. Transitioning to bone metastases segmentation (Co. 6), a Double U-Net model enhances precision and sensitivity. A revolutionary note emerges in Co. 7, where a one-stage model (YOLOv5) redefines coronary lesion detection, excelling in specific lesion types. Co. 8 delves into autism classification, shedding light on the nuanced effectiveness of 3D augmentation techniques.

Ocular health comes to the fore both in Co. 9 and Co. 11. Co. 9 presents an improved ResNet-50 model for Diabetic Retinopathy diagnosis with remarkable accuracy, while Co. 11 investigates the application of AI in glaucoma diagnosis. Co. 10 introduces a novel semantic segmentation approach for liver tumors, outperforming existing models, particularly in segmenting small objects. Co. 12, an umbrella review, delves into fMRI and AI integration for autism diagnosis, recognizing potential and addressing challenges.

The last contribution, Co. 13 provides a perspective, underscoring the enhancement achieved through 3D augmentation, AI, and fMRI integration. This fusion refines diagnostic accuracy and unravels nuanced insights into advanced clinical medical imaging techniques, marking a moment in the evolution of medical diagnostics.

3.2. Suggestions for a Broader Investigation and Key Emerging Themes

From the overview, it is also possible to detect the emerging themes and the suggestions for a broader investigation.

The collective contributions (Co. 2–13) encompass diverse facets of medical imaging, showcasing the evolving landscape of artificial intelligence in healthcare. Lin et al. (Co. 2) illuminate lumbar disc issues through machine learning, prompting collaborative endeavors across orthopedics and technology. Stanojević Pirković's work (Co. 3) on cardiovascular diseases encourages merging datasets for a holistic approach. Rao et al. (Co. 4) advocate for transparent kidney tumor segmentation models, emphasizing interpretability to instill trust. Efficient Brain Tumor Classification (Co. 5) prompts exploration of real-world applications, while ESRNet (Co. 6) advocates personalized medicine integration.

Chen et al. (Co. 7) propose one-stage models for coronary lesion detection, urging longitudinal studies. Jönemo's insights (Co. 8) on autism classification with 3D CNNs suggest collaborative human–AI analysis. Bhimavarapu's study (Co. 9) emphasizes scalable AI models for Diabetic Retinopathy screening. Ethical considerations in liver tumor detection (Co. 10) underscore the need for responsible AI use. Glaucoma diagnosis (Co. 11) pushes for patient-centric AI integration, acknowledging diverse perspectives. The Umbrella Review (Co. 12) highlights the potential of fusing fMRI and AI in autism with calls for ethical healthcare integration. The comment (Co. 13) applauds the synergy of 3D augmentation, AI, and fMRI, envisioning nuanced insights into medical imaging's intricacies.

Through this experience, we identified noteworthy dominant themes, which are detailed in Table 1, along with the reference contributions. These discerned themes can serve as valuable inspiration for fellow researchers delving into this field.

Table 1. Dominant emerging theme by article.

Themes	Description	Studies
Spinal and Skeletal Insights	Machine Learning for Lumbar Disc Height Correlation on X-rays. Bone Metastases Segmentation on Breast Cancer Bone Scans.	(Co. 2) (Co. 6)
Cardiovascular Precision	Fractional Flow Reserve-Based Patient Risk Classification. One-Stage Detection for Multi-Type Coronary Lesions with Deep Learning.	(Co. 3) (Co. 7)
Renal and Hepatic tumor detection/segmentation	Efficient Kidney Tumor Segmentation with UNet-PWP Deep-Learning Model on CT Scan Images. Coarse-to-Fine Fusion Network for Small Liver Tumor Detection.	(Co. 4) (Co.10)
Neurological Exploration	ESRNet for Efficient Brain Tumor Classification. Augmentation Methods for Autism Classification with 3D CNN. AI-Enabled Fusion for Enhanced Autism Spectrum Disorder Diagnosis.	(Co. 5) (Co. 8) (Co. 13)
Ocular Health Focus	Co. 9: Automatic Diabetic Retinopathy Detection with CNN. Co. 11: Advancements in AI for Glaucoma Diagnosis	(Co. 9) (Co. 11)
AI and fMRI	Umbrella Review of fMRI and AI Fusion in Autism	(Co. 12)

4. Conclusions

In conclusion, the evolution of artificial intelligence technologies in the field of medical imaging offers promising prospects for enhancing diagnosis and treatment. The studies presented in this editorial highlight the growing intersection between medicine and artificial intelligence, addressing challenges from early spinal pathology diagnosis to Efficient Brain Tumor Classification. The research emphasizes the crucial aspects of interpretability and encourages multidisciplinary collaboration, providing valuable insights for further ethical investigations and practical applications.

The Special Issue curated significant contributions in various domains, identifying both emerging and established themes and delineating intriguing directions for future advancements. This initiative underscores the importance of these tools as a central hub for scholarly exchange and discussions among researchers worldwide.

Conflicts of Interest: The authors declare no conflict of interest.

List of Contributions

1. Pirrera, A.; Giansanti, D. Human–Machine Collaboration in Diagnostics: Exploring the Synergy in Clinical Imaging with Artificial Intelligence. *Diagnostics* 2023, *13*, 2162. https://doi.org/10.3390/diagnostics13132162.
2. Lin, P.-C.; Chang, W.-S.; Hsiao, K.-Y.; Liu, H.-M.; Shia, B.-C.; Chen, M.-C.; Hsieh, P.-Y.; Lai, T.-W.; Lin, F.-H.; Chang, C.-C. Development of a Machine Learning Algorithm to Correlate Lumbar Disc Height on X-rays with Disc Bulging or Herniation. *Diagnostics* 2024, *14*, 134. https://doi.org/10.3390/diagnostics14020134.
3. Stanojević Pirković, M.; Pavić, O.; Filipović, F.; Saveljić, I.; Geroski, T.; Exarchos, T.; Filipović, N. Fractional Flow Reserve-Based Patient Risk Classification. *Diagnostics* 2023, *13*, 3349. https://doi.org/10.3390/diagnostics13213349.
4. Rao, P.K.; Chatterjee, S.; Janardhan, M.; Nagaraju, K.; Khan, S.B.; Almusharraf, A.; Alharbe, A.I. Optimizing Inference Distribution for Efficient Kidney Tumor Segmentation Using a UNet-PWP Deep-Learning Model with XAI on CT Scan Images. *Diagnostics* 2023, *13*, 3244. https://doi.org/10.3390/diagnostics13203244.
5. Kaur, M.; Singh, D.; Roy, S.; Amoon, M. Efficient Skip Connections-Based Residual Network (ESRNet) for Brain Tumor Classification. *Diagnostics* 2023, *13*, 3234. https://doi.org/10.3390/diagnostics13203234.
6. Chen, Y.-Y.; Yu, P.-N.; Lai, Y.-C.; Hsieh, T.-C.; Cheng, D.-C. Bone Metastases Lesion Segmentation on Breast Cancer Bone Scan Images with Negative Sample Training. *Diagnostics* 2023, *13*, 3042. https://doi.org/10.3390/diagnostics13193042.

7. Wu, H.; Zhao, J.; Li, J.; Zeng, Y.; Wu, W.; Zhou, Z.; Wu, S.; Xu, L.; Song, M.; Yu, Q.; et al. One-Stage Detection without Segmentation for Multi-Type Coronary Lesions in Angiography Images Using Deep Learning. *Diagnostics* **2023**, *13*, 3011. https://doi.org/10.3390/diagnostics13183011.
8. Jönemo, J.; Abramian, D.; Eklund, A. Evaluation of Augmentation Methods in Classifying Autism Spectrum Disorders from fMRI Data with 3D Convolutional Neural Networks. *Diagnostics* **2023**, *13*, 2773. https://doi.org/10.3390/diagnostics13172773.
9. Bhimavarapu, U.; Chintalapudi, N.; Battineni, G. Automatic Detection and Classification of Diabetic Retinopathy Using the Improved Pooling Function in the Convolution Neural Network. *Diagnostics* **2023**, *13*, 2606. https://doi.org/10.3390/diagnostics13152606.
10. Wu, S.; Yu, H.; Li, C.; Zheng, R.; Xia, X.; Wang, C.; Wang, H. A Coarse-to-Fine Fusion Network for Small Liver Tumor Detection and Segmentation: A Real-World Study. *Diagnostics* **2023**, *13*, 2504. https://doi.org/10.3390/diagnostics13152504.
11. Bragança, C.P.; Torres, J.M.; Macedo, L.O.; Soares, C.P.D.A. Advancements in Glaucoma Diagnosis: The Role of AI in Medical Imaging. *Diagnostics* **2024**, *14*, 530.
12. Giansanti, D. An Umbrella Review of the Fusion of fMRI and AI in Autism. *Diagnostics* **2023**, *13*, 3552. https://doi.org/10.3390/diagnostics13233552.
13. Giansanti, D. AI-Enabled Fusion of Medical Imaging, Behavioral Analysis and Other Systems for Enhanced Autism Spectrum Disorder. Comment on Jönemo et al. Evaluation of Augmentation Methods in Classifying Autism Spectrum Disorders from fMRI Data with 3D Convolutional Neural Networks. *Diagnostics* **2023**, *13*, 2773; reprinted in *Diagnostics* **2023**, *13*, 3545. https://doi.org/10.3390/diagnostics13233545.

References

1. Albano, D.; Galiano, V.; Basile, M.; Di Luca, F.; Gitto, S.; Messina, C.; Cagetti, M.G.; Del Fabbro, M.; Tartaglia, G.M.; Sconfienza, L.M. Artificial intelligence for radiographic imaging detection of caries lesions: A systematic review. *BMC Oral Health* **2024**, *24*, 274. [CrossRef] [PubMed]
2. Bai, A.; Si, M.; Xue, P.; Qu, Y.; Jiang, Y. Artificial intelligence performance in detecting lymphoma from medical imaging: A systematic review and meta-analysis. *BMC Med. Inform. Decis. Mak.* **2024**, *24*, 13. [CrossRef] [PubMed]
3. Akazawa, M.; Hashimoto, K. Artificial intelligence in gynecologic cancers: Current status and future challenges—A systematic review. *Artif. Intell. Med.* **2021**, *120*, 102164. [CrossRef] [PubMed]
4. Grignaffini, F.; Barbuto, F.; Troiano, M.; Piazzo, L.; Simeoni, P.; Mangini, F.; De Stefanis, C.; Muda, A.O.; Frezza, F.; Alisi, A. The Use of Artificial Intelligence in the Liver Histopathology Field: A Systematic Review. *Diagnostics* **2024**, *14*, 388. [CrossRef] [PubMed]
5. Furriel, B.C.R.S.; Oliveira, B.D.; Prôa, R.; Paiva, J.Q.; Loureiro, R.M.; Calixto, W.P.; Reis, M.R.C.; Giavina-Bianchi, M. Artificial intelligence for skin cancer detection and classification for clinical environment: A systematic review. *Front. Med.* **2024**, *10*, 1305954. [CrossRef] [PubMed]
6. Fernandes, J.R.N.; Teles, A.S.; Fernandes, T.R.S.; Lima, L.D.B.; Balhara, S.; Gupta, N.; Teixeira, S. Artificial Intelligence on Diagnostic Aid of Leprosy: A Systematic Literature Review. *J. Clin. Med.* **2023**, *13*, 180. [CrossRef] [PubMed]
7. Marks, D.; Kitcher, S.; Attrazic, E.; Hing, W.; Cottrell, M. The Health Economic Impact of Musculoskeletal Physiotherapy Delivered by Telehealth: A Systematic Review. *Int. J. Telerehabil.* **2022**, *14*, e6524. [CrossRef] [PubMed]
8. Singh, K.; Kaur, N.; Prabhu, A. Combating COVID-19 Crisis using Artificial Intelligence (AI) Based Approach: Systematic Review. *Curr. Top. Med. Chem.* **2024**, *24*, 1–17. [CrossRef] [PubMed]

Disclaimer/Publisher's Note: The statements, opinions and data contained in all publications are solely those of the individual author(s) and contributor(s) and not of MDPI and/or the editor(s). MDPI and/or the editor(s) disclaim responsibility for any injury to people or property resulting from any ideas, methods, instructions or products referred to in the content.

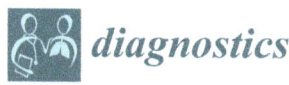

Editorial

Human–Machine Collaboration in Diagnostics: Exploring the Synergy in Clinical Imaging with Artificial Intelligence

Antonia Pirrera and Daniele Giansanti *

Centre TISP, ISS, 00166 Rome, Italy
* Correspondence: daniele.giansanti@iss.it

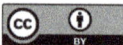

Citation: Pirrera, A.; Giansanti, D. Human–Machine Collaboration in Diagnostics: Exploring the Synergy in Clinical Imaging with Artificial Intelligence. *Diagnostics* **2023**, *13*, 2162. https://doi.org/10.3390/diagnostics13132162

Received: 20 June 2023
Accepted: 21 June 2023
Published: 25 June 2023

Copyright: © 2023 by the authors. Licensee MDPI, Basel, Switzerland. This article is an open access article distributed under the terms and conditions of the Creative Commons Attribution (CC BY) license (https://creativecommons.org/licenses/by/4.0/).

Advancements in artificial intelligence (AI), thanks to IT developments during the COVID-19 pandemic, have revolutionized the field of diagnostics, particularly in clinical imaging [1–3]. Diagnostic imaging, whether it is applied *inside the human body for organs* [4] *or functional diagnostics* [5], in *tissues or within cells* [6,7], *or outside in the dermis*, is having fabulous developments thanks to AI [8]. With the advent of digital health and digital radiology (DR), digital pathology (DP), and digital dermatology (DD), healthcare professionals have gained powerful tools that enable faster, more accurate diagnoses. Increasingly innovative algorithms are developed in the medical imaging sector by researchers in basic data science research and implemented by IT specialists in increasingly innovative tools. These tools are increasingly used, and much is expected from them.

The DR, DP, and DD have evolved differently due to: (1) the different peculiarities of clinical diagnostics. (2) The different evolutions and developments of the digitization of the standardization of images (DR, for example, later than the DP [9–12]), which is the basis of the development and implementation of AI algorithms. (3) The different roles of the patient (for example, more operator-technologists in DD, more passive in DP and DR) [13,14].

DR has transformed [15] how medical images are captured, stored, and analyzed. It refers not only to traditional radiology but also to all the other fields of *organ and functional* imaging, ranging from echography to positron emission tomography. For example, traditional film-based X-rays in radiology and videotape recordings in echography have given way to digital imaging technologies, improving physicians' workflow. Integrating AI algorithms with digital radiology has unlocked immense potential, empowering radiologists with intelligent systems that aid in detecting and interpreting abnormalities. Preliminary to this important development was the early development of the DICOM [11] standard, which facilitated the integration of these tools in every area and consequently made available a vast amount of image data for developing medical knowledge on AI.

Digital pathology [16] has emerged as a game-changer in histopathology and cytopathology, enabling the digitization and analysis of tissue and cell samples. By converting glass slides into digital slides and storing them into PACS (pathologists and cytologists) can interact easily through virtual scopes to discuss cases and for training.

However, this digitization has different characteristics in the two sectors of histology and cytology. The second one is more complex since the cytologist must use the focus function in the cytology, and its digital imitation requires an extension of the file. Compared to digital radiology, digital pathology has had greater inertia as regards standardization. The specialized DICOM for digital pathology, DICOM Whole Slide Image (WSI) [12], has had a much longer release time and a more articulated adaptation of the manufacturers. All this has meant that AI in digital pathology has certainly had a less rapid start.

DD has revolutionized the field of skin disease diagnosis and management [17–19]. Dermatologists now have access to powerful imaging technologies that capture high-resolution images of skin lesions and conditions. AI algorithms can assist in analyzing these images, identifying patterns, and suggesting potential diagnoses or treatment options. All this is also done thanks to mHealth mobile applications directly in the hands of the citizen integrated with the smartphone, who also becomes an *operator-technologist*. This aspect is new compared to DR and DP and opens a new paradigm in *Digital Health*.

Targeted searches on Pubmed give us an idea of the growth in the volume of studies, since the first applications of AI on the imaging at the date of this study.

Regarding the applications of AI in Pathology, the search with the key reported in *Box 1, position 1*, highlights 683 studies starting from 1989. Of these studies, 607 (*88.9%*) were carried out starting 1 January 2020. In all, there are 277 reviews (systematic and non-systematic).

Regarding the applications of AI in Dermatology, the search with the key reported in *Box 1, position 2*, highlights 97 studies starting from 2006. Of these studies, 83 (*85.6%*) were carried out starting 1 January 2020. In all, there are 42 reviews (systematic and not).

The DR includes, as explained, many sectors. To get an idea, we considered radiology and magnetic resonance.

Regarding the applications of AI in radiology imaging, the search with the key reported in *Box 1, position 3*, highlights 779 studies starting from 1983. Of these studies, 647 (*83.1%*) were carried out starting 1 January 2020. In all, there are 346 reviews (systematic and non-systematic).

Regarding the applications of AI in Magnetic Resonance imaging, the search with the key reported in *Box 1, position 4*, highlights 1132 studies starting from 1990. Of these studies, 1015 (*89.7%*) were carried out starting 1 January 2020. In all, there are 455 reviews (systematic and non-systematic).

This brief overview highlights how in these sectors: (1) scientific production and interest have accelerated during the COVID-19 pandemic. (2) The greatest production is in the DR sector. (3) There is a good percentage of review studies, indicating good progress in the stabilization process of topics of scientific interest (Figure 1).

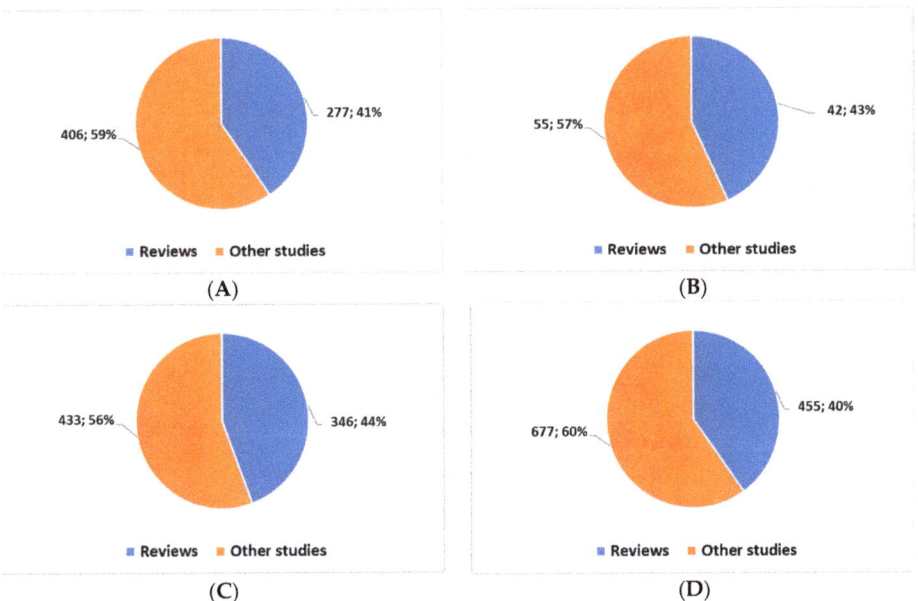

Figure 1. The volume of publications (at the date of this study) for the field of Pathology and AI (**A**); for the field of Dermatology and AI (**B**); for the field of radiology and AI (**C**); for the field of magnetic resonance and AI (**D**).

Box 1. The composite key used for the searches in Pubmed.

((pathology[Title/Abstract]) AND ((image[Title/Abstract]) OR (imaging[Title/Abstract]))) AND (Artificial Intelligence[Title/Abstract])

((dermatology[Title/Abstract]) AND ((image[Title/Abstract]) OR (imaging[Title/Abstract]))) AND (Artificial Intelligence[Title/Abstract])

((radiology[Title/Abstract]) AND ((image[Title/Abstract]) OR (imaging[Title/Abstract]))) AND (Artificial Intelligence[Title/Abstract])

((magnetic resonance[Title/Abstract]) AND ((image[Title/Abstract]) OR (imaging[Title/Abstract]))) AND (Artificial Intelligence[Title/Abstract])

These developments can streamline the health domain processes and change the role and workflow of the professionals already involved in the decision-making process, such as radiologists, pathologists, cytologists, histologists, and dermatologists. However, other professional figures will also be able to make use of AI in the workflow, such as the medical radiology technician, the biological laboratory technician, and even the tattoo artists, who will be able to interact with other professional figures in diagnostics to monitor any problems [20] of this widespread practice [21].

However, a real integration has not yet been achieved in DR, DP, and DD, which implies acceptance of the actors, robust guidelines and stable regulations at an implementation and legislative level, well-defined workflows, adequacy for cyber security aspects, and ethical issues (the last two in some cases also interlaced), a better understanding of the AI algorithms of the actors though an explainable AI to have better control of the process and, more generally, consensus initiatives acting on multiple domains and involving all the actors and experts in the field [15,16,19]. There is a great need to discuss this area to exchange and share experiences with a 360-degree perspective, encapsulating opportunities, problems, and even failures. With this in mind, the Special Issue "Artificial Intelligence in Clinical Medical Imaging" [22] was launched.

Conclusions

The COVID-19 pandemic has led to a terrifying acceleration in research and development on the application of AI. This applies to DP, DR, and DD.

However, creating ever more up-to-date tools based on increasingly performing innovative algorithms must be followed by initiatives in health domain integration that act on multiple domains. There is an increasing need for studies focused on AI in clinical imaging, also through synergistic initiatives, such as collections or Special Issues such as this one, which touch on successes and failures, opportunities, and bottlenecks.

Funding: This research received no external funding.

Institutional Review Board Statement: Not applicable.

Informed Consent Statement: Not applicable.

Data Availability Statement: Not applicable.

Conflicts of Interest: The authors declare no conflict of interest.

References

1. Alhasan, M.; Hasaneen, M. Digital imaging, technologies and artificial intelligence applications during COVID-19 pandemic. *Comput. Med. Imaging Graph.* **2021**, *91*, 101933. [CrossRef] [PubMed]
2. Barragán-Montero, A.; Javaid, U.; Valdés, G.; Nguyen, D.; Desbordes, P.; Macq, B.; Willems, S.; Vandewinckele, L.; Holmström, M.; Löfman, F.; et al. Artificial intelligence and machine learning for medical imaging: A technology review. *Phys. Medica* **2021**, *83*, 242–256. [CrossRef] [PubMed]
3. Giger, M.L. Machine Learning in Medical Imaging. *J. Am. Coll. Radiol.* **2018**, *15 Pt B*, 512–520. [CrossRef]
4. Jaudet, C.; Weyts, K.; Lechervy, A.; Batalla, A.; Bardet, S.; Corroyer-Dulmont, A. The Impact of Artificial Intelligence CNN Based Denoising on FDG PET Radiomics. *Front. Oncol.* **2021**, *11*, 3136. [CrossRef] [PubMed]

5. Grenier, P.A.; Brun, A.L.; Mellot, F. The Potential Role of Artificial Intelligence in Lung Cancer Screening Using Low-Dose Computed Tomography. *Diagnostics* **2022**, *12*, 2435. [CrossRef] [PubMed]
6. Houri, O.; Gil, Y.; Gemer, O.; Helpman, L.; Vaknin, Z.; Lavie, O.; Ben Arie, A.; Amit, A.; Levy, T.; Namazov, A.; et al. Prediction of endometrial cancer recurrence by using a novel machine learning algorithm: An Israeli gynecologic oncology group study. *J. Gynecol. Obstet. Hum. Reprod.* **2022**, *51*, 102466. [CrossRef] [PubMed]
7. Qiao, Y.; Zhao, L.; Luo, C.; Luo, Y.; Wu, Y.; Li, S.; Bu, D.; Zhao, Y. Multi-modality artificial intelligence in digital pathology. *Briefings Bioinform.* **2022**, *23*, bbac367. [CrossRef] [PubMed]
8. Du-Harpur, X.; Watt, F.; Luscombe, N.; Lynch, M. What is AI? Applications of artificial intelligence to dermatology. *Br. J. Dermatol.* **2020**, *183*, 423–430. [CrossRef] [PubMed]
9. Shah, A.; Muddana, P.S.; Halabi, S. A Review of Core Concepts of Imaging Informatics. *Cureus* **2022**, *14*, e32828. [CrossRef] [PubMed]
10. Boeken, T.; Feydy, J.; Lecler, A.; Soyer, P.; Feydy, A.; Barat, M.; Duron, L. Artificial intelligence in diagnostic and interventional radiology: Where are we now? *Diagn. Interv. Imaging* **2023**, *104*, 1–5. [CrossRef] [PubMed]
11. DICOM, Digital Imaging and COmmunications in Medicine. Available online: https://www.dicomstandard.org/ (accessed on 16 June 2023).
12. DICOM Whole Slide Imaging (WSI). NEMA. Available online: http://dicom.nema.org/Dicom/DICOMWSI/ (accessed on 6 July 2021).
13. Hadeler, E.; Hong, J.; Mosca, M.; Hakimi, M.; Brownstone, N.; Bhutani, T.; Liao, W. Perspectives on the Future Development of Mobile Applications for Dermatology Clinical Research. *Dermatol. Ther.* **2021**, *11*, 1451–1456. [CrossRef] [PubMed]
14. Chin, Y.P.H.; Huang, I.H.; Hou, Z.Y.; Chen, P.Y.; Bassir, F.; Wang, H.H.; Lin, Y.T.; Li, Y.C.J. User satisfaction with a smartphone-compatible, artificial intelligence-based cutaneous pigmented lesion evaluator. *Comput. Methods Programs Biomed.* **2020**, *195*, 105649. [CrossRef] [PubMed]
15. Giansanti, D.; Di Basilio, F. The Artificial Intelligence in Digital Radiology: Part 1: The Challenges, Acceptance and Consensus. *Healthcare* **2022**, *10*, 509. [CrossRef] [PubMed]
16. Giovagnoli, M.R.; Giansanti, D. Artificial Intelligence in Digital Pathology: What Is the Future? Part 1: From the Digital Slide Onwards. *Healthcare* **2021**, *9*, 858. [CrossRef] [PubMed]
17. Young, A.T.; Xiong, M.; Pfau, J.; Keiser, M.J.; Wei, M.L. Artificial Intelligence in Dermatology: A Primer. *J. Investig. Dermatol.* **2020**, *140*, 1504–1512. [CrossRef] [PubMed]
18. Pasquali, P.; Sonthalia, S.; Moreno-Ramirez, D.; Sharma, P.; Agrawal, M.; Gupta, S.; Kumar, D.; Arora, D. Teledermatology and its current perspective. *Indian Dermatol. Online J.* **2020**, *11*, 12–20. [CrossRef] [PubMed]
19. Giansanti, D. The Artificial Intelligence in Teledermatology: A Narrative Review on Opportunities, Perspectives, and Bottlenecks. *Int. J. Environ. Res. Public Health* **2023**, *20*, 5810. [CrossRef] [PubMed]
20. Pirrera, A.; Giansanti, D.; Renzoni, A. Can the Use of Digital Technologies Enhance the Safety of Tattooing Practice? Available online: https://wctp2023.org/fileadmin/user_upload/WCTP/WCTP2023/WCTP_2023_ALL_Poster_abstracts_NEW.pdf (accessed on 16 June 2023).
21. Giulbudagian, M.; Schreiver, I.; Singh, A.V.; Laux, P.; Luch, A. Safety of tattoos and permanent make-up: A regulatory view. *Arch. Toxicol.* **2020**, *94*, 357–369. [CrossRef] [PubMed]
22. Special Issue "Artificial Intelligence in Clinical Medical Imaging". Available online: https://www.mdpi.com/journal/diagnostics/special_issues/3FXN9682V0 (accessed on 16 June 2023).

Disclaimer/Publisher's Note: The statements, opinions and data contained in all publications are solely those of the individual author(s) and contributor(s) and not of MDPI and/or the editor(s). MDPI and/or the editor(s) disclaim responsibility for any injury to people or property resulting from any ideas, methods, instructions or products referred to in the content.

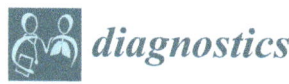

Review

Advancements in Glaucoma Diagnosis: The Role of AI in Medical Imaging

Clerimar Paulo Bragança [1,2,*], José Manuel Torres [1,3], Luciano Oliveira Macedo [2] and Christophe Pinto de Almeida Soares [1,3]

1. ISUS Unit, Faculty of Science and Technology, University Fernando Pessoa, 4249-004 Porto, Portugal; jtorres@ufp.edu.pt (J.M.T.); csoares@ufp.edu.pt (C.P.d.A.S.)
2. Department of Ophthalmology, Eye Hospital of Southern Minas Gerais State, Rua Joaquim Rosa 14, Itanhandu 37464-000, MG, Brazil; lucianoomacedo@gmail.com
3. Artificial Intelligence and Computer Science Laboratory, LIACC, University of Porto, 4100-000 Porto, Portugal
* Correspondence: 39270@ufp.edu.pt

Abstract: The progress of artificial intelligence algorithms in digital image processing and automatic diagnosis studies of the eye disease glaucoma has been growing and presenting essential advances to guarantee better clinical care for the population. Given the context, this article describes the main types of glaucoma, traditional forms of diagnosis, and presents the global epidemiology of the disease. Furthermore, it explores how studies using artificial intelligence algorithms have been investigated as possible tools to aid in the early diagnosis of this pathology through population screening. Therefore, the related work section presents the main studies and methodologies used in the automatic classification of glaucoma from digital fundus images and artificial intelligence algorithms, as well as the main databases containing images labeled for glaucoma and publicly available for the training of machine learning algorithms.

Keywords: deep learning; glaucoma; image analysis; artificial intelligence

Citation: Bragança, C.P.; Torres, J.M.; Macedo, L.O.; Soares, C.P.d.A. Advancements in Glaucoma Diagnosis: The Role of AI in Medical Imaging. *Diagnostics* **2024**, *14*, 530. https://doi.org/10.3390/diagnostics14050530

Academic Editors: Jae-Ho Han and Daniele Giansanti

Received: 30 November 2023
Revised: 17 February 2024
Accepted: 23 February 2024
Published: 1 March 2024

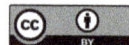

Copyright: © 2024 by the authors. Licensee MDPI, Basel, Switzerland. This article is an open access article distributed under the terms and conditions of the Creative Commons Attribution (CC BY) license (https://creativecommons.org/licenses/by/4.0/).

1. Introduction

Glaucoma is a multifactorial neuropathy that can affect the fundus of the eye, causing gradual loss of vision and, in severe cases, blindness. Traditionally, the diagnosis of glaucoma is applied with the help of readily available ophthalmological teams and highly specialized equipment. The sensitivity of the diagnosis is generally high, as tests applied in ophthalmology offices have the clinical potential to identify virtually all cases of the disease. However, despite this sophisticated diagnostic scenario, the silent and slow evolution of the disease, the costs of exams and consultations, and the lack of access to public ophthalmological services in many cases prevent thousands of people from consulting an ophthalmologist during the early stages of this neuropathy. This contributes to the fact that around 70% of the patients are self-diagnosed, that is, alerted by their own visual impairment and not by an appropriate early diagnosis [1,2].

Glaucoma is considered a global problem; even in developed countries, it is estimated that at least 50% of patients with glaucoma do not know of their condition. This percentage is even worse in low-income countries [3]. It is considered a progressive, chronic, and incurable pathology; however, it can generally be efficiently controlled when treatment begins in the early stages of the disease.

There are several types of glaucoma: open-angle glaucoma, angle-closure glaucoma, congenital glaucoma and secondary glaucoma [4,5]. However, they all cause damage to the optic nerve, which in most cases occurs slowly, initially leading to the loss of midperipheral vision. In advanced stages, it affects central vision, leading to irreversible blindness.

Damage to the optic nerve can be analyzed using fundus examinations, also known as ophthalmoscopy or fundoscopy. The ophthalmoscopy examination is performed on the back part of the eye (fundus), which includes the retina, optic disc, choroid, and blood vessels. The funduscopic examination can be performed with a variety of equipment, such as direct ophthalmoscopy, indirect ophthalmoscopy, and slit lamp ophthalmoscopy. Found in almost all ophthalmology offices, these devices offer ophthalmologists a detailed view of the eyeball. As shown in Figure 1, the brightest part of the retina represents the optic disc (OD), which contains an excavation known as the optical cup (OC), depicted by the whitest part of the interior of the optic disc. Therefore, if the size of the optic cup increases, it is considered one of the main indicators of glaucoma [2,6–8].

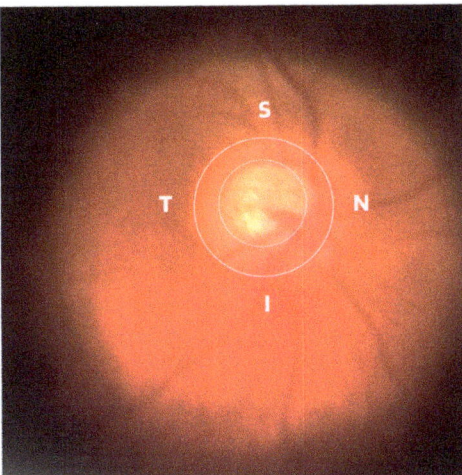

Figure 1. ISNT (Inferior (I), Superior (S), Nasal (N) and Temporal (T)) Rule.

In terms of the basic and traditional methods of diagnosing glaucoma, in addition to the fundus examination to examine the optic disc and the retinal nerve fiber layer (RNFL), ophthalmologists generally use tonometry and visual field tests as adjuncts. Tonometry is an exam to assess the degree of dysfunction and measures intraocular pressure (IOP) in millimeters of mercury (mmHg). The common eye pressure range is 10 to 21 mmHg, which is based on the average eye pressure level of a normal person. Although tonometry examination is very important in the management and treatment of glaucoma, it cannot be considered a diagnosis due to the presence of cases of normal pressure glaucoma [9]. Perimetry through the perimetry or campimetry exam, as is also known, the degree of functional impairment resulting from the disease is examined through the results of the obtained visual field map. In clinical practice, visual field testing identifies so-called blind spots (scotomas) and their locations in human vision and is therefore widely used as the gold standard to assess whether a patient suffers from typical functional glaucomatous damage [10].

Although the demographic and clinical characteristics associated with glaucoma are relatively well known, there is still no uniform definition of the diagnosis of this disease by ophthalmologists. In this way, many international efforts have been made to develop such a definition, but no real consensus standard has been reached. Therefore, those with an IOP greater than 21 mmHg, accompanied by characteristic damage to the optic disc or defects in the visual field compatible with glaucoma, are generally included as glaucomatous [11]. Due to this particularity, it is important to assess and document the appearance of an increase in the cup-to-disc ratio as a way of evaluating possible structural damage caused by the disease, as well as accompanying the patient to treatment or routine appointments. Therefore, from ophthalmoscopy images, ophthalmologists can evaluate at least four important informative characteristics of glaucoma, such as cup/disc ratio, inferior (I), superior (S), nasal (N), and temporal (T) rule (ISNT), cup asymmetry, and in addition other structural damage caused to the optic disc, namely the following:

- Cup-to-Disc Ratio (CDR): An abnormal increase in disc cupping is important in the diagnosis of glaucoma; however, many people may have increased nerve cupping and not necessarily have glaucoma. This is especially true for myopic people, who tend to have a larger optical disc and consequently a larger optical cup. Therefore, during the diagnosis of glaucoma, it is important to assess not only the optical cup but also the cup-to-disc ratio (CDR). For better understanding, the CDR measurement is calculated from the relationship between the vertical diameter of the excavation (VCD) and the vertical diameter of the disc (VDD), as shown in Figure 2.
  To calculate the CDR ratio, the optical disc must be divided into 10 equal parts, as in Figure 3, and then the excavation scope must be taken into account in each division made. Therefore, it is considered a fractional percentage measurement, generally made horizontally, and can vary greatly between normal individuals. However, optical excavations greater than 0.65 indicate possible abnormalities, suggesting further investigation [2,12].
- ISNT Rule: The border formed between the optic cup and the optic disc, called the neuroretinal ring or neural ring, is also considered an indication of glaucoma, for which there is a rule called ISNT, which alludes to the orientation (inferior, superior, nasal, and temporal) of the edges in the image of the fundus, as shown in Figure 1. When considering the ISNT rule, in nonglaucomatous eyes, it is suggested that the thickness of the neural ring should be greatest in the inferior quadrant, followed by the superior, nasal, and temporal quadrants. Misalignment in the guidelines of this rule leads to suspicion of glaucoma [13].
- Cup-to-disc ratio (CDR) asymmetry: The CDR relationship between both eyes is symmetric in most people, and asymmetry is an important sign of suspected glaucomatous damage. This is due to the observation that 1% to 6% normal adults may have a discrepancy of 0.2 in the cup/disc ratio, while 1% of the general population may have an asymmetry of 0.3. Therefore, cup asymmetry is a finding on ophthalmological examination that requires additional tests to rule out the presence of glaucoma or other possible complications [14,15].
- Other structural damage to the optic disc: The main descriptions of these types of damage related to glaucoma are as follows [2,16,17]:
  1. Changes in RNFL: the presence of defects located in the retinal nerve fiber layer is called Hoyt's sign and is characterized by a dark area that extends and widens from the optic disc, exhibiting an arched shape.
  2. Peripapillary atrophy: According to the ophthalmological appearance, peripapillary atrophy can be divided into a peripheral alpha zone and a central beta zone. The alpha zone is characterized by patchy hypopigmentation and thinning of the layers of the chorioretinal tissue. It is laterally adjacent to the retina and medially in contact with the beta area, with the sclera and large choroidal vessels visible. In normal eyes, the alpha and beta areas are usually located in the temporal area, followed by the inferior and superior areas. In glaucomatous eyes, the beta area is more present in the temporal region and its extension is associated with thinning of the RNFL.
  3. Excavation of the optic disc: In addition to disc excavation, the neuroretinal ring or neural rim must also be observed, as excavation is influenced by the size of the optic disc.
  4. Disc hemorrhage: The presence of peripapillary hemorrhages is an important sign in both the diagnosis and the monitoring of glaucoma. Therefore, vessel deflection and nasal excavation must be examined.
  5. Denudation of the lamina, cribriform: the presence of visible extinction of the cribriform lamina to the edge of the optic disc is called a notch, which represents

the evolution of a defect located in the neural rim until there is a complete absence of tissue in the region, which exposes the cribriform lamina and allows visualization of its pores. Although it is very suggestive of glaucoma, this sign is not characteristic of the disease.

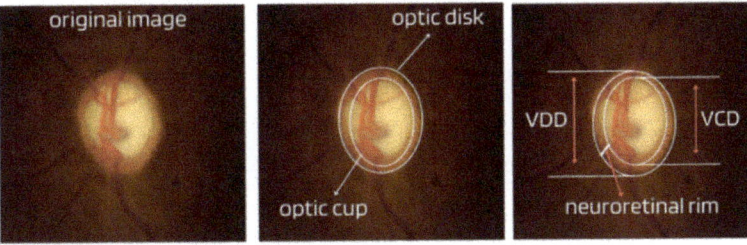

Figure 2. Measures considered in the CDR calculation.

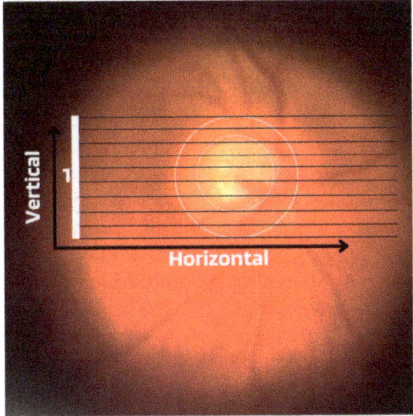

Figure 3. Example of CDR calculation with figure showing excavation of 0.6.

Regarding the difficulties associated with the diagnosis of glaucoma, it is considered that in cases in the moderate or advanced stages of the disease, the diagnosis is usually more simplified. However, the best way is to detect early glaucoma, which is essential for adequate treatment, mainly because quality of life can be altered even with slight loss of visual field [18]. However, the early identification of this disease, although important, can be challenging for several reasons, including glaucomatous characteristics that can be ambiguous in the optic disc region, RNFL, or visual field results at the beginning of the disease.

Over the years, more sensitive tests have been developed to more reliably identify early loss of visual function in patients with glaucoma, and more sophisticated imaging devices have been created to identify the first signs of disease-induced structural damage to aid in precocious diagnosis. Among these devices, optical coherence tomography (OCT), laser scanning polarimetry, and confocal laser scanning ophthalmoscopy stand out [19,20]. Although devices have demonstrated a good ability to assist ophthalmologists in the diagnosis of glaucoma, few studies have specifically examined the use of such technologies early in the disease, making the early diagnosis of glaucoma a difficult task for specialists, even with the aid of sophisticated equipment [19].

Given the difficulties in diagnosing glaucoma early, what ophthalmology clinics have done to try to overcome this difficulty is a combination of functional and structural exams. Although functional changes may be detected before structural changes, in many cases the first detectable manifestation of glaucoma is a structural abnormality change in the optic disc and RNFL, which therefore requires that the tests be combined to establish probability levels of the presence or absence of the disease [9,12,18].

2. Epidemiology

According to the World Health Organization (WHO), at least 2.2 billion people around the world suffer from some type of visual impairment. In almost half of the cases, this deficiency could have been avoided or has not yet been treated. When considering these data, it is inferred that today millions of people live with visual impairment or blindness that could have been avoided but unfortunately were not.

Although the exact number is unknown, it is estimated that 11.9 million people worldwide have moderate or severe visual impairment or blindness due to eye diseases such as glaucoma, trachoma (an inflammatory condition that affects the conjunctiva and cornea), and diabetic retinopathy, a chronic complication of diabetes mellitus [21–23].

Visual impairment and blindness can have a major impact on the daily lives of people affected by such disabilities, since vision is the dominant sense for humans at all stages of life. However, research estimates that by 2030, around 95.4 million people worldwide will have glaucoma.

Visual impairment, in addition to being detrimental to patient quality of life, also presents a huge global financial burden, as demonstrated by previous research that estimated the costs of lost productivity. These costs can be divided into direct costs and indirect costs. Direct costs include medications, surgeries, medical consultations, hospitalizations, and complementary examinations. Indirect medical costs include mainly the economic impacts caused by visual impairment on work productivity.

Although glaucoma generally progresses slowly and is underdiagnosed worldwide, it is the most common cause of irreversible blindness globally, yet it can be prevented. The disease is considered preventable because, if detected early, there are ways to control it, but global statistics show that due to underdiagnosis, the result is a large number of blind people. This problem can be even more serious in low-income or underdeveloped countries, such as Brazil, considered by the World Inequality Lab report in 2018 [24] as one of the countries with the highest social and income inequality in the world, marked by extreme levels for many consecutive years.

Although statistical numbers of underdiagnosis in the general population combined with the need for early diagnosis to prevent blindness may suggest that glaucoma is a good candidate for population screening, studies have shown that, at least in countries such as the United Kingdom and Finland, the detection of population-based glaucoma using traditional diagnostic methods is not feasible due to the high cost of implementation and maintenance and the relatively low prevalence of the disease in the general population, which is approximately 3.5% [25,26]. Similarly, the US Preventive Services Task Force [27], with the support of the American Academy of Family Physicians [28], does not recommend screening for glaucoma in the primary care setting, citing insufficient evidence to assess its implications, benefits, or harms.

3. Scientific and Technological Advances in Artificial Intelligence

In recent years, scientific and technological advances have opened up a wide range of clinical and research opportunities in the field of ophthalmological care, which can help combat glaucoma. In this way, artificial intelligence technologies have proven effective in areas of medicine such as radiology, pathology, dermatology, etc. All of these studies are in related areas that share parallels with ophthalmology because of their deep roots in diagnostic imaging.

The term artificial intelligence is a technology that covers several areas of knowledge and generally refers to the development of computational systems capable of performing tasks that mimic human intelligence. More recently, through machine learning and algorithms known as artificial neural networks (ANN) and deep neural networks (DNN) many advances have been possible [29,30].

The concept of machine learning encompasses a variety of methodologies, such as random forests [31], K-nearest neighbors (KNN) [32], support vector machines (SVM) [33], naive bayes [34], and artificial neural networks [29]. All of these technologies are aimed at pattern recognition, statistical regression, and data classification processes. Among machine learning algorithms, deep learning technology stands out, which has been at the forefront of the development and advances in computing and big data in recent years, mainly with the introduction and development of convolutional neural network (CNN) networks, proposed by researcher Yann LeCun [35] and especially used in the areas of pattern recognition and digital image classification.

The networks presented are algorithms that require a lot of data for training, but often there are not enough data, especially when considering clinical information. Therefore, a widely used technique that allows neural networks to be applied to small data sets is the process of transfer learning, considered the method of transferring knowledge acquired during training in a certain domain (a database) to be applied in another domain, that is, another similar problem. In view of this, algorithms that offer this technology are called pre-trained. One of the conveniences of using pre-trained networks is that they already have defined weights; that is, the weights are initialized with values obtained from already completed training.

Still in transfer learning, the ImageNet Large Scale Visual Recognition Challenge (ILSVRC) is an annual competition run by the ImageNet team since 2010, in which research teams evaluate the performance of computer vision and machine learning algorithms on various transfer learning tasks. visual recognition, such as object classification and localization [36]. ImageNet is a project aiming to provide large libraries of images for use in pre-training algorithms to be used in various other tasks and has been fundamental for advancing research in computer vision and deep learning. This database contains more than 14 million images, divided into more than 20,000 categories.

Due to data deficiency and other purposes, generative adversarial networks (GANs) also emerged, a machine learning architecture that consists of two networks that 'fight' against each other (damage to the environment). The potential of GANs is enormous because they can learn to imitate any data distribution in the following way: First, a neural network called a generator generates new data instances, while another neural network called a discriminator evaluates their authenticity. In this way, the generator produces false images in the hope that the false images will even be considered real by the discriminator. With this exchange of information, the generator learns to generate plausible data, while the discriminator learns to distinguish false data from the generator. The discriminator penalizes the generator for producing concrete results, and with this, the generator improves more and more.

Training of GANs networks is carried out using real data instances as positive and fake data instances created by the generator as negative. After training, the classifier classifies the real and fake generator data and propagates the discriminator loss through the discriminator network to update the weights [37].

All these artificial intelligence technologies, regardless of the difficulty in finding large sets of public data or the algorithmic model used, show the great commitment of researchers to spread scientific growth seeking to find valid and effective solutions in the diagnosis of glaucoma. In this way, with respect to the application of artificial intelligence to ophthalmology, in addition to studies aimed at the automatic diagnosis of glaucoma, this technology also focuses on studies on the diagnosis of diseases such as cataracts, age-related macular degeneration, diabetic retinopathy, and others, showing that there is a set of ophthalmological diseases that can receive greater attention considering the use of deep learning.

Regarding the ophthalmological scenario of glaucoma, the use of artificial intelligence appears as an auxiliary tool in the diagnosis of the disease by detecting changes present in the OCT results, the results of the visual field exam, and mainly in the images of the fundus. This is because, despite the potential to apply automation to different types of ophthalmic images, fundus images (i.e., images obtained with conventional ophthalmic equipment) have gained prominence in many related works due to the availability, quality, and cost effectiveness of acquisition.

4. Related Works

To prepare this review, the manuscripts were selected based on the titles and summaries of the artificial intelligence methods used to classify glaucoma from digital fundus images, therefore presenting some of the relevant scientific works published in recent years. The search for articles was applied to the main data platforms (Scopus, Web of Science, Google Scholar, Scielo and Medline). Due to the scope of this study, the search was limited to algorithms developed to analyze digital fundus images, mainly with the aid of CNN algorithms. Before presenting methods using deep learning, we describe the main public databases containing fundus images used by many of the related works described as instances for training and testing the classifiers, which are mostly supervised.

4.1. Main Public Databases

Table 1 describes some publicly found databases for work focused on classifying glaucoma using deep learning and digital images of the fundus obtained by conventional retinography with cameras. The viewing angle of each database is also described, as it determines the amount of fundus area that will appear close to the optical disc. Furthermore, to fill in the data in the table, only images labeled glaucoma and nonglaucoma from each reported database were considered.

Table 1. Public and labeled databases for glaucoma.

Database	Glaucoma	Normal	Total	Viewing Angle
Acrima [38]	396	396	700	30 a 50°
Drions [39]	55	55	110	30 a 50°
Drishti-Gs1 [40]	50	51	101	30°
Drive [41]	34	6	40	45°
Glaucoma DB [42]	85	35	120	30 a 50°
Hrf [43]	15	15	30	45°
sjchoi86-Frf [44]	101	300	401	30 a 50°
Messidor [?]	28	72	100	45°
Origa [46]	168	482	650	30 a 50°
Papila [47]	155	333	488	30 a 50°
Refuge [48]	120	1080	1200	30 a 50°
G1020 [49]	296	724	1020	45°
BrG [50]	1000	1000	2000	25°
Rim-one DL [51]	172	313	485	30 a 50°

4.2. Approaches Using Deep Learning

Based on the analysis of the literature that constitutes the related studies, it was observed that artificial intelligence models used in studies of this disease based on digital fundus images are generally applied in two specific ways: calculating CDR or identifying glaucoma patterns in the optic disc region.

CDR calculation: One of the ways that glaucoma classification models have used has been through the calculation of the CDR measurement, generally obtained from the segmentation of the disc and optical cup structures; see Figure 4. The algorithms then, using the calculated CDR, estimate the presence or absence of glaucoma.

Although many algorithms, such as [52,53], have shown a high accuracy rate in segmenting these structures, this method can only be considered an indication of glaucoma and the need for a more detailed evaluation, since the diagnosis of this neuropathy is made by examination of the entire structure of the optic disc and not just excavation. Furthermore, although increased cupping suggests glaucoma, not all optic nerve cupping is related to this disease, as there are other conditions that can cause increased cupping of the optic nerve, such as neuritis, tumors, multiple sclerosis, etc.

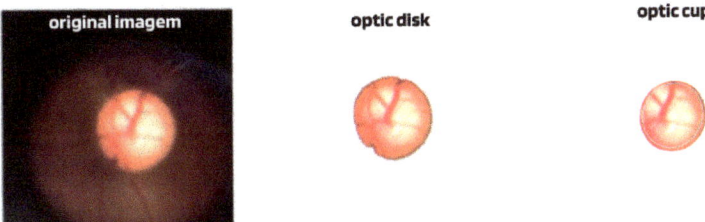

Figure 4. Example of image with segmentation of the disc and optical cup.

Recognition of glaucomatous patterns: Although the CDR calculation algorithms only evaluate the excavation of the optic disc, this pattern recognition methodology seeks to evaluate the entire region of the optic disc in search of characteristics that could lead to the recognition of glaucoma. According to the context of deep learning and the analysis of related work described in this section, this type of application can be operated by at least four different methodologies, such as the following:

1. Feature vector extraction and classification: In this type of application, various image processing and feature extraction techniques can be used on digital images; however, a classifier will be the part of the system responsible for the categorization task, or that is, it will apply the decision process on which category a given image belongs to. Among the algorithms that work in this way are SVM, KNN, Naive Bayes, etc. Works such as these have been published by several authors and have appeared in [54,55].
2. Use of CNN networks: This approach eliminates the need to extract feature vectors, since CNN networks can extract such features through feature maps with their convolutional layers. Considered the gold standard of digital image processing, this methodology was applied in works such as those consulted in [38,56,57], using public and private databases.
3. Use of GANs networks: This involves discovering regularities and patterns in the input data and learning them automatically. Examples of these algorithms in glaucoma classification can be found in [58–60].
4. Use of multitechnologies: This type of modeling seeks to achieve the desired objective using a combination of techniques, such as KNN, SVM, CNN, etc. Numerous researchers, such as [61–63], have opted for this type of application, which is shown to be a valid way to recognize glaucomatous patterns.

Table 2 presents some of the various relevant works published in recent years as presented in reviews as available in Zedan et al. [64].

Table 2. Examples of work related to glaucoma classification using artificial intelligence algorithms.

Paper	Algorithm	Dataset	Accuracy/Precision
Dias et al. [38]	multilevel CNN	Private	99.4%
Bragança et al. [50]	Ensemble CNN	BrG	90.0%
Singh et al. [54]	SVM, KNN e Naive Bayes	STARE e MESSIDOR	95.0%
Shiny et al. [55]	SVM	DRISHTI	95.3%
Shinde et al. [61]	Le-Net e modelo U-Net CNN	RIM-ONE, DRISHTI-GS, DRIONS-DB, JSIEC e DRIVE	100%
Sreng et al. [62]	VGG16-19,Xception, ResNet50 e InceptionV3	ACRIMA, DRISHTI GS1, HRF, RIM-ONE,	96.5%
Santos et al. [63]	DeepLabv3+ and MobileNet	RIM-ONE, ORIGA,ACRIMA, DRISHTI-GS1 and REFUGE	95.59
Zulfira et al. [65]	SVM, KNN e Naive Bayes	DRIONS-DB	98.6%
Yunitasari et al. [66]	Dynamic Ensemble	RIM-ONE	91.0%

Table 2. Cont.

Paper	Algorithm	Dataset	Accuracy/Precision
Wang et al. [67]	SVM	DRISHTI	95.0%
Gheisari et al. [68]	VGG e AlexNet	DRIONS-DB, HRF, RIM-ONE e DRISHTI-GS1	94.3%
Li et al. [69]	VGG, ResNet e RNN	Private	95.0%
Liu et al. [70]	ResNet	Private	95.0%
Nawaz et al. [71]	ResNet	Private	96.2%
Kim et al. [72]	EficienteNet-B0	ORIGA	97.2%
Hemelings et al. [73]	VGG,Inception e ResNet	Private	96.2%
Alghamdi et al. [74]	ResNet	Private	98.0%
Aamir et al. [75]	VGG-16	RIM-ONE e RIGA	93.0%

The benefits sought for these possible applications are varied, from the potential reduction in costs associated with the traditional diagnosis of glaucoma to assistance in population screening applications aimed at early diagnosis and reducing the rate of underdiagnosis of the disease.

5. Discussion and Conclusions

Significant progress has been made in the development of glaucoma classification algorithms, which have shown remarkable success in differentiating between digital fundoscopic images of glaucoma and nonglaucoma. According to the work of Phene et al. [76] in experiments using artificial intelligence in glaucoma classification, these algorithms have even shown higher precision compared to classifications made by experienced ophthalmologists. However, despite the consensus among various studies that artificial intelligence algorithms can be utilized as a supportive tool for the diagnosis of glaucoma, currently there is no software available for real clinical applications. This suggests that further theoretical and practical efforts are required to enhance the usability and effectiveness of such algorithms.

The machine learning methodology to achieve more representative tests faces challenges due to the limited number of images in the databases. In addition, the labeling process of these images can negatively affect the classification algorithms. In relation to database labeling, the studies discussed in this review generally required assessors (specifically ophthalmologists) to annotate labels by only examining retinal images to determine the presence or absence of glaucoma. However, a study involving six glaucoma specialists assigned to diagnose the disease solely on photographs of the ocular fundus revealed that their agreement was only 49% [77]. This finding highlights the fact that labeling the database solely based on fundus image observation can be detrimental to the classifier's final results, as it is highly prone to errors. Consequently, training algorithms with inaccurately labeled data can compromise the overall quality of classifier results. To minimize errors in database insertion through image labeling, it is important to incorporate certain practices. One of such practice involves ensuring the presence of experienced ophthalmologists and adhering to the standard for the diagnosis of glaucoma, which entails a combination of functional and structural exams. Achieving this level of quality is often considered challenging. Consequently, some authors, such as Ting et al. [57] and Phene et al. [76] who work with large private datasets, have opted not to label their databases against a diagnostic gold standard. Instead, they have relied on a labeling consensus evaluated by experienced ophthalmologists. However, it should be noted that their databases were still labeled solely based on visual information obtained from fundus images.

The availability of images labeled with glaucoma in publicly accessible databases is limited in terms of quantity and diversity. These databases often consist of small sample sizes that are racially or clinically homogeneous, which may not accurately represent the entire population under study. Consequently, the applicability of algorithms to a broader context may be hindered. To address this limitation, researchers have explored the use of Generative Adversarial Networks (GANs) to generate synthetic images that resemble the original images. However, even if these networks produce satisfactory results, the generated images may not effectively address the issue of data homogeneity with respect to race or variations in the manifestation of glaucomatous damage. In light of these challenges, many authors opt to combine or merge multiple databases to improve the classification of glaucoma.

The exclusion of people with multiple eye injuries is an important consideration in the development of databases and glaucoma classification studies. Many authors have reported that they specifically removed individuals with ocular diseases other than glaucoma from their training and testing datasets. They also excluded images that were compromised by systemic diseases that could directly impact the optic nerve or visual field. However, this type of exclusion can be seen as a negative aspect, as it may manipulate the real-world scenario in favor of algorithmic precision. Furthermore, the racial homogeneity of the datasets contrasts with the diverse population, making it challenging to generalize the algorithms to populations beyond those observed in the dataset. However, when considering the quality of the databases and their construction, several key characteristics can be observed.

- The databases were obtained using high-resolution retinal cameras, except for the BrG set, which was obtained using a smartphone connected to a portable ophthalmoscope.
- With the exception of the refuge and Rim-one-dl datasets, which were formed using two digital fundus cameras, all other datasets were obtained using only one digital retinal camera.
- Most databases were labeled based on ophthalmological opinions solely by examining fundus images. Only a few databases were labeled with ophthalmic care and the gold standard for diagnosing glaucoma.
- All publicly available databases are considered too small to train classification algorithms from scratch, which means without using transfer learning.
- Publicly available databases generally have a homogeneous ethnic composition in the collected population.

In addition to the limitations of the database, deep learning algorithms face challenges in accurately classifying glaucoma due to the absence of consistent and objective diagnostic criteria. Consequently, researchers exploring the application of artificial intelligence in this field have had to establish their own definitions for categorizing instances as "yes" or "no" for glaucoma. As a result, various approaches have been pursued, such as texture analysis, analysis of the CDR ratio, ISNT rules, and others. This divergence in methods is mainly attributed to the absence of specific and quantifiable biomarkers to define the disease. Consequently, many researchers have attempted to predict similar diagnostic results for glaucoma, but have employed different methodologies, making it challenging to compare the performance of different studies. These biomarkers are essential not only to provide a definitive diagnosis, but also to justify the reasoning behind the diagnosis.

In light of this medical necessity, numerous authors, such as Ting et al. [57], have demonstrated the importance of identifying crucial image regions in order to validate the results obtained by deep learning algorithms when used for the classification of glaucoma. This approach serves as a justification for the results achieved by the methodology, at least until the healthcare community fully accepts these algorithms.

In the given context, it is important to note that the main objective of the previous studies was not to develop a market-ready algorithm, but rather to showcase the essential components required to achieve satisfactory results in glaucoma classification using fundus images. These findings may be valuable for potential future applications. As a result, for further advancement of such research, it is recommended to label databases based on the diagnostic gold standard in order to enhance the utilization of deep learning algorithms. In addition, there should be a clear distinction between training and test sets, with a diverse range of images captured by different devices, involving patients from various ethnic backgrounds. Furthermore, the databases should include images captured under different lighting conditions, contrast levels, noise levels, etc. [51,78].

After analyzing the databases identified, it can be observed that they only partially fulfill the requirements outlined in this study. However, they still play an important role in the training of various algorithms and driving technological advancement. In terms of the algorithms themselves, although some scientific research has demonstrated their high accuracy in distinguishing between glaucomatous and nonglaucomatous images, further clinical trials and in-depth studies are needed to identify and address potential factors that may hinder the integration of such algorithms into practical clinical applications. With continued efforts in this area, it is anticipated that future advances in artificial intelligence will greatly contribute to the diagnosis of eye diseases, including glaucoma.

Author Contributions: Conceptualization, C.P.B.; methodology, C.P.B.; data curation, C.P.B.; writing—original draft preparation, C.P.B.; supervision. J.M.T. and C.P.d.A.S.; reviewing, J.M.T., C.P.d.A.S. and L.O.M.; investigation, J.M.T. and C.P.d.A.S.; visualization, L.O.M. All authors have read and agreed to the published version of the manuscript.

Funding: This research was funded by Fundação Ensino e Cultura Fernando Pessoa (FECFP), and supported by the Artificial Intelligence and Computer Science Laboratory, LIACC.

Institutional Review Board Statement: The study was submitted and reviewed by the National Ethics Committee in Brazil, according to CAAE: 29983120.0.0000.8078–Number: 4056930.

Informed Consent Statement: Not applicable.

Data Availability Statement: This study explores the possibility of using artificial intelligence algorithms to help reduce the underdiagnosis of glaucoma. Therefore, a more general analysis of the state of the art is carried out, taking into account the subject discussed.

Acknowledgments: Work was in partnership with Fundação Ensino e Cultura Fernando Pessoa (FECFP), represented here by its R&D group Intelligent Sensing and Ubiquitous Systems (ISUS), and supported by the Artificial Intelligence and Computer Science Laboratory, LIACC.

Conflicts of Interest: The authors declare no conflicts of interest.

References

1. Tan, N.Y.; Friedman, D.S.; Stalmans, I.; Ahmed, I.I.K.; Sng, C.C. Current opinion in ophthalmology. *Curr. Opin. Ophthalmol.* **2020**, *31*, 91–100. [CrossRef]
2. Bragança, C.P.; Torres, J.M.; De Almeida Soares, C.P. Inteligência artificial e diagnóstico do glaucoma. *Braz. Appl. Sci. Rev.* **2023**, *7*, 683–707. [CrossRef]
3. Heijl, A.; Bengtsson, B.; Oskarsdottir, S.E. Prevalence and severity of undetected manifest glaucoma: Results from the early manifest glaucoma trial screening. *Ophthalmology* **2013**, *120*, 1541–1545. [CrossRef]
4. Salmon, J.F. *Clinical Ophthalmology: A Systematic Approach*, 10th ed.; Elsevier Health Sciences: Amsterdam, The Netherlands, 2024.
5. NIH National Library of Medicine. Medical Encyclopedia [Internet]. Medical Encyclopedia: Glaucoma. 2023. Available online: https://medlineplus.gov/ency/article/001620.htm (accessed on 20 February 2024).
6. Giorgis, A.T.; Alemu, A.M.; Arora, S.; Gessesse, G.W.; Melka, F.; Woldeyes, A.; Amin, S.; Kassam, F.; Kurji, A.K.; Damji, K.F. Results from the first teleglaucoma pilot project in Addis Ababa, Ethiopia. *J. Glaucoma* **2019**, *28*, 701–707. [CrossRef]
7. Smith, A.M.; Czyz, C.N. Neuroanatomy, cranial nerve 2 (Optic). In *StatPearls [Internet]*; StatPearls Publishing: Treasure Island, FL, USA, 2022.
8. Sociedade Brasileira de Glaucoma (SBC). Manual De Exame Em Glaucoma. 2015. Available online: https://www.sbglaucoma.org.br/medico/wp-content/uploads/2016/05/folder.pdf (accessed on 20 February 2024).
9. Oshika, T.; Yoshitomi, F.; Oki, K. The pachymeter guide: A new device to facilitate accurate corneal thickness measurement. *Jpn. J. Ophthalmol.* **1997**, *41*, 426–427. [CrossRef]
10. Li, F.; Wang, Z.; Qu, G.; Song, D.; Yuan, Y.; Xu, Y.; Gao, K.; Luo, G.; Xiao, Z.; Lam, D.S.; et al. Automatic differentiation of Glaucoma visual field from non-glaucoma visual filed using deep convolutional neural network. *BMC Med. Imaging* **2018**, *18*, 1–7. [CrossRef]
11. Garway-Heath, D.F. Early diagnosis in glaucoma. *Prog. Brain Res.* **2008**, *173*, 47–57. [PubMed]
12. Schuster, A.K.; Erb, C.; Hoffmann, E.M.; Dietlein, T.; Pfeiffer, N. The diagnosis and treatment of glaucoma. *Dtsch. äRzteblatt Int.* **2020**, *117*, 225. [CrossRef] [PubMed]
13. Khalil, T.; Usman Akram, M.; Khalid, S.; Jameel, A. Improved automated detection of glaucoma from fundus image using hybrid structural and textural features. *IET Image Process.* **2017**, *11*, 693–700. [CrossRef]
14. Arvind, H.; George, R.; Raju, P.; Ve, R.S.; Mani, B.; Kannan, P.; Vijaya, L. Optic Disc Dimensions and Cup-Disc Ratios among Healthy South Indians: The Chennai Glaucoma Study. *Ophthalmic Epidemiol.* **2011**, *18*, 189–197. [CrossRef]

15. Qiu, M.; Boland, M.V.; Ramulu, P.Y. Cup-to-Disc Ratio Asymmetry in U.S. Adults: Prevalence and Association with Glaucoma in the 2005–2008 National Health and Nutrition Examination Survey. *Ophthalmology* **2017**, *124*, 1229–1236. [CrossRef]
16. Tinku, R.S.J.; Diniz Filho, A. *Simplificando o Diagnóstico e Tratamento do Glaucoma*; Cultura Médica: Rio de Janeiro, Brazil, 2019.
17. Jung, K.I.; Jeon, S.; Park, C.K. Lamina Cribrosa Depth is Associated With the Cup-to-Disc Ratio in Eyes With Large Optic Disc Cupping and Cup-to-Disc Ratio Asymmetry. *J. Glaucoma* **2016**, *25*, e536–e545. [CrossRef]
18. Tatham, A.J.; Weinreb, R.N.; Medeiros, F.A. Strategies for improving early detection of glaucoma: The combined structure–function index. *Clin. Ophthalmol.* **2014**, *8*, 611–621.
19. Topouzis, F.; Anastasopoulos, E. Glaucoma—The Importance of Early Detection and Early Treatment. *J.-Glaucoma Importance Early Detect. Early Treat.* **2007**, *1*, 13.
20. Camara, J.; Neto, A.; Pires, I.M.; Villasana, M.V.; Zdravevski, E.; Cunha, A. A Comprehensive Review of Methods and Equipment for Aiding Automatic Glaucoma Tracking. *Diagnostics* **2022**, *12*, 935. [CrossRef]
21. World Health Organization. World Report on Vision. 2019. Available online: https://www.who.int/docs/default-source/documents/publications/world-vision-report-accessible.pdf (accessed on 20 February 2024).
22. da Silva Negreiros, E.C.M.; dos Santos Silva, L.C.; de Araújo, A.C.R.; Dias, L.R.C.; de Moura, L.V.M.; Santa Rosa, I.M.; de Menezes Filho, J.M.; Marques, C.P.C. Mortalidade por Diabetes Mellitus no nordeste do Brasil no período de 2014 a 2018. *Braz. J. Health Rev.* **2023**, *6*, 14138–14155. [CrossRef]
23. Reis, T.M.; de Moraes Ramos, Y.T.; da Silva, Y.R.M.; Silva, R.A.; de Araújo, M.R.A.; de Araújo, W.M.; Beserra, I.Â.; da Cunha, A.D.R.; Silva, M.B.A. Análise de um triênio dos casos de tracoma em escolares residentes do município de Moreno. *Braz. J. Health Rev.* **2019**, *2*, 2273–2286.
24. Alvaredo, F.; Chancel, L.; Piketty, T.; Saez, E.; Zucman, G. *World Inequality Report 2018*; Belknap Press: Cambridge, MA, USA, 2018.
25. Vaahtoranta-Lehtonen, H.; Tuulonen, A.; Aronen, P.; Sintonen, H.; Suoranta, L.; Kovanen, N.; Linna, M.; Läärä, E.; Malmivaara, A. Cost effectiveness and cost utility of an organized screening programme for glaucoma. *Acta Ophthalmol. Scand.* **2007**, *85*, 508–518. [CrossRef] [PubMed]
26. Zaleska-Żmijewska, A.; Szaflik, J.P.; Borowiecki, P.; Pohnke, K.; Romaniuk, U.; Szopa, I.; Pniewski, J.; Szaflik, J. A new platform designed for glaucoma screening: Identifying the risk of glaucomatous optic neuropathy using fundus photography with deep learning architecture together with intraocular pressure measurements. *Klin. Oczna/Acta Ophthalmol. Pol.* **2020**, *122*, 1–6. [CrossRef]
27. Mangione, C.M.; Barry, M.J.; Nicholson, W.K.; Cabana, M.; Chelmow, D.; Coker, T.R.; Davis, E.M.; Donahue, K.E.; Epling, J.W.; Jaén, C.R.; et al. Screening for primary open-angle glaucoma: US Preventive Services Task Force recommendation statement. *JAMA* **2022**, *327*, 1992–1997. [PubMed]
28. Gedde, S.J.; Vinod, K.; Wright, M.M.; Muir, K.W.; Lind, J.T.; Chen, P.P.; Li, T.; Mansberger, S.L. Primary open-angle glaucoma preferred practice pattern®. *Ophthalmology* **2021**, *128*, P71–P150. [CrossRef]
29. McCarthy, J.; Minsky, M.L.; Rochester, N.; Shannon, C.E. A proposal for the dartmouth summer research project on artificial intelligence, August 31, 1955. *AI Mag.* **2006**, *27*, 12.
30. Russell, S.; Norvig, P. *Artificial Intelligence: A Modern Approach*, 4th ed.; Pearson: London, UK, 2020.
31. Breiman, L. Random forests. *Mach. Learn.* **2001**, *45*, 5–32. [CrossRef]
32. Cover, T.; Hart, P. Nearest neighbor pattern classification. *IEEE Trans. Inf. Theory* **1967**, *13*, 21–27. [CrossRef]
33. Cortes, C.; Vapnik, V. Support-vector networks. *Mach. Learn.* **1995**, *20*, 273–297. [CrossRef]
34. Saritas, M.M.; Yasar, A. Performance analysis of ANN and Naive Bayes classification algorithm for data classification. *Int. J. Intell. Syst. Appl. Eng.* **2019**, *7*, 88–91. [CrossRef]
35. LeCun, Y.; Bottou, L.; Bengio, Y.; Haffner, P. Gradient-based learning applied to document recognition. *Proc. IEEE* **1998**, *86*, 2278–2324. [CrossRef]
36. Russakovsky, O.; Deng, J.; Su, H.; Krause, J.; Satheesh, S.; Ma, S.; Huang, Z.; Karpathy, A.; Khosla, A.; Bernstein, M.; et al. Imagenet large scale visual recognition challenge. *Int. J. Comput. Vis.* **2015**, *115*, 211–252. [CrossRef]
37. Goodfellow, I.; Pouget-Abadie, J.; Mirza, M.; Xu, B.; Warde-Farley, D.; Ozair, S.; Courville, A.; Bengio, Y. Generative adversarial networks. *Commun. ACM* **2020**, *63*, 139–144. [CrossRef]
38. Diaz-Pinto, A.; Morales, S.; Naranjo, V.; Köhler, T.; Mossi, J.M.; Navea, A. CNNs for automatic glaucoma assessment using fundus images: An extensive validation. *Biomed. Eng. Online* **2019**, *18*, 1–19. [CrossRef]
39. Carmona, E.J.; Rincón, M.; García-Feijoó, J.; Martínez-de-la Casa, J.M. Identification of the optic nerve head with genetic algorithms. *Artif. Intell. Med.* **2008**, *43*, 243–259. [CrossRef] [PubMed]
40. Sivaswamy, J.; Krishnadas, S.; Joshi, G.D.; Jain, M.; Tabish, A.U.S. Drishti-gs: Retinal image dataset for optic nerve head (onh) segmentation. In Proceedings of the 2014 IEEE 11th International Symposium on Biomedical Imaging (ISBI), Beijing, China, 29 April–2 May 2014; pp. 53–56.
41. Staal, J.; Abràmoff, M.D.; Niemeijer, M.; Viergever, M.A.; Van Ginneken, B. Ridge-based vessel segmentation in color images of the retina. *IEEE Trans. Med. Imaging* **2004**, *23*, 501–509. [CrossRef] [PubMed]
42. Ramani, R.G.; Shanthamalar, J.J. Improved image processing techniques for optic disc segmentation in retinal fundus images. *Biomed. Signal Process. Control* **2020**, *58*, 101832. [CrossRef]

43. Budai, A.; Bock, R.; Maier, A.; Hornegger, J.; Michelson, G. Robust vessel segmentation in fundus images. *Int. J. Biomed. Imaging* **2013**, *2013*, 154860. [CrossRef] [PubMed]
44. Abbas, Q. Glaucoma-Deep: Detection of Glaucoma Eye Disease on Retinal Fundus Images using Deep Learning. *Int. J. Adv. Comput. Sci. Appl.* **2017**, *8*. [CrossRef]
45. Decencière, E.; Zhang, X.; Cazuguel, G.; Lay, B.; Cochener, B.; Trone, C.; Gain, P.; Ordonez, R.; Massin, P.; Erginay, A.; et al. Feedback on a publicly distributed image database: The Messidor database. *Image Anal. Stereol.* **2014**, *33*, 231–234. [CrossRef]
46. Zhang, Z.; Yin, F.S.; Liu, J.; Wong, W.K.; Tan, N.M.; Lee, B.H.; Cheng, J.; Wong, T.Y. Origa-light: An online retinal fundus image database for glaucoma analysis and research. In Proceedings of the 2010 Annual International Conference of the IEEE Engineering in Medicine and Biology, Buenos Aires, Argentina, 31 August–4 September 2010; pp. 3065–3068.
47. Kovalyk, O.; Morales-Sánchez, J.; Verdú-Monedero, R.; Sellés-Navarro, I.; Palazón-Cabanes, A.; Sancho-Gómez, J.L. PAPILA: Dataset with fundus images and clinical data of both eyes of the same patient for glaucoma assessment. *Sci. Data* **2022**, *9*, 291. [CrossRef]
48. Orlando, J.I.; Fu, H.; Breda, J.B.; Van Keer, K.; Bathula, D.R.; Diaz-Pinto, A.; Fang, R.; Heng, P.A.; Kim, J.; Lee, J.; et al. Refuge challenge: A unified framework for evaluating automated methods for glaucoma assessment from fundus photographs. *Med. Image Anal.* **2020**, *59*, 101570. [CrossRef]
49. Bajwa, M.N.; Singh, G.A.P.; Neumeier, W.; Malik, M.I.; Dengel, A.; Ahmed, S. G1020: A benchmark retinal fundus image dataset for computer-aided glaucoma detection. In Proceedings of the 2020 International Joint Conference on Neural Networks (IJCNN), Glasgow, UK, 19–24 July 2020; pp. 1–7.
50. Bragança, C.P.; Torres, J.M.; Soares, C.P.d.A.; Macedo, L.O. Detection of glaucoma on fundus images using deep learning on a new image set obtained with a smartphone and handheld ophthalmoscope. *Healthcare* **2022**, *10*, 2345. [CrossRef] [PubMed]
51. Batista, F.J.F.; Diaz-Aleman, T.; Sigut, J.; Alayon, S.; Arnay, R.; Angel-Pereira, D. Rim-one dl: A unified retinal image database for assessing glaucoma using deep learning. *Image Anal. Stereol.* **2020**, *39*, 161–167. [CrossRef]
52. Sevastopolsky, A.; Drapak, S.; Kiselev, K.; Snyder, B.M.; Keenan, J.D.; Georgievskaya, A. Stack-u-net: Refinement network for image segmentation on the example of optic disc and cup. *arXiv* **2018**, arXiv:1804.11294.
53. Gupta, N.; Garg, H.; Agarwal, R. A robust framework for glaucoma detection using CLAHE and EfficientNet. *Vis. Comput.* **2021**, *38*, 2315–2328. [CrossRef]
54. Singh, L.K.; Pooja.; Garg, H.; Khanna, M.; Bhadoria, R.S. An enhanced deep image model for glaucoma diagnosis using feature-based detection in retinal fundus. *Med. Biol. Eng. Comput.* **2021**, *59*, 333–353. [CrossRef]
55. Shiny Christobel, J.; Vimala, D.; Joshan Athanesious, J.; Christopher Ezhil Singh, S.; Murugan, S. Effectiveness of Feature Extraction by PCA-Based Detection and Naive Bayes Classifier for Glaucoma Images. *Int. J. Digit. Multimed. Broadcast.* **2022**, *2022*, 5. [CrossRef]
56. Li, L.; Xu, M.; Liu, H.; Li, Y.; Wang, X.; Jiang, L.; Wang, Z.; Fan, X.; Wang, N. A large-scale database and a CNN model for attention-based glaucoma detection. *IEEE Trans. Med. Imaging* **2019**, *39*, 413–424. [CrossRef] [PubMed]
57. Ting, D.S.W.; Cheung, C.Y.L.; Lim, G.; Tan, G.S.W.; Quang, N.D.; Gan, A.; Hamzah, H.; Garcia-Franco, R.; San Yeo, I.Y.; Lee, S.Y.; et al. Development and validation of a deep learning system for diabetic retinopathy and related eye diseases using retinal images from multiethnic populations with diabetes. *JAMA* **2017**, *318*, 2211–2223. [CrossRef] [PubMed]
58. Singh, V.K.; Rashwan, H.; Akram, F.; Pandey, N.; Sarker, M.M.K.; Saleh, A.; Abdulwahab, S.; Maaroof, N.; Romani, S.; Puig, D. Retinal Optic Disc Segmentation using Conditional Generative Adversarial Network. *arXiv* **2018**, arXiv:cs.CV/1806.03905.
59. Chang, C.W.; Chang, C.Y.; Lin, Y.Y.; Su, W.W.; Chen, H.S.L. A Glaucoma Detection System Based on Generative Adversarial Network and Incremental Learning. *Appl. Sci.* **2023**, *13*, 2195. [CrossRef]
60. Jain, S.; Indora, S.; Atal, D.K. Rider manta ray foraging optimization-based generative adversarial network and CNN feature for detecting glaucoma. *Biomed. Signal Process. Control* **2022**, *73*, 103425. [CrossRef]
61. Shinde, R. Glaucoma detection in retinal fundus images using U-Net and supervised machine learning algorithms. *Intell.-Based Med.* **2021**, *5*, 100038. [CrossRef]
62. dos Santos Ferreira, M.V.; de Carvalho Filho, A.O.; de Sousa, A.D.; Silva, A.C.; Gattass, M. Deep learning for optic disc segmentation and glaucoma diagnosis on retinal images. *Appl. Sci.* **2020**, *10*, 4916.
63. Vinícius dos Santos Ferreira, M.; Oseas de Carvalho Filho, A.; Dalília de Sousa, A.; Corrêa Silva, A.; Gattass, M. Convolutional neural network and texture descriptor-based automatic detection and diagnosis of glaucoma. *Expert Syst. Appl.* **2018**, *110*, 250–263. [CrossRef]
64. Zedan, M.J.; Zulkifley, M.A.; Ibrahim, A.A.; Moubark, A.M.; Kamari, N.A.M.; Abdani, S.R. Automated glaucoma screening and diagnosis based on retinal fundus images using deep learning approaches: A comprehensive review. *Diagnostics* **2023**, *13*, 2180. [CrossRef] [PubMed]
65. Zulfira, F.Z.; Suyanto, S.; Septiarini, A. Segmentation technique and dynamic ensemble selection to enhance glaucoma severity detection. *Comput. Biol. Med.* **2021**, *139*, 104951. [CrossRef] [PubMed]
66. Yunitasari, D.A.; Sigit, R.; Harsono, T. Glaucoma detection based on cup-to-disc ratio in retinal fundus image using support vector machine. In Proceedings of the 2021 International Electronics Symposium (IES), Surabaya, Indonesia, 29–30 September 2021; pp. 368–373.
67. Wang, P.; Yuan, M.; He, Y.; Sun, J. 3D augmented fundus images for identifying glaucoma via transferred convolutional neural networks. *Int. Ophthalmol.* **2021**, *41*, 2065–2072. [CrossRef] [PubMed]

68. Gheisari, S.; Shariflou, S.; Phu, J.; Kennedy, P.J.; Agar, A.; Kalloniatis, M.; Golzan, S.M. A combined convolutional and recurrent neural network for enhanced glaucoma detection. *Sci. Rep.* **2021**, *11*, 1945. [CrossRef] [PubMed]
69. Li, F.; Yan, L.; Wang, Y.; Shi, J.; Chen, H.; Zhang, X.; Jiang, M.; Wu, Z.; Zhou, K. Deep learning-based automated detection of glaucomatous optic neuropathy on color fundus photographs. *Graefe'S Arch. Clin. Exp. Ophthalmol.* **2020**, *258*, 851–867. [CrossRef] [PubMed]
70. Liu, H.; Li, L.; Wormstone, I.M.; Qiao, C.; Zhang, C.; Liu, P.; Li, S.; Wang, H.; Mou, D.; Pang, R.; et al. Development and validation of a deep learning system to detect glaucomatous optic neuropathy using fundus photographs. *JAMA Ophthalmol.* **2019**, *137*, 1353–1360. [CrossRef] [PubMed]
71. Nawaz, M.; Nazir, T.; Javed, A.; Tariq, U.; Yong, H.S.; Khan, M.A.; Cha, J. An efficient deep learning approach to automatic glaucoma detection using optic disc and optic cup localization. *Sensors* **2022**, *22*, 434. [CrossRef]
72. Kim, M.; Han, J.C.; Hyun, S.H.; Janssens, O.; Van Hoecke, S.; Kee, C.; De Neve, W. Medinoid: Computer-aided diagnosis and localization of glaucoma using deep learning. *Appl. Sci.* **2019**, *9*, 3064. [CrossRef]
73. Hemelings, R.; Elen, B.; Barbosa-Breda, J.; Lemmens, S.; Meire, M.; Pourjavan, S.; Vandewalle, E.; Van de Veire, S.; Blaschko, M.B.; De Boever, P.; et al. Accurate prediction of glaucoma from colour fundus images with a convolutional neural network that relies on active and transfer learning. *Acta Ophthalmol.* **2020**, *98*, e94–e100. [CrossRef] [PubMed]
74. Alghamdi, M.; Abdel-Mottaleb, M. A comparative study of deep learning models for diagnosing glaucoma from fundus images. *IEEE Access* **2021**, *9*, 23894–23906. [CrossRef]
75. Aamir, M.; Irfan, M.; Ali, T.; Ali, G.; Shaf, A.; Al-Beshri, A.; Alasbali, T.; Mahnashi, M.H. An adoptive threshold-based multi-level deep convolutional neural network for glaucoma eye disease detection and classification. *Diagnostics* **2020**, *10*, 602. [CrossRef] [PubMed]
76. Phene, S.; Dunn, R.C.; Hammel, N.; Liu, Y.; Krause, J.; Kitade, N.; Schaekermann, M.; Sayres, R.; Wu, D.J.; Bora, A.; et al. Deep Learning and Glaucoma Specialists: The Relative Importance of Optic Disc Features to Predict Glaucoma Referral in Fundus Photographs. *Ophthalmology* **2019**, *126*, 1627–1639. [CrossRef]
77. Lee, E.B.; Wang, S.Y.; Chang, R.T. Interpreting deep learning studies in glaucoma: Unresolved challenges. *Asia-Pac. J. Ophthalmol.* **2021**, *10*, 261–267. [CrossRef]
78. Camara, J.; Neto, A.; Pires, I.M.; Villasana, M.V.; Zdravevski, E.; Cunha, A. Literature Review on Artificial Intelligence Methods for Glaucoma Screening, Segmentation, and Classification. *J. Imaging* **2022**, *8*, 19. [CrossRef]

Disclaimer/Publisher's Note: The statements, opinions and data contained in all publications are solely those of the individual author(s) and contributor(s) and not of MDPI and/or the editor(s). MDPI and/or the editor(s) disclaim responsibility for any injury to people or property resulting from any ideas, methods, instructions or products referred to in the content.

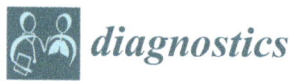

Article

Development of a Machine Learning Algorithm to Correlate Lumbar Disc Height on X-rays with Disc Bulging or Herniation

Pao-Chun Lin [1,2], Wei-Shan Chang [3,4], Kai-Yuan Hsiao [3,4], Hon-Man Liu [5], Ben-Chang Shia [3,4], Ming-Chih Chen [3,4], Po-Yu Hsieh [6], Tseng-Wei Lai [6], Feng-Huei Lin [1] and Che-Cheng Chang [7,8,*]

1. Department of Biomedical Engineering, National Taiwan University, Taipei City 10617, Taiwan; killer-ryan-lin@hotmail.com (P.-C.L.); double@ntu.edu.tw (F.-H.L.)
2. Department of Neurosurgery, Fu Jen Catholic University Hospital, Fu Jen Catholic University, New Taipei City 24352, Taiwan
3. Graduate Institute of Business Administration, College of Management, Fu Jen Catholic University, New Taipei City 24352, Taiwan; sanchangai@gmail.com (W.-S.C.); st880005@gmail.com (K.-Y.H.); 025674@mail.fju.edu.tw (B.-C.S.); 081438@mail.fju.edu.tw (M.-C.C.)
4. Artificial Intelligence Development Center, Fu Jen Catholic University, New Taipei City 24352, Taiwan
5. Department of Radiology, Fu Jen Catholic University Hospital, Fu Jen Catholic University, New Taipei City 24352, Taiwan; 138583@mail.fju.edu.tw
6. Industrial Technology Research Institute (ITRI), Hsinchu City 310401, Taiwan; poyu429@itri.org.tw (P.-Y.H.); lai51613@gmail.com (T.-W.L.)
7. Department of Neurology, Fu Jen Catholic University Hospital, Fu Jen Catholic University, New Taipei City 24352, Taiwan
8. PhD Program in Nutrition and Food Science, Fu Jen Catholic University, New Taipei City 24352, Taiwan
* Correspondence: changcc75@gmail.com; Tel.: +886-2-8512-8888

Citation: Lin, P.-C.; Chang, W.-S.; Hsiao, K.-Y.; Liu, H.-M.; Shia, B.-C.; Chen, M.-C.; Hsieh, P.-Y.; Lai, T.-W.; Lin, F.-H.; Chang, C.-C. Development of a Machine Learning Algorithm to Correlate Lumbar Disc Height on X-rays with Disc Bulging or Herniation. *Diagnostics* 2024, 14, 134. https://doi.org/10.3390/diagnostics14020134

Academic Editor: Daniele Giansanti

Received: 2 December 2023
Revised: 28 December 2023
Accepted: 2 January 2024
Published: 6 January 2024

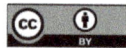

Copyright: © 2024 by the authors. Licensee MDPI, Basel, Switzerland. This article is an open access article distributed under the terms and conditions of the Creative Commons Attribution (CC BY) license (https://creativecommons.org/licenses/by/4.0/).

Abstract: Lumbar disc bulging or herniation (LDBH) is one of the major causes of spinal stenosis and related nerve compression, and its severity is the major determinant for spine surgery. MRI of the spine is the most important diagnostic tool for evaluating the need for surgical intervention in patients with LDBH. However, MRI utilization is limited by its low accessibility. Spinal X-rays can rapidly provide information on the bony structure of the patient. Our study aimed to identify the factors associated with LDBH, including disc height, and establish a clinical diagnostic tool to support its diagnosis based on lumbar X-ray findings. In this study, a total of 458 patients were used for analysis and 13 clinical and imaging variables were collected. Five machine-learning (ML) methods, including LASSO regression, MARS, decision tree, random forest, and extreme gradient boosting, were applied and integrated to identify important variables for predicting LDBH from lumbar spine X-rays. The results showed L4-5 posterior disc height, age, and L1-2 anterior disc height to be the top predictors, and a decision tree algorithm was constructed to support clinical decision-making. Our study highlights the potential of ML-based decision tools for surgeons and emphasizes the importance of L1-2 disc height in relation to LDBH. Future research will expand on these findings to develop a more comprehensive decision-supporting model.

Keywords: lumbar disc bulging; herniated intervertebral disc; disc height; machine learning; decision tree; plain radiography; magnetic resonance imaging

1. Introduction

Lumbar disc bulging or herniation (LDBH) is one of the most common degenerative spinal disorders, leading to nerve compression and radiculopathy [1]. Approximately 10% of patients experiencing low-back pain are diagnosed with LDBH [2]. Large herniated discs can result in severe compression of nerve roots and spinal stenosis, leading to lower-extremity neuralgia, weakness, and numbness and potentially causing various disabilities [3]. To prevent irreversible neurological complications, surgical intervention is needed for patients with severe neurological symptoms [4–10]. Diagnostic imaging, including X-rays and magnetic resonance imaging (MRI), is often employed to assess the degree of nerve root compression caused by disc herniation and to identify the level of LDBH before surgical intervention [4]. Simple spinal X-rays can offer insights into the parameters of the bony structure; nevertheless, for accurate confirmation of disc herniation and the severity of nerve root compression, spinal MRI is typically necessary [8,11]. MRI offers clear visualization of various spinal structures, including ligaments, facet joints, and discs, making it especially effective for soft-tissue assessment. As a result, MRI is commonly the preferred preoperative evaluation tool for surgeons [12]. However, MRI has limitations, including time consumption, limited accessibility (due to insufficient facilities), and high cost.

Plain radiography (X-ray) is the most commonly used and accessible imaging technique due to its cost-effectiveness and ease of use [13]. Spinal X-rays provide rapid visualization of conditions such as spine fractures, spondylolisthesis, spur formation, and structural deformities. Some degree of soft-tissue degeneration can also be inferred from changes in bony structure [14]. For example, a decreased intervertebral space may suggest degenerative disc changes, and severe spondylolisthesis often coexists with spinal stenosis. Despite advances in imaging technology, the accuracy of X-ray-based diagnostic imaging for LDBH remains questionable [15]. Literature reviews have even noted discrepancies between imaging findings and clinical parameters [16]. Additionally, there is a lack of standardized methods for interpreting the lumbar X-ray images of patients with LDBH. Therefore, the utilization of simple lumbar X-ray imaging to establish an effective method to assist physicians in rapid interpretation is an important yet still poorly understood area.

The emergence of machine learning (ML) has introduced a new perspective for addressing healthcare challenges in medicine and surgical decision-making [17]. Current medical practices incorporate ML methods, which play a crucial role by extracting valuable insights from data without the need for predefined human rules [18–20]. ML also aids healthcare professionals in enhancing the quality of care and making precise decisions based on data analysis and interpretation [18]. ML is already extensively employed by physicians and surgeons, encompassing applications in surgical decision support, computer-assisted navigation, and robot-assisted procedures, which have become standard in surgical practice [21,22]. In the current medical landscape, ML algorithms are not only utilized for constructing quantitative classification models but are also widely adopted for medical image interpretation. Various neural network architectures, for instance, have been applied to the interpretation of high-quality CT scans, contributing to image enhancement, restoration, and the generation of 2D/3D medical imagery [23–26]. These advancements provide healthcare professionals with diverse decision-making references.

Deep learning techniques have initially demonstrated success in the automatic detection and classification of spinal scoliosis. Transfer learning methods, for example, have been proposed to automatically detect and classify spinal scoliosis from spinal X-rays, achieving a level of high accuracy in practical applications [27]. Deep learning techniques have also been applied to identify conditions such as osteopenia and osteoporosis from lumbar X-rays [28]. Natural language processing (NLP) techniques have shown their potential value in spine image analysis. Research has employed the noninvasive identification of curve types in spinal scoliosis from a patient's 3D back surface, exhibiting a level of high accuracy when compared to expert evaluations from X-ray images [29]. Additionally, NLP techniques have been utilized to identify lumbar spine imaging findings related to low back pain, demonstrating performance comparisons with traditional statistical analysis methods [30]. The diagnosis and treatment of osteoporosis have also benefited from ML techniques. ML models have been employed to predict the T score and identify osteoporotic vertebrae based solely on conventional CT Hounsfield unit (HU) measurements, aiding spine surgeons in accurately assessing osteoporotic spines preoperatively [31]. Furthermore, ML techniques have achieved high levels of accuracy in the classification of conditions such as spondylolisthesis and lumbar lordosis [32].

The use of ML techniques in spine image analysis has increased substantially, showing their potential in enhancing diagnostic accuracy and predictive capabilities across various studies [28,33–35]. However, to our knowledge, there is a dearth of research addressing the interpretation or prediction of LDBH outcomes and the relationship between MRI and plain lumbar X-ray. This prospective study aimed to achieve the following objectives: (1) utilize ML techniques to establish the connection between lumbar disc-height measurements from X-ray images and the presence of LDBH detected through MRI scans; and (2) based on this connection, develop a decision-support system capable of predicting LDBH exclusively using X-ray images and basic patient information, including age and sex. This system was designed to develop a decision-support algorithm for clinical practitioners. It aims to identify potential candidates for surgical intervention while minimizing subjective factors and human interference. This process facilitates prompt MRI scheduling for individuals in need of surgical treatment.

2. Materials and Methods

2.1. Participants and Study Design

A total of 662 patients who underwent lumbar spine MRI at Fu Jen Catholic University Hospital, Taipei, Taiwan, between January 2020 and December 2020 were retrospectively analyzed. Patients were included if they had undergone both lumbar spine MRI studies and X-rays, with the time interval between the two not exceeding 3 months. Patients were excluded if they lacked lumbar spine X-rays or had undergone previous lumbar fixation or fusion surgery. Patients with pathological factors, including vertebral fracture and spondylodiscitis, were also excluded from this study. All imaging was performed using the same equipment and imaging site. A total of 662 patients who underwent both lumbar spine MRI and X-ray were eventually included in this study. Sixty-eight patients with incomplete studies, 37 with previous spine surgery, 21 with vertebral body fractures, 3 patients with extremely blurred X-ray, and 8 patients with spondylodiscitis or other congenital spine diseases were all excluded. Moreover, X-rays from 67 patients were also excluded due to potential interference, such as severe scoliosis, excessive obesity, and issues with imaging quality. These interferences resulted in errors in the image segmentation produced by the measurement software, leading to the exclusion of certain measurement data that exceeded the upper limits of normal anatomical structures. The L1-2, L2-3, L3-4, L4-5, and L5-S1 anterior and posterior disc heights of the included patients were measured from the lateral view of their spinal X-rays, and the measurements were rechecked by one experienced neurosurgeon and one neurologist. Finally, a total of 458 patients were used for analysis (Figure 1). In total, 13 clinical and imaging variables were collected. The protocol of this study was evaluated and deemed acceptable by the Research Ethics Review Committee of the Fu Jen Catholic University Hospital (No. FJUH110121).

2.2. Definition of Disc Bulging, Protrusion, and Herniated Disc

Disc bulging and protrusion are defined as the presence of fibrous tissue on the dorsal side of the disc annulus that extends beyond the posterior edge of the vertebral endplates, leading to a reduction in the volume of the spinal canal or the occupation of the foramen space. In addition, the migration of disc material, including the nucleus pulposus, endplate cartilage, and annulus fibrosus, can also cause a reduction in the neural canal space. In clinical practice, we commonly use MRI to diagnose intervertebral disc protrusion and to assess whether there is any compression of the nerves. When a patient's lumbar spine MRI showed disc protrusion and compression on the spinal canal in any segment from L1-S1, the patient was classified into the LDBH group.

2.3. Definition and Measurement of Disc Height

In this study, disc height was defined as the distance between the corner point of the vertebral body and the point of its orthogonal projection on the endplate of the adjacent vertebral body (Figure 2). For example, in the figure, the distance between corner point

C and its orthogonal projection point E is defined as the anterior disc height. In the same way, the length from corner point B to its projection point F is defined as the posterior disc height. The anterior height and posterior height were measured separately at the L1-2, L2-3, L3-4, L4-5, and L5-S1 levels. Consequently, 10 measurement data points were collected from every included patient. In most studies, disc height is preferentially measured as the length between adjacent corner points (bd or ac), but in severe spondylolisthesis patients, the length may be overestimated [36–41].

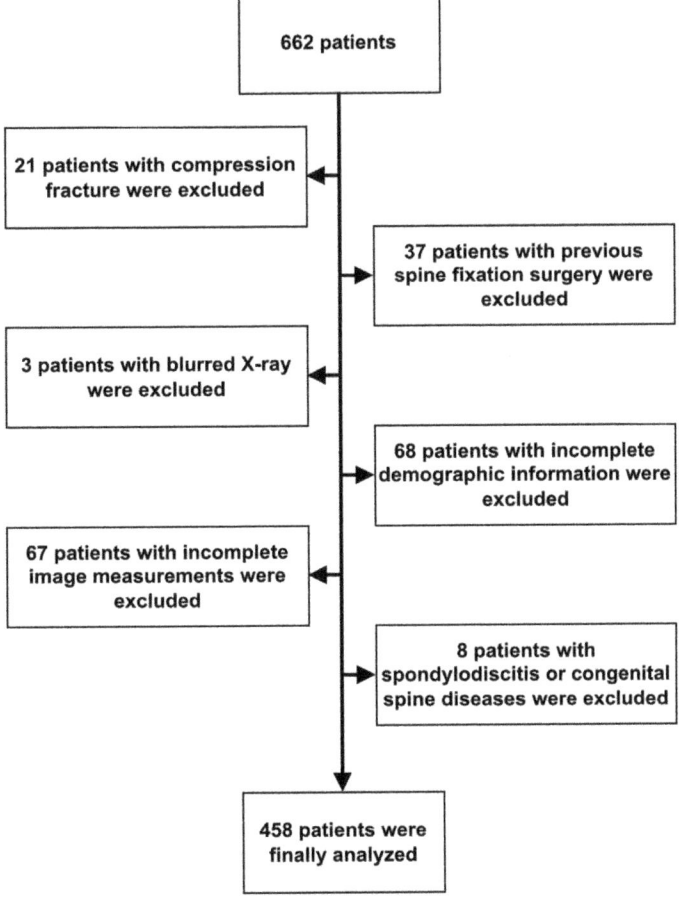

Figure 1. Algorithm of case identification.

Measurement of Disc Height with BiLuNet

BiLuNet is a novel multipath convolutional neural network designed for semantic segmentation in X-ray images, and it has been employed in medical applications such as lumbar vertebrae, sacrum, and femoral head segmentation. One of the significant benefits of BiLuNet is its capability to produce a high level of accuracy in segmenting and shape fitting lumbar vertebrae, sacrum, and femoral heads on X-ray images [42]. This study employs BiLuNet for the localization of intervertebral discs in X-ray images and measures their heights. The measured values are then applied in the subsequent machine learning workflow (Figure 3).

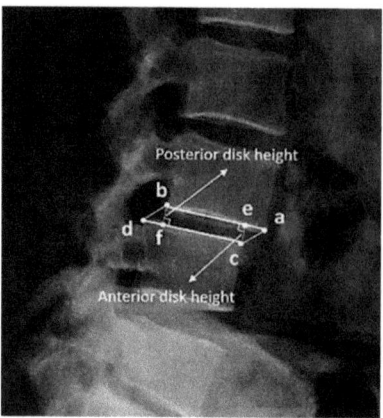

Figure 2. (a–d) are the corner points of the adjacent vertebral body. (e) is the orthogonal projection point on the endplate (a and b) of (c), and (f) is the orthogonal projection point of (b). The disc height is defined as the distance between the corner point of the vertebral body and the point of its orthogonal projection on the endplate of the adjacent vertebral body. For example, the anterior disc height is the length from (e) to (c), and the posterior disc height is the length from (b) to (f).

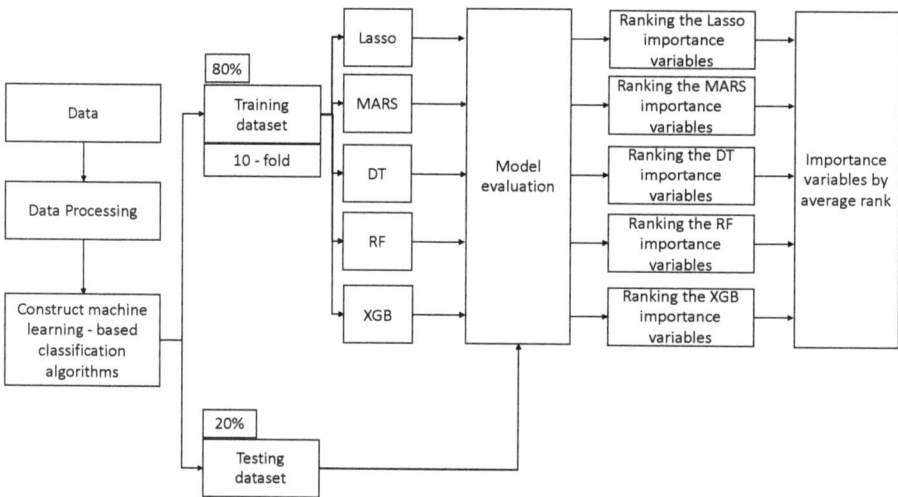

Figure 3. Machine learning (ML) analytical workflow in our study.

2.4. Statistical Analysis

This study used five ML algorithms, namely, least absolute shrinkage and selection operator (LASSO), multivariate adaptive regression splines (MARS), decision tree, random forest, and extreme gradient boosting (XGBoost), to construct predictive models for classifying LDBH patients and to evaluate the importance of different measurements of disc height.

2.4.1. LASSO

LASSO is one of the best regression methods for both variable selection and regularization for addressing the overfitting problem and obtaining accurate results. It uses a penalty parameter to shrink small coefficients toward zero during model estimation [43,44].

2.4.2. MARS

The MARS technique, standing for multivariate adaptive regression splines, represents a sophisticated and nonlinear approach to spline regression, a variant of regression analysis. This method distinctively employs a multitude of piecewise linear segments, commonly known as splines, each characterized by varying slopes or gradients. In its operation, MARS treats every data sample as a 'knot', segmenting the dataset into multiple parts. This partitioning facilitates the execution of linear regression analysis in a stepwise manner, focusing on each divided section individually. The process of knot determination in MARS is twofold: initially, a forward selection procedure is employed. This step involves the comprehensive screening of all potential basic functions along with their respective knots. Following this, a backward elimination strategy is implemented, where these basic functions are systematically removed. The aim of this backward phase is to refine and optimize the combinations of the remaining knots, ensuring that the most effective and representative model is achieved [45].

2.4.3. Decision Tree

A decision tree is a supervised learning method in which a tree-like structure is used to draw conclusions about some observations. Numerous different trees can be developed: regressive binary partition trees use an algorithm that can perform classification for regression problems; models where the target variables are continuous data are called regression trees; and models where the target variables are discrete data are known as classification trees [46]. The latter form was used in this study.

2.4.4. Random Forest

Random forest is an ML model in which the integration of multiple decision trees can improve the high variability in the original decision tree model. A random forest is constructed by first generating multiple decision trees [47]. Then, the final prediction is obtained by voting for the result of the resulting decision tree.

2.4.5. Extreme Gradient Boosting

XGBoost is a popular algorithm for both regression and classification tasks. It improves the integration of the gradient boosting algorithm to obtain better performance in ML tasks. The XGBoost algorithm uses parallel, distributed learning via fast, well-optimized, and scalable algorithms [48]. Ensemble algorithms can enhance the model's performance through the addition of new models until the performance of the model no longer advances.

2.4.6. ML Workflow and Implementation Details

In this study, all methods were conducted in R software version 4.0.3 and RStudio version 1.4.1103. The algorithms for the methods are based on the relevant R packages. LASSO was implemented using the "glmnet" package, version 4.1-1. MARS was implemented using the "earth" package, version 5.3.2. The decision tree was implemented using the "rpart" package, version 4.1-15. Random forest was implemented with the "randomForest" package, version 4.6-14. XGBoost was implemented with the "XGBoost" package, version 1.5.0.1. The "caret" package, version 6.0-90, was used to evaluate the importance of different factors in each method.

This research introduced a structured machine learning workflow (Figure 3), primarily aimed at evaluating and ranking the importance of features. Initially, the raw data underwent preprocessing to ensure its quality and integrity. After this preprocessing phase, the dataset was partitioned into training and testing sets, with the training set accounting for 80% of the total data and the testing set accounting for the remaining 20%. Subsequently, several classification models were employed, and each model was subjected to 10-fold cross-validation to assess its performance. The 10-fold cross-validation method was adopted to determine the optimal hyperparameters for each model, as this approach provides a more consistent evaluation of various methods. This study assessed the performance of these machine learning algorithms using metrics such as accuracy, recall, specificity, precision, and F1 score.

To estimate the best parameter set for the development of the five models, the "caret" package in R was utilized to tune the relevant hyperparameters. The initial models were constructed using default settings. Afterward, feature importance was extracted independently from each model. An average ranking method was then applied, considering the outputs from all models, to offer a comprehensive and objective assessment of feature significance. This study employed the "varImp" function from the caret package to ascertain the relative significance of predictors in each model. Through this function, we sorted the predictors based on their relative contribution to the importance of variables for every model.

3. Results

The 12 variables considered as impact factors for LDBH (Y) in patients are shown in Table 1. The average age of patients who had LDBH was 60.00 ± 14.00 years, while the average age of the non-LDBH patients was 58.98 ± 14.14 years. In the LDBH group, there were 133 males (51.4%) and 126 females (48.6%). In the non-LDBH group, 100 patients (50.3%) were male, and 99 patients (49.7%) were female. The anterior and posterior mean disc heights from L1/2 to L5/S1 were measured and are listed in Table 1.

Table 1. Subject demographics and clinical characteristics.

	LDBH $n = 259$	Non-LDBH $n = 199$
Age (mean ± SD)	60.00 ± 14.00	58.98 ± 14.14
Sex = Male (%)	133 (51.4)	100 (50.3)
BMI (mean ± SD)	25.76 ± 4.09	26.33 ± 4.21
Disc height measurement (mean ± SD) (mm)		
Disc height L1-2 anterior	9.69 ± 2.12	9.36 ± 2.19
Disc height L1-2 posterior	7.46 ± 1.60	7.33 ± 1.50
Disc height L2-3 anterior	10.74 ± 2.40	10.26 ± 2.16
Disc height L2-3 posterior	8.04 ± 2.04	7.68 ± 1.79
Disc height L3-4 anterior	11.83 ± 2.68	11.44 ± 2.78
Disc height L3-4 posterior	8.96 ± 2.74	8.28 ± 2.12
Disc height L4-5 anterior	12.88 ± 8.90	11.47 ± 3.76
Disc height L4-5 posterior	10.99 ± 9.53	9.68 ± 5.99
Disc height L5-S1 anterior	15.10 ± 7.27	14.57 ± 7.92
Disc height L5-S1 posterior	9.59 ± 9.31	8.51 ± 5.28

Abbreviations: LDBH: lumbar disc bulging or herniation.

This study used LASSO, MARS, decision tree, random forest, and XGBoost to construct predictive models to evaluate the measured parameters. Table 2 shows the model performance of the five methods with the validation dataset and testing dataset. The average F1 score values of the LASSO, MARS, decision tree, random forest, and XGBoost models were 0.706, 0.778, 0.569, 0.729, and 0.706 with the testing dataset, respectively. The MARS model provided the highest average F1 score value, followed by the random forest, LASSO, XGBoost, and decision tree models.

The importance ranking of each variable generated by the LASSO, MARS, decision tree, random forest, and XGBoost methods is shown in Figure 4. In this figure, it can be seen that each model provides a different sequence for the relative importance ranking of each variable. For example, the posterior L3-4 disc height is the most important variable in the model constructed with LASSO regression, and the second most important variable is anterior L4-5 disc height. Computing the average rank to explore the importance of the variables shows that the three most relatively important variables are the anterior L4-5 disc height, anterior L1-2 disc height, and posterior L1-2 disc height, which can provide certain insights into their role in LDBH.

Table 2. Performance of the LASSO, MARS, decision tree, random forest, and XGBoost methods.

Method	Avg_Accuracy	Avg_Recall	Avg_Precision	Avg_Specificity	Avg_F1
		Testing Dataset			
LASSO Regression	0.615	0.857	0.600	0.333	0.706
MARS	0.689	0.924	0.676	0.357	0.778
Decision Tree	0.516	0.592	0.547	0.429	0.569
Random Forest	0.655	0.794	0.675	0.458	0.729
XGBoost	0.615	0.857	0.600	0.333	0.706

Abbreviations: avg: average.

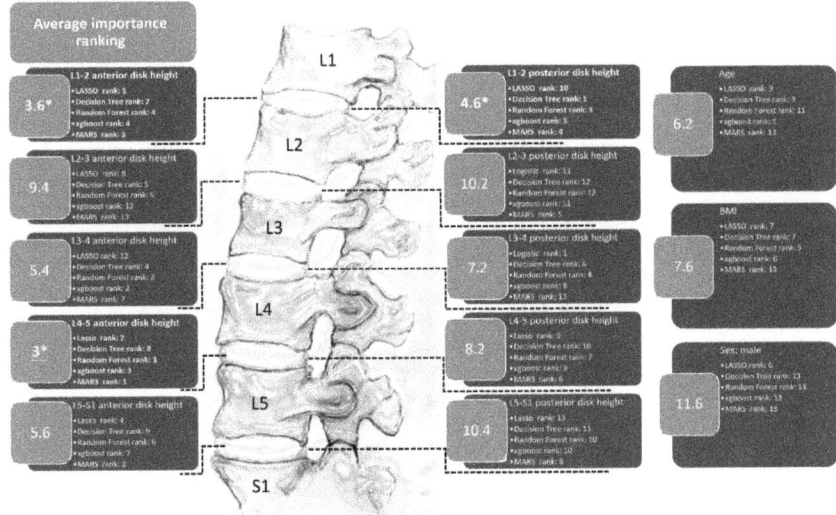

Figure 4. The importance rankings of each variable using the LASSO, ridge, decision tree, random forest, XGBoost, and MARS methods. This figure reveals that the anterior L4-5 and the anterior and posterior L1-2 disc heights are the three most important variables in terms of average ranking. * The top three most important variables.

4. Discussion

To our knowledge, few studies have attempted to use ML methods to predict lumbar disc diseases from spinal X-rays. This study revealed that the L4-5 anterior disc height and L1-2 anterior and posterior disc heights were the top three parameters that helped us to best predict LDBH using plain lumbar X-ray imaging. The classification and regression tree (CART) method generated the best and most promising classification results and provided an output of six clinical features that were critical for the prediction of LDBH. Decision rules for the prediction of LDBH according to the plain X-ray findings were also constructed, as shown in Figure 5.

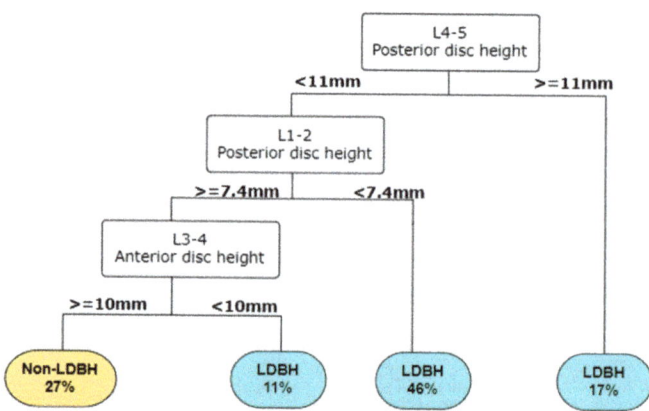

Figure 5. A decision tree can be built in RStudio according to the importance of the input parameters. For example, according to this decision tree, a patient has a 46% risk of LDBH if his posterior L4-5 disc height is less than 11 mm and his L1-2 posterior disc height is less than 7.4 mm. This decision tree helps identify the risk of lumbar disc bulging, or herniation simply from information derived from lumbar spine X-ray. Abbreviations: LDBH: Lumbar disc bulging or herniation.

Disc bulging, protrusion, and even herniated intervertebral discs (HIVDs) are the most common spinal degenerative diseases and can only be confirmed by spinal MRI. Disc degeneration is the beginning stage of LDBH and is strongly associated with facet degeneration, foramen, and lateral recess narrowing, spondylolisthesis, and spinal stenosis. As the degeneration worsens, the symptoms can change from low-back pain to severe neuralgia, claudication, and even cauda equina syndrome. Access to facilities and the costs of MRI limit early detection. This delay may result in irreversible neurological deficits. Decreased disc height, spur formation, spondylolisthesis, and an abnormal range of motion between adjacent vertebral bodies are features of disc degeneration on spinal X-ray, but it is difficult to diagnose LDBH and its related neural structure compression. In this situation, ML can help clinicians construct a decision tree model to predict LDBH simply with plain lumbar X-ray findings and gain new insights for future studies. In areas without access to MRI, such as remote or primary care clinics, this decision-support system may assist high-risk patients in receiving timely examination and treatment.

The strength of artificial intelligence (AI) has grown in the field of neurosurgery. ML can help clinicians via automated computer systems that predict outputs through mathematics [49]. Currently, ML applications in spinal surgery include image classification (e.g., the detection of compression fractures on CT or MRI [50–52], the construction of risk models, and decision support tools) and diagnostic assistance [53–57]. Trinh et al. [58] reported that several deep learning methods can be used to develop a diagnostic algorithm for automatically recognizing spondylolisthesis based on lumbar X-ray images. In one retrospective cohort study, a deep learning method was applied to predict adolescent idiopathic scoliosis (AIS) with standing posteroanterior X-rays [59].

However, few studies have focused on using plain X-ray findings to identify potential patients who need further MRI studies or surgical intervention due to LDBH. The relationship between disc degenerative diseases and disc height remains controversial. One in vitro study with partial discectomy of 15 human lumbar discs demonstrated that the change in disc height was associated with the mass of central disc tissue, and disc height decreases were also related to radial disc bulge. Another study showed that the influences of disc level and degree of degeneration on mechanical behavior are not significant [60,61]. However, in another retrospective study, researchers investigated the relationship between disc morphology and bulging by using MRI scans. They revealed that disc height/depth was significantly associated with the outcome of disc herniation, especially at the L3-4 and L4-5 levels [37]. Our study, which differed from previous methods, attempted to identify possible significant measurements of different disc heights on spine X-rays using ML methods. The age, sex, BMI, and anterior and posterior disc heights at L1-2, L2-3, L3-4, L4-5, and L5-S1 were measured and analyzed using ML methods. The performance of the ML methods, listed in Table 2, demonstrates that these methods are not inferior to traditional LASSO regression.

The importance of the anterior and posterior disc height at different levels was ranked by the five ML methods and is listed in Figure 4. The parameter with the highest average rank was the anterior disc height of L4-5. This finding is compatible with previous studies and clinical MRI results [61]. Disc degeneration can occur at any lumbar spine level but is more commonly found at L4-5 [61]. In the context of this study, age, gender, and BMI are relatively ranked in the middle to lower range in terms of average importance for predicting overall LDBH risks. This suggests that the predictive significance of age, sex, and BMI for LDBH may not be as substantial as is commonly perceived. When only considering patient X-ray information, the measurement of disc height for each segment appears to hold more reference value in predicting LDBH compared to the actual measurements of age, sex, and BMI.

Disc degeneration mainly occurs at L3-4, 4-5, and L5-S1 and frequently results in LDBH. Clinical physicians can easily and directly diagnose disc degeneration through degenerative findings at these three levels on spinal X-rays. However, the average ranking from the ML methods revealed that the height at L1-2 was a potentially more predictive factor than the heights at L3-4 and L5-S1. ML methods may uncover the importance of disc height at L1-2 to predict overall LDBH risks. ML methods may uncover the importance of disc height at L1-2 to predict overall LDBH risks. This unconventional finding seems to have clinical relevance as well. Decreased disc height is always present from the beginning of disc degeneration, and the L1-2 disc degeneration rate is the lowest among all levels in the lumbar discs. More severe degeneration in L1-2 hints at a higher risk of other levels of disc bulging or herniation. The thoracolumbar junction, particularly the segment from T12 to L2, is considered a transition zone between the relatively less mobile thoracic vertebrae and the more mobile lumbar vertebrae. Segments within this region bear significant stress, contributing to over 60% of compressive fractures occurring in the vertebral bodies of T12-L2 [62]. The reduced disc height at L1-2 may also suggest that patients' spines experience greater stress, leading to an accelerated rate of degeneration in the lumbar region compared to normal individuals. This could explain the close relationship between L1-2 disc height and the overall lumbar disc body height.

In the past, plain X-ray could only be used to identify simple bone structure problems, such as spondylosis, spondylolisthesis or compression fractures. The advantages of X-ray over other imaging modalities are that it is less expensive, and its images can be assessed and judged more easily and faster. Our study results, although preliminary, show the development of a novel decision-support system that enables clinical physicians in remote or primary care clinics lacking access to MRI to use simple and fast spinal X-ray screening to identify high-risk patients and promptly refer them to hospitals with MRI capabilities. The purpose and results of this study do not replace the critical role of MRI in diagnosing lumbar degenerative diseases. However, from the perspective of diagnostic assistance and decision support, it can be seen as a valuable contribution.

4.1. Clinical Implications

This pilot study has some clinical implications. First, our study aimed to provide a tool for identifying potential parameters to rapidly identify the possible risk of LDBH based on X-ray findings. By analyzing the results, we provided a potential method for physicians to quickly refer patients in a timely manner. Although previous studies have provided controversial conclusions about the correlation between the parameters found in spinal X-rays and the definite diagnosis found in MRI, this study still used multiple analysis methods, including ML methods, to clarify the relationship between X-ray findings and

MRI diagnosis. If a reliable decision tree can be made in the future, X-rays can identify high-risk patients in rural areas and shorten the MRI waiting list in medical centers. Although the patient number is limited, the result is positive and hints that X-rays can potentially provide more information. Second, this study used ML methods to assess LDBH and revealed a new perspective. Using this method could improve the diagnosis of LDBH and allow hospitals with insufficient equipment or long MRI schedules to select potential high-risk patients. In future works, the model can be combined with other clinical parameters, including occupation, and any other information from plain X-rays. This pilot study recommends the model as a potential primary benchmarking tool for use in the screening of LDBH in outpatient clinics.

4.2. Limitations and Work in Progress

This study presents several limitations. Primarily, the sample size we utilized is not very large and is sourced exclusively from a single institution. In addition to the data processing discussed, our research employed a range of statistical techniques pertinent to ML. As outlined in Section 2.4, our approach integrated methods such as LASSO, ridge regression, decision trees, random forests, and XGBoost. We further incorporated a 10-fold cross-validation approach to ensure a more stable evaluation of our models. The amalgamation of these methodologies reinforces the robustness and credibility of our findings. Second, our analysis focused exclusively on disc height, sex, BMI, and age. To broaden the scope of future investigations, it is imperative to explore a more extensive array of parameters that can be derived from X-rays. Consequently, the generalizability of our findings should be interpreted with caution, and further studies are warranted. In recognition of these constraints, we are actively pursuing several enhancements to address these limitations. These include the following: (1) Expanding the sample size to bolster the reliability and comprehensiveness of our results. (2) Collaborating with multiple institutions to access a more diverse and representative dataset. (3) Integrating additional parameters for a more in-depth analysis, including the clinical sign and symptoms of each induvial to enhance the accuracy of predicting MRI outcomes. Our ongoing efforts are dedicated to fortifying the robustness and applicability of our study in the pursuit of more extensive and generalizable insights.

5. Conclusions

Our study utilized ML-based methods to correlate lumbar disc height on X-rays with LDBH and attempted to construct a potential clinical decision-making tool to support the diagnosis of LDBH based on X-ray imaging parameters. The results revealed that the anterior L4-5 and anterior L1-2 disc heights, as well as posterior L1-2 disc heights, were the three most important variables in diagnosing potential LDBH. The importance of the L1-2 disc height was also revealed for the first time in this study. While still only preliminary, the current study attempts to correlate lumbar disc height on X-rays with LDBH and construct a potential algorithm for screening high-risk LDBH patients. Our results represent an exploratory study of LDBH risk using MRI as the gold standard, and further studies will include more patients and analyze more parameters to construct a more reliable decision-supporting model.

Author Contributions: Data curation: P.-C.L., K.-Y.H., W.-S.C., T.-W.L. and P.-Y.H.; writing original draft: P.-C.L., C.-C.C., K.-Y.H. and W.-S.C.; supervision: B.-C.S., H.-M.L. and M.-C.C.; project administration: P.-C.L.; conceptualization: P.-C.L., C.-C.C. and W.-S.C.; methodology: P.-C.L., K.-Y.H. and W.-S.C.; validation: P.-C.L., K.-Y.H. and W.-S.C.; visualization: P.-C.L., K.-Y.H. and W.-S.C.; resources: H.-M.L., B.-C.S. and F.-H.L.; review and editing: C.-C.C. and H.-M.L. All authors have read and agreed to the published version of the manuscript.

Funding: This research was funded by Fu Jen Catholic University Hospital (PL-202108030-V).

Institutional Review Board Statement: The protocol of this study was evaluated and deemed acceptable by the Institutional Review Board of the Fu Jen Catholic University Hospital (No. FJUH110121).

Informed Consent Statement: Patient consent was waived due to the retrospective nature of the study, which was approved by the Institutional Review Board of Fu Jen Catholic University Hospital.

Data Availability Statement: Data are available upon reasonable request from the authors with the permission of the local ethics committee.

Acknowledgments: We gratefully acknowledge the radiology department of Fu Jen Catholic University Hospital and Artificial Intelligence Development Center of Fu Jen Catholic University.

Conflicts of Interest: The authors declare no conflicts of interest.

References

1. Deyo, R.A.; Loeser, J.D.; Bigos, S.J. Herniated lumbar intervertebral disk. *Ann. Intern. Med.* **1990**, *112*, 598–603. [CrossRef] [PubMed]
2. Murray, C.J.; Barber, R.M.; Foreman, K.J.; Abbasoglu Ozgoren, A.; Abd-Allah, F.; Abera, S.F.; Aboyans, V.; Abraham, J.P.; Abubakar, I.; Abu-Raddad, L.J.; et al. Global, regional, and national disability-adjusted life years (DALYs) for 306 diseases and injuries and healthy life expectancy (HALE) for 188 countries, 1990–2013: Quantifying the epidemiological transition. *Lancet* **2015**, *386*, 2145–2191. [CrossRef] [PubMed]
3. Humphreys, S.C.; Eck, J.C. Clinical evaluation and treatment options for herniated lumbar disc. *Am. Fam. Physician* **1999**, *59*, 575–582, 578–587. [PubMed]
4. Takahashi, K.; Kagechika, K.; Takino, T.; Matsui, T.; Miyazaki, T.; Shima, I. Changes in epidural pressure during walking in patients with lumbar spinal stenosis. *Spine* **1995**, *20*, 2746–2749. [CrossRef] [PubMed]
5. Rydevik, B. Neurophysiology of cauda equina compression. *Acta Orthop. Scand. Suppl.* **1993**, *251*, 52–55. [CrossRef] [PubMed]
6. Baker, A.R.; Collins, T.A.; Porter, R.W.; Kidd, C. Laser Doppler study of porcine cauda equina blood flow. The effect of electrical stimulation of the rootlets during single and double site, low pressure compression of the cauda equina. *Spine* **1995**, *20*, 660–664. [CrossRef] [PubMed]
7. Ooi, Y.; Mita, F.; Satoh, Y. Myeloscopic study on lumbar spinal canal stenosis with special reference to intermittent claudication. *Spine* **1990**, *15*, 544–549. [CrossRef] [PubMed]
8. Wassenaar, M.; van Rijn, R.M.; van Tulder, M.W.; Verhagen, A.P.; van der Windt, D.A.; Koes, B.W.; de Boer, M.R.; Ginai, A.Z.; Ostelo, R.W. Magnetic resonance imaging for diagnosing lumbar spinal pathology in adult patients with low back pain or sciatica: A diagnostic systematic review. *Eur. Spine J.* **2012**, *21*, 220–227. [CrossRef]
9. Ikawa, M.; Atsuta, Y.; Tsunekawa, H. Ectopic firing due to artificial venous stasis in rat lumbar spinal canal stenosis model: A possible pathogenesis of neurogenic intermittent claudication. *Spine* **2005**, *30*, 2393–2397. [CrossRef]
10. Kaiser, M.C.; Capesius, P.; Roilgen, A.; Sandt, G.; Poos, D.; Gratia, G. Epidural venous stasis in spinal stenosis. CT appearance. *Neuroradiology* **1984**, *26*, 435–438. [CrossRef]
11. Jarvik, J.G.; Deyo, R.A. Diagnostic evaluation of low back pain with emphasis on imaging. *Ann. Intern. Med.* **2002**, *137*, 586–597. [CrossRef] [PubMed]
12. Taylor, J.A.; Bussières, A. Diagnostic imaging for spinal disorders in the elderly: A narrative review. *Chiropr. Man. Ther.* **2012**, *20*, 16. [CrossRef] [PubMed]
13. Jarvik, J.G.; Hollingworth, W.; Martin, B.; Emerson, S.S.; Gray, D.T.; Overman, S.; Robinson, D.; Staiger, T.; Wessbecher, F.; Sullivan, S.D.; et al. Rapid magnetic resonance imaging vs radiographs for patients with low back pain: A randomized controlled trial. *JAMA* **2003**, *289*, 2810–2818. [CrossRef] [PubMed]
14. Steurer, J.; Roner, S.; Gnannt, R.; Hodler, J. Quantitative radiologic criteria for the diagnosis of lumbar spinal stenosis: A systematic literature review. *BMC Musculoskelet. Disord.* **2011**, *12*, 175. [CrossRef]
15. Deyo, R.A.; Bigos, S.J.; Maravilla, K.R. Diagnostic imaging procedures for the lumbar spine. *Ann. Intern. Med.* **1989**, *111*, 865–867. [CrossRef]
16. Mostofi, K.; Karimi Khouzani, R. Reliability of the Path of the Sciatic Nerve, Congruence between Patients' History and Medical Imaging Evidence of Disc Herniation and Its Role in Surgical Decision Making. *Asian Spine J.* **2015**, *9*, 200–204. [CrossRef]
17. Liu, Y.; Chen, P.C.; Krause, J.; Peng, L. How to Read Articles That Use Machine Learning: Users' Guides to the Medical Literature. *JAMA* **2019**, *322*, 1806–1816. [CrossRef] [PubMed]
18. Rajkomar, A.; Dean, J.; Kohane, I. Machine Learning in Medicine. *N. Engl. J. Med.* **2019**, *380*, 1347–1358. [CrossRef]
19. Qadri, S.F.; Lin, H.; Shen, L.; Ahmad, M.; Qadri, S.; Khan, S.; Khan, M.; Zareen, S.S.; Akbar, M.A.; Bin Heyat, M.B.; et al. CT-Based Automatic Spine Segmentation Using Patch-Based Deep Learning. *Int. J. Intell. Syst.* **2023**, *2023*, 2345835. [CrossRef]
20. Ahmad, M.; Ding, Y.; Furqan Qadri, S.; Yang, J. Convolutional-neural-network-based feature extraction for liver segmentation from CT images. In Proceedings of the Eleventh International Conference on Digital Image Processing (ICDIP 2019), Guangzhou, China, 10–13 May 2019; p. 159.
21. Katsos, K.; Johnson, S.E.; Ibrahim, S.; Bydon, M. Current Applications of Machine Learning for Spinal Cord Tumors. *Life* **2023**, *13*, 520. [CrossRef]
22. Chang, M.; Canseco, J.A.; Nicholson, K.J.; Patel, N.; Vaccaro, A.R. The Role of Machine Learning in Spine Surgery: The Future Is Now. *Front. Surg.* **2020**, *7*, 54. [CrossRef] [PubMed]

23. Zhuang, Y.; Chen, S.; Jiang, N.; Hu, H. An Effective WSSENet-Based Similarity Retrieval Method of Large Lung CT Image Databases. *KSII Trans. Internet Inf. Syst.* **2022**, *16*, 2359–2376. [CrossRef]
24. Cao, Z.; Wang, Y.; Zheng, W.; Yin, L.; Tang, Y.; Miao, W.; Liu, S.; Yang, B. The algorithm of stereo vision and shape from shading based on endoscope imaging. *Biomed. Signal Process. Control* **2022**, *76*, 103658. [CrossRef]
25. Liu, Y.; Tian, J.; Hu, R.; Yang, B.; Liu, S.; Yin, L.; Zheng, W. Improved Feature Point Pair Purification Algorithm Based on SIFT During Endoscope Image Stitching. *Front. Neurorobot.* **2022**, *16*, 840594. [CrossRef] [PubMed]
26. Liu, S.; Yang, B.; Wang, Y.; Tian, J.; Yin, L.; Zheng, W. 2D/3D Multimode Medical Image Registration Based on Normalized Cross-Correlation. *Appl. Sci.* **2022**, *12*, 2828. [CrossRef]
27. Amin, A.; Abbas, M.; Salam, A.A. Automatic Detection and classification of Scoliosis from Spine X-rays using Transfer Learning. In Proceedings of the 2022 2nd International Conference on Digital Futures and Transformative Technologies (ICoDT2), Rawalpindi, Pakistan, 24–26 May 2022; pp. 1–6.
28. Zhang, B.; Yu, K.; Ning, Z.; Wang, K.; Dong, Y.; Liu, X.; Liu, S.; Wang, J.; Zhu, C.; Yu, Q.; et al. Deep learning of lumbar spine X-ray for osteopenia and osteoporosis screening: A multicenter retrospective cohort study. *Bone* **2020**, *140*, 115561. [CrossRef] [PubMed]
29. Adankon, M.M.; Dansereau, J.; Labelle, H.; Cheriet, F. Non invasive classification system of scoliosis curve types using least-squares support vector machines. *Artif. Intell. Med.* **2012**, *56*, 99–107. [CrossRef] [PubMed]
30. Tan, W.K.; Hassanpour, S.; Heagerty, P.J.; Rundell, S.D.; Suri, P.; Huhdanpaa, H.T.; James, K.; Carrell, D.S.; Langlotz, C.P.; Organ, N.L.; et al. Comparison of Natural Language Processing Rules-based and Machine-learning Systems to Identify Lumbar Spine Imaging Findings Related to Low Back Pain. *Acad. Radiol.* **2018**, *25*, 1422–1432. [CrossRef]
31. Jin, M.; Schröder, M.; Staartjes, V.E. 15—Artificial Intelligence and Machine Learning in Spine Surgery. In *Robotic and Navigated Spine Surgery*; Veeravagu, A., Wang, M.Y., Eds.; Elsevier: New Delhi, India, 2023; pp. 213–229.
32. Masood, R.F.; Taj, I.A.; Khan, M.B.; Qureshi, M.A.; Hassan, T. Deep Learning based Vertebral Body Segmentation with Extraction of Spinal Measurements and Disorder Disease Classification. *Biomed. Signal Process. Control* **2022**, *71*, 103230. [CrossRef]
33. Jujjavarapu, C.; Pejaver, V.; Cohen, T.A.; Mooney, S.D.; Heagerty, P.J.; Jarvik, J.G. A Comparison of Natural Language Processing Methods for the Classification of Lumbar Spine Imaging Findings Related to Lower Back Pain. *Acad. Radiol.* **2022**, *29* (Suppl. 3), S188–S200. [CrossRef]
34. Nam, K.H.; Seo, I.; Kim, D.H.; Lee, J.I.; Choi, B.K.; Han, I.H. Machine Learning Model to Predict Osteoporotic Spine with Hounsfield Units on Lumbar Computed Tomography. *J. Korean Neurosurg. Soc.* **2019**, *62*, 442–449. [CrossRef] [PubMed]
35. D'Antoni, F.; Russo, F.; Ambrosio, L.; Vollero, L.; Vadalà, G.; Merone, M.; Papalia, R.; Denaro, V. Artificial Intelligence and Computer Vision in Low Back Pain: A Systematic Review. *Int. J. Environ. Res. Public Health* **2021**, *18*, 10909. [CrossRef] [PubMed]
36. Onishi, F.J.; de Paiva Neto, M.A.; Cavalheiro, S.; Centeno, R.S. Morphometric analysis of 900 lumbar intervertebral discs: Anterior and posterior height analysis and their ratio. *Interdiscip. Neurosurg.* **2019**, *18*, 100523. [CrossRef]
37. Hung, I.Y.-J.; Shih, T.T.-F.; Chen, B.-B.; Guo, Y.L. Prediction of Lumbar Disc Bulging and Protrusion by Anthropometric Factors and Disc Morphology. *Int. J. Environ. Res. Public Health* **2021**, *18*, 2521. [CrossRef] [PubMed]
38. Wáng, J.Q.; Kaplar, Z.; Deng, M.; Griffith, J.F.; Leung, J.C.; Kwok, A.W.; Kwok, T.; Leung, P.C.; Wáng, Y.X. Thoracolumbar intervertebral disc area morphometry in elderly Chinese men and women: Radiographic quantifications at baseline and changes at year-4 follow-up. *bioRxiv* **2017**, 139402. [CrossRef] [PubMed]
39. Muellner, M.; Wang, Z.; Hu, Z.; Hardt, S.; Pumberger, M.; Becker, L.; Haffer, H. Hip replacement improves lumbar flexibility and intervertebral disc height—A prospective observational investigation with standing and sitting assessment of patients undergoing total hip arthroplasty. *Int. Orthop.* **2022**, *46*, 2195–2203. [CrossRef]
40. Lv, X.; Liu, Y.; Zhou, S.; Wang, Q.; Gu, H.; Fu, X.; Ding, Y.; Zhang, B.; Dai, M. Correlations between the feature of sagittal spinopelvic alignment and facet joint degeneration: A retrospective study. *BMC Musculoskelet. Disord.* **2016**, *17*, 341. [CrossRef]
41. Kumar, N.; Shah, S.M.; Ng, Y.H.; Pannierselvam, V.K.; Dasde, S.; Shen, L. Role of coflex as an adjunct to decompression for symptomatic lumbar spinal stenosis. *Asian Spine J.* **2014**, *8*, 161–169. [CrossRef]
42. Tran, V.L.; Lin, H.Y.; Liu, H.W.; Jang, F.J.; Tseng, C.H. BiLuNet: A Multi-path Network for Semantic Segmentation on X-ray Images. In Proceedings of the 2020 25th International Conference on Pattern Recognition (ICPR), Milan, Italy, 10–15 January 2021; pp. 10034–10041.
43. Tibshirani, R. Regression Shrinkage and Selection via the Lasso. *J. R. Stat. Soc. Ser. B* **1996**, *58*, 267–288. [CrossRef]
44. Kwon, S.; Lee, S.; Na, O. Tuning parameter selection for the adaptive LASSO in the autoregressive model. *J. Korean Stat. Soc.* **2017**, *46*, 285–297. [CrossRef]
45. Tsai, M.H.; Jhou, M.J.; Liu, T.C.; Fang, Y.W.; Lu, C.J. An integrated machine learning predictive scheme for longitudinal laboratory data to evaluate the factors determining renal function changes in patients with different chronic kidney disease stages. *Front. Med.* **2023**, *10*, 1155426. [CrossRef]
46. Che, D.; Liu, Q.; Rasheed, K.; Tao, X. Decision tree and ensemble learning algorithms with their applications in bioinformatics. *Adv. Exp. Med. Biol.* **2011**, *696*, 191–199. [CrossRef]
47. Sarica, A.; Cerasa, A.; Quattrone, A. Random Forest Algorithm for the Classification of Neuroimaging Data in Alzheimer's Disease: A Systematic Review. *Front. Aging Neurosci.* **2017**, *9*, 329. [CrossRef] [PubMed]
48. Torlay, L.; Perrone-Bertolotti, M.; Thomas, E.; Baciu, M. Machine learning-XGBoost analysis of language networks to classify patients with epilepsy. *Brain Inform.* **2017**, *4*, 159–169. [CrossRef] [PubMed]
49. Jordan, M.I.; Mitchell, T.M. Machine learning: Trends, perspectives, and prospects. *Science* **2015**, *349*, 255–260. [CrossRef]

50. Burns, J.E.; Yao, J.; Summers, R.M. Vertebral Body Compression Fractures and Bone Density: Automated Detection and Classification on CT Images. *Radiology* **2017**, *284*, 788–797. [CrossRef] [PubMed]
51. Bar, A.; Wolf, L.; Bergman Amitai, O.; Toledano, E.; Elnekave, E. Compression fractures detection on CT. In Proceedings of the Society of Photo-Optical Instrumentation Engineers (SPIE) Conference Series, Orlando, FL, USA, 1 March 2017; p. 1013440.
52. Frighetto-Pereira, L.; Rangayyan, R.M.; Metzner, G.A.; de Azevedo-Marques, P.M.; Nogueira-Barbosa, M.H. Shape, texture and statistical features for classification of benign and malignant vertebral compression fractures in magnetic resonance images. *Comput. Biol. Med.* **2016**, *73*, 147–156. [CrossRef] [PubMed]
53. Karhade, A.V.; Thio, Q.; Ogink, P.T.; Shah, A.A.; Bono, C.M.; Oh, K.S.; Saylor, P.J.; Schoenfeld, A.J.; Shin, J.H.; Harris, M.B.; et al. Development of Machine Learning Algorithms for Prediction of 30-Day Mortality After Surgery for Spinal Metastasis. *Neurosurgery* **2019**, *85*, E83–E91. [CrossRef]
54. Ogink, P.T.; Karhade, A.V.; Thio, Q.; Gormley, W.B.; Oner, F.C.; Verlaan, J.J.; Schwab, J.H. Predicting discharge placement after elective surgery for lumbar spinal stenosis using machine learning methods. *Eur. Spine J.* **2019**, *28*, 1433–1440. [CrossRef]
55. Ramkumar, P.N.; Karnuta, J.M.; Navarro, S.M.; Haeberle, H.S.; Iorio, R.; Mont, M.A.; Patterson, B.M.; Krebs, V.E. Preoperative Prediction of Value Metrics and a Patient-Specific Payment Model for Primary Total Hip Arthroplasty: Development and Validation of a Deep Learning Model. *J. Arthroplasty* **2019**, *34*, 2228–2234.e2221. [CrossRef]
56. Stopa, B.M.; Robertson, F.C.; Karhade, A.V.; Chua, M.; Broekman, M.L.D.; Schwab, J.H.; Smith, T.R.; Gormley, W.B. Predicting nonroutine discharge after elective spine surgery: External validation of machine learning algorithms. *J. Neurosurg. Spine* **2019**, *31*, 742–747. [CrossRef] [PubMed]
57. Thio, Q.; Karhade, A.V.; Ogink, P.T.; Raskin, K.A.; De Amorim Bernstein, K.; Lozano Calderon, S.A.; Schwab, J.H. Can Machine-learning Techniques Be Used for 5-year Survival Prediction of Patients With Chondrosarcoma? *Clin. Orthop. Relat. Res.* **2018**, *476*, 2040–2048. [CrossRef] [PubMed]
58. Trinh, G.M.; Shao, H.C.; Hsieh, K.L.; Lee, C.Y.; Liu, H.W.; Lai, C.W.; Chou, S.Y.; Tsai, P.I.; Chen, K.J.; Chang, F.C.; et al. Detection of Lumbar Spondylolisthesis from X-ray Images Using Deep Learning Network. *J. Clin. Med.* **2022**, *11*, 5450. [CrossRef] [PubMed]
59. Wang, H.; Zhang, T.; Cheung, K.M.; Shea, G.K. Application of deep learning upon spinal radiographs to predict progression in adolescent idiopathic scoliosis at first clinic visit. *EClinicalMedicine* **2021**, *42*, 101220. [CrossRef]
60. Brinckmann, P.; Grootenboer, H. Change of disc height, radial disc bulge, and intradiscal pressure from discectomy. An in vitro investigation on human lumbar discs. *Spine* **1991**, *16*, 641–646. [CrossRef]
61. Nachemson, A.L.; Schultz, A.B.; Berkson, M.H. Mechanical properties of human lumbar spine motion segments. Influence of age, sex, disc level, and degeneration. *Spine* **1979**, *4*, 1–8. [CrossRef]
62. Alexandru, D.; So, W. Evaluation and management of vertebral compression fractures. *Perm. J.* **2012**, *16*, 46–51. [CrossRef]

Disclaimer/Publisher's Note: The statements, opinions and data contained in all publications are solely those of the individual author(s) and contributor(s) and not of MDPI and/or the editor(s). MDPI and/or the editor(s) disclaim responsibility for any injury to people or property resulting from any ideas, methods, instructions or products referred to in the content.

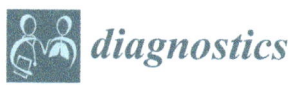

Article

A Coarse-to-Fine Fusion Network for Small Liver Tumor Detection and Segmentation: A Real-World Study

Shu Wu [1], Hang Yu [2], Cuiping Li [1], Rencheng Zheng [2], Xueqin Xia [2], Chengyan Wang [3,*] and He Wang [2,3,4,5,*]

[1] Zhiyu Software Information Co., Ltd., Shanghai 200030, China
[2] Institute of Science and Technology for Brain-Inspired Intelligence, Fudan University, Shanghai 200433, China
[3] Human Phenome Institute, Fudan University, Shanghai 200433, China
[4] Department of Neurology, Zhongshan Hospital, Fudan University, Shanghai 200032, China
[5] Key Laboratory of Computational Neuroscience and Brain-Inspired Intelligence (Fudan University), Ministry of Education, Shanghai 200433, China
* Correspondence: wangcy@fudan.edu.cn (C.W.); hewang@fudan.edu.cn (H.W.)

Abstract: Liver tumor semantic segmentation is a crucial task in medical image analysis that requires multiple MRI modalities. This paper proposes a novel coarse-to-fine fusion segmentation approach to detect and segment small liver tumors of various sizes. To enhance the segmentation accuracy of small liver tumors, the method incorporates a detection module and a CSR (convolution-SE-residual) module, which includes a convolution block, an SE (squeeze and excitation) module, and a residual module for fine segmentation. The proposed method demonstrates superior performance compared to conventional single-stage end-to-end networks. A private liver MRI dataset comprising 218 patients with a total of 3605 tumors, including 3273 tumors smaller than 3.0 cm, were collected for the proposed method. There are five types of liver tumors identified in this dataset: hepatocellular carcinoma (HCC); metastases of the liver; cholangiocarcinoma (ICC); hepatic cyst; and liver hemangioma. The results indicate that the proposed method outperforms the single segmentation networks 3D UNet and nnU-Net as well as the fusion networks of 3D UNet and nnU-Net with nnDetection. The proposed architecture was evaluated on a test set of 44 images, with an average Dice similarity coefficient (DSC) and recall of 86.9% and 86.7%, respectively, which is a 1% improvement compared to the comparison method. More importantly, compared to existing methods, our proposed approach demonstrates state-of-the-art performance in segmenting small objects with sizes smaller than 10 mm, achieving a Dice score of 85.3% and a malignancy detection rate of 87.5%.

Keywords: dynamic contrast-enhanced imaging; segmentation; lesion detection; small liver tumor; convolutional neural network; deep learning

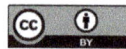

1. Introduction

According to the World Health Organization (WHO), liver cancer ranks as one of the most prevalent forms of cancer globally, resulting in a significant number of fatalities annually [1]. Hepatocellular carcinoma (HCC), the most common primary liver cancer type, stands as the fifth most widespread malignancy and the third leading cause of cancer-related death worldwide. In general, accurate segmentation of the liver and liver tumor is an important prerequisite before surgery to help physicians make accurate assessments and treatment plans. Traditionally, liver and liver-tumor segmentation rely on manual annotation by radiologists [2], which is time-consuming and susceptible to personal subjective experience. Therefore, there is an urgent need for automated liver and tumor segmentation methods for healthcare professionals in clinical practice. Recently, deep learning has achieved remarkable results in liver tumor segmentation, and most of the top-ranked methods in the 2017 Liver Tumor Segmentation (LiTS) Challenge were based on deep learning [3]; however, the accurate automatic segmentation of small liver tumors is still very challenging.

In complex and diverse real-world scenarios, detection and segmentation of large targets often work well but are not satisfactory for small targets such as early tumors and vascular plaque [4]. The main difficulties for the accurate detection and segmentation of small objects in medical images are as follows: small object region to be detected; few extractable features for small objects; and susceptibility to noise interference [5]. At present, there is still relatively little research dedicated to these problems, so it is an important research direction to explore how to improve the mainstream detection and segmentation algorithms to make them effective for small object detection and the segmentation of medical images [6]. Research on small object detection will help promote the development of the target detection field, broaden the application scenarios of target detection in the real world, improve the level of scientific and technological innovation, and accelerate the pace of the world's overall step into an era of intelligence [7]. Though further fine segmentation may bring more value, and quantifying small objects may once again promote the progress of AI in medicine [8], little research has combined small object detection and segmentation for medical images, and most of the research almost only does detection, for example, lung-nodule detection in medicine [9].

In this paper, we propose a multi-network fusion segmentation framework to comprehensively detect and segment benign and malignant liver tumors and, in particular, to improve the performance of the model on small tumor segmentation. The end-to-end network is more difficult to detect and segment tumors comprehensively as liver tumors vary in size and types of features. Whereas multi-network fusion and coarse-to-fine segmentation can compensate for the shortcomings of end-to-end networks in this regard, the proposed method can learn features and fuse tumors in high and low dimensions of the image; moreover, the fusion network combines detection and segmentation to complement each other to improve the detection rate and segmentation performance simultaneously. The proposed model was evaluated on an MRI liver tumor dataset containing different sizes and different types of liver tumors, and we innovatively provided evaluation methods for this fusion method in terms of detection and segmentation metrics. Our proposed multi-stage coarse-to-fine fusion segmentation method refines the coarse segmentation results at different stages of the network architecture and innovatively includes a detection module as well as a CSR module—consisting of a convolutional block, SE module, and residual module—at the tumor fine segmentation stage. For specific information on the CSR module and SE module, see the CSR-UNet paragraph. The proposed method shows superior performance compared to the segmentation capability of single-stage end-to-end network architecture.

Related Work

To improve the tumor segmentation efficacy on MRI, much of the related research is directed at the improvement of neural network structures or related parameters. Jin et al. [10] proposed a 3D hybrid residual attention-aware segmentation method, i.e., RA-UNet, to precisely extract the liver region and segment tumors from the liver. Two-dimensional convolutions cannot fully leverage the spatial information along the third dimension, while 3D convolutions suffer from high computational costs and high GPU memory consumption. Although deep convolutional neural networks (DCNNs) have contributed to many breakthroughs in image segmentation, the task still remains challenging since 2D DCNNs are incapable of exploring the inter-slice information and 3D DCNNs are too complex to be trained with the available small dataset. Tang et al. [11] proposed a two-stage framework for 2D liver and tumor segmentation. Umer et al. [12] applied a simpler and faster one-stage detector RetinaNet for the localization of liver tumors on LiTS17, and the proposed method precisely detects one or more tumors. Ayalew et al. [13] propose a liver and tumor segmentation method using a UNet architecture as a baseline. Due to the heterogeneity and low contrast of biomedical images, current state-of-the-art tumor-segmentation approaches are facing the challenge of the insensitive detection of small tumor regions. To tackle this problem, Wong et al. [14] proposed a network architecture and the corresponding loss function, which improved the segmentation of very small structures. Kofler et al. [15] proposed a novel family of loss functions, nicknamed blob loss, primarily aimed at maximizing instance-level detection metrics, such as F1 score and sensitivity. Isensee et al. proposed the nnU-Net [16], which as a benchmark medical image segmentation method provides 2D and 3D models based on U-Net, and also provides a variety of image preprocessing and enhancement methods.

In addition, some multi-stage deep network models have been proposed and proven to be effective. Li et al. [17] proposed a new three-stage curriculum learning approach for training deep networks to tackle this small object segmentation problem. It is a challenging task since the tumors are small against the background. The experimental results show that compared with the traditional U-Net, the Dice index of liver and tumor segmentations with the improved model increased by 5.14% and 2.63%, respectively, and the recall rate increased by 1.8% and 9.05% [18]. Luan et al. [19] proposed a neural network (S-Net) that can incorporate attention mechanisms for end-to-end segmentation of liver tumors from CT images. Li et al. [20] proposed a Liver and Tumor Segmentation Network (LiTS-Net) framework. Yang et al. [21] aimed to improve liver tumor detection performance by proposing a dual-path feature-extracting strategy and employing Swin Transformer. Fan et al. [22] provided a multiscale nested U-net (MSN-UNet) for liver segmentation. The MSN-Unet contains multiscale context fusion (MSCF) blocks that acquire multiscale semantic data and obtain multilevel feature maps, and the Res block exploits residual connectivity. Tang et al. [23] proposed an enhanced region CNN (R-CNN) and DeepLab for liver segmentation. The deep learning method was applied to the detection and segmentation steps of the liver to reduce the influence of human factors on the segmentation. The principle of residual learning is also utilized to fuse and extract multi-level information from the network using a jump structure.

2. Materials and Methods

2.1. Data

2.1.1. Patient Inclusion

We developed and evaluated our model based on a private dataset from Shanghai Public Health Clinical Center (Affiliated with Fudan University) and Shanghai ZhiYu Software Technology Co., Ltd., Shanghai, China. This dataset has a total of 218 abdominal MRI scans of liver cancer patients, and we used the sequence of DCE imaging delayed phase. This data set included 100 women and 118 men with an average age of 45 years. The liver tumor categories were Hepatocellular carcinoma (HCC), metastases of liver, Cholangiocarcinoma (ICC), hepatic cyst, and liver hemangioma.

2.1.2. Dataset

MRI was performed on a 3.0 T clinical scanner (Ingenia, Philips Medical System). Gadopentetate dimeglumine (Magnevist; Bayer Healthcare, Leverkusen, Germany, 0.1 mmol kg^{-1}) was injected at a rate of 2 mL s^{-1} followed by a saline flush with a maximum volume of 20 mL. The images of hepatic arterial, portal, and delay phases were obtained at 25–30 s, 60–90 s, and 180 s after contrast medium injection, respectively.

The recorded pixel sizes of our datasets were 640 × 640 × 60 corresponding to a spatial resolution of 0.5938 × 0.5938 × 5.0 mm^3. The main target of our study was detection and segmentation of small liver tumors, and the main object of this study was the differentiation of space-occupying tumors with long diameters from 5 mm to 30 mm and tumor category from benign to malignant.

The dataset was labeled by Shanghai ZhiYu Software Technology Co., Ltd., according to the category of the tumor, and the distribution of liver tumors in terms of size and type as shown in Figure 1. Specifically, a total of 3605 liver tumors were counted, of which the type occupying the major proportion was hepatocellular carcinoma. The benign types were hepatic cysts and liver hemangioma, and the malignant types were HCC, metastases of liver, and ICC, with more than half of the malignant types. For tumor size, more than 50% of the tumors were between 10 and 30 mm, while a slightly lower percentage were between 5 and 10 mm. Since the slice thickness of MRI was more than 5 mm, it was not possible to quantify the occupancies smaller than 5 mm, so they were classified as 5–10 mm in this paper. Our main subject, small liver tumors smaller than 30 mm, occupied the majority of this dataset with 90.7%. Some delay phases with their ground truth are shown in Figure 2.

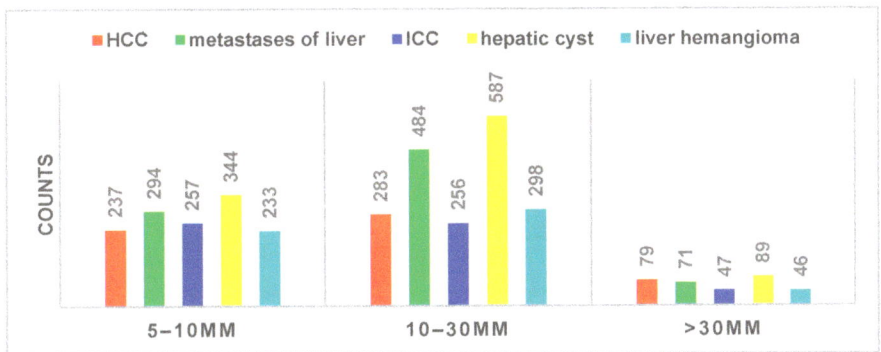

Figure 1. Class and size distribution of different tumors in the dataset.

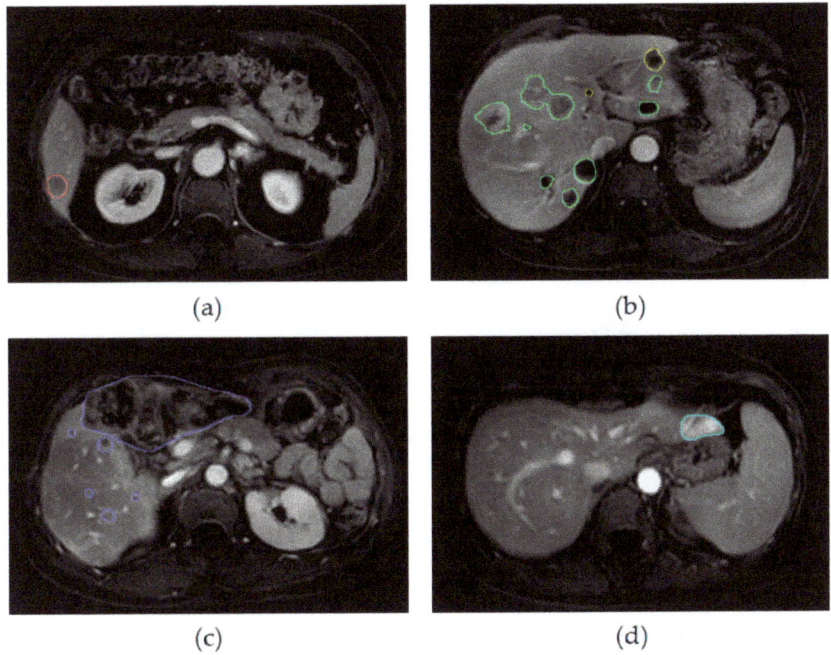

Figure 2. The five types of liver tumors with the ground truth: (**a**) HCC (red); (**b**) metastases of liver (green) and hepatic cyst (yellow); (**c**) ICC (dark blue); (**d**) liver hemangioma (light blue).

2.2. Methods

2.2.1. Architecture

The model architecture mainly includes three steps: preprocessing and liver segmentation; tumor detection by nnDetection model; coarse-to-fine segmentation through CSR-UNet and merging, shown in Figure 3.

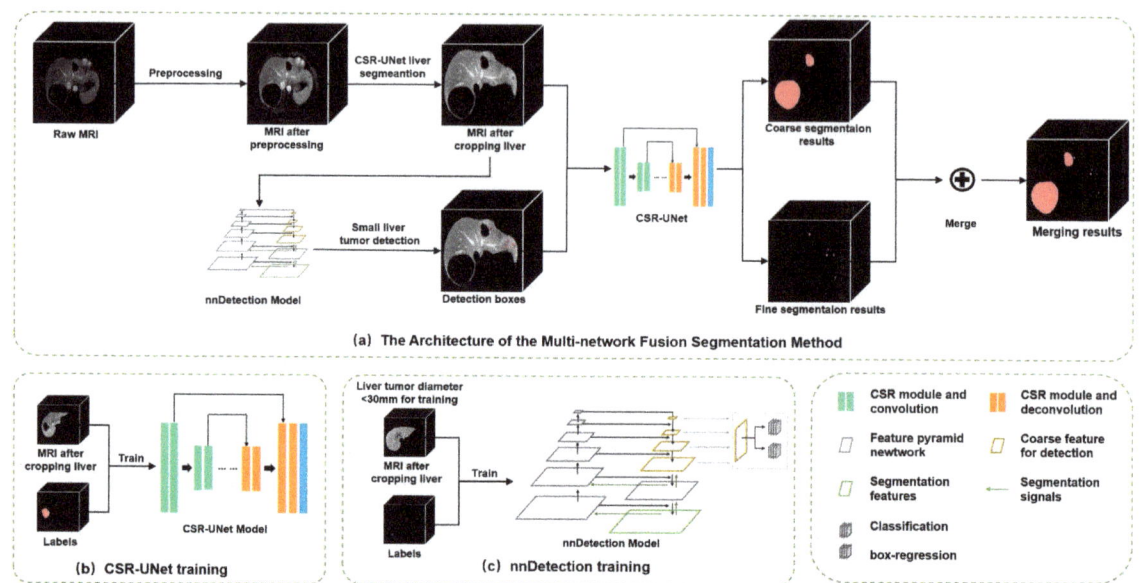

Figure 3. The architecture of the proposed coarse-to-fine fusion network. This present study utilized the raw MR images to extract the liver region via the implementation of a 3D CSR-UNet liver segmentation module. Following this, the region of interest (ROI) was subjected to two subsequent processes: Tumor coarse segmentation and tumor detection. The former was achieved through the use of a 3D CSR-UNet coarse segmentation module, whereas the latter was accomplished via training and inference with the Retina U-Net model utilizing the nnDetection detection module. The detected tumors were fine-segmented via the application of a 2.5D CSR tumor fine segmentation module and subsequently integrated with the coarse segmentation output, leading to the final segmentation results.

Firstly, in the preprocessing process, each slice of 3D MRI data was resampled into a size of 512 × 512 [24]. Specifically, bilinear interpolation was used for original images, and the nearest neighbor interpolation method was used for liver and tumor labels. Every five slices were saved into a 3D patch and values from 0.5 to 99.5% were retained to obtain better contrast within the liver. and then normalized from 0 to 1. Various online data augmentation methods such as flip, rotate, and crop were performed during training [25]. Liver segmentation was performed using CSR-UNet to obtain the liver region; the main purpose of this step was to remove extra-hepatic interference information. The predicted liver region was regarded as the initial ROI for tumor coarse segmentation by 3D CSR-UNet model. Specifically, the segmented liver data were partitioned into multiple patches of size 192 × 192 × 80 and normalized before training [26]. Tumor coarse segmentation was trained using adaptive approach, and the prediction was performed by means of a sliding window with the patch overlapping mechanism. The results of multiple patches were assembled into an overall coarse segmentation result. Through this tumor coarse-segmentation module, most of the tumors larger than 30 mm could be segmented.

In order to improve the segmentation accuracy of small objects, detection module and CSR-UNet are added to the architecture to refine small tumor segmentation. The detection module based on nnDetection model [27] is used to detect only the space-occupying tumors smaller than 30 mm. nnDetection is a novel detection approach that employs Retina U-Net network [28], exhibiting exceptional segmentation performance in complex image scenes, with high precision and accuracy. In this step, tumors smaller than 30 mm were chosen for model training and validation. The detected tumors were cropped into a uniform size of $64 \times 64 \times 5$ before inputting into the CSR-UNet network for tumor fine segmentation.

The final tumor segmentation result is a combination of the coarse-to-fine segmentation results. In specific, large tumor segmentation is achieved by coarse segmentation, while for small tumors, the initial ROI is further reduced with the help of a detection module, and fine segmentation is achieved. By fusing the results of coarse segmentation and fine segmentation, the final segmentation results of liver tumors can be obtained.

2.2.2. CSR-UNet

Figure 4 shows the network architecture of CSR-UNet. CSR-UNet incorporates CSR module into the commonly used UNet framework. The difference between 3D and 2.5D CSR-UNet networks is whether the input is a 3D or a 5-layer 2D matrix, and the former uses 3D convolution while the latter is 2D convolution. The CSR module comprises dual 3×3 convolutional block with batch normalization, combined with an SE module and a residual module [29], as shown in Figure 3 on the left top. Batch normalization is the regularization during training to reduce generalization errors and overfitting. The main function of the SE module is to increase the attention perception of important regions, while the residual module reduces the difficulty of deep network training and improves the segmentation accuracy.

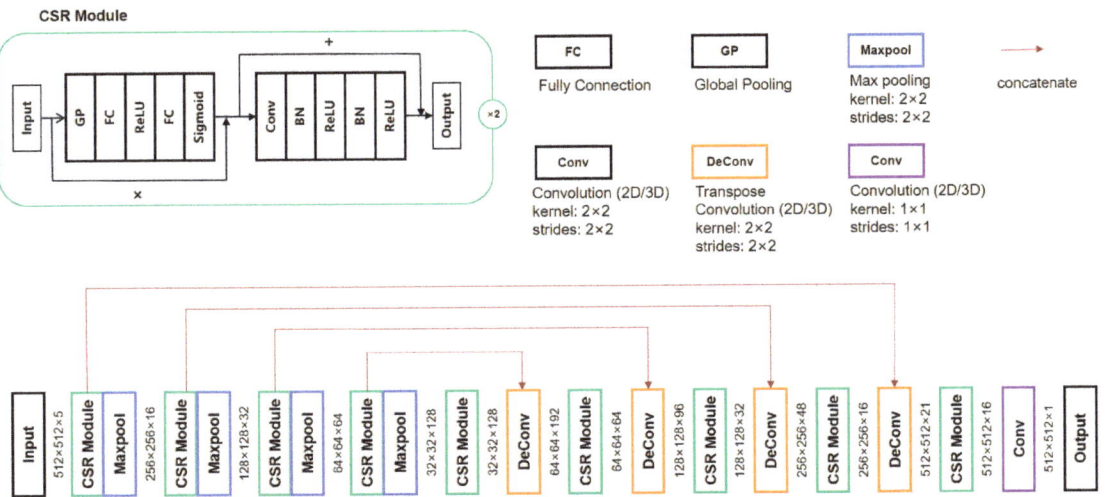

Figure 4. Overview of CSR-UNet in the coarse-to-fine fusion network.

2.2.3. Preprocessing and Adaptive Network Parameters

In order to obtain better network performance, a sliding augmentation module, random online augmentation module, and adaptive network parameters module are added to the CSR-UNet framework. These three modules are used to preprocess the data and generate the hyperparameters of the network before inputting them into the network. In the sliding augmentation module, we performed a sliding window crop for each input data matrix in each dimension [29]. The weights of the cropped input images are also different, giving higher weights to the positions corresponding to the images and labels that the network needs to focus on. The random online augmentation module is image augmentation of the input data, and different image augmentation methods are randomly occurring. These image augmentation methods include image rotation, image flipping, and image scaling. The adaptive network parameters module can consider the performance of the whole network, including the configuration of different patch sizes, learning rates, batch-size settings, etc. Through the complementary roles of these three modules, the data is then fed into the configured network for training iterations.

2.2.4. Loss Function

Focal Tversky Loss is used in our network. Tversky coefficient is a generalization of Dice and Jaccard coefficients [30]. Similar to Focal loss, which focuses on difficult examples by reducing the weight of easy-to-use or common losses, Focal Tversky Loss also tries to learn difficult examples such as in the case of small ROIs (regions of interest) with the help of parameter coefficients [31].

Focal Tversky Loss is an improved version of the Tversky loss function, which is designed to address the issue of class imbalance in medical image analysis. In many medical imaging tasks, such as liver cancer detection, the number of abnormal pixels may be much smaller than the number of normal pixels, making it challenging to train deep neural networks to accurately recognize these abnormalities. Focal Tversky Loss introduces a focus parameter that allows the network to concentrate on difficult samples during training, thereby improving its ability to recognize abnormal pixels in small liver cancers; moreover, the loss function can be adjusted to balance the impact of classification errors on the overall loss, which further enhances the model's performance in liver cancer recognition. Overall, Focal Tversky Loss is suitable for addressing small liver cancer recognition problems, as it helps the network learn relevant features and improve accuracy and robustness.

2.2.5. Implementation Details

Both CSR-UNet and nnDetection are with optimal hyperparameters computed by an adaptive framework. CSR-UNet is implemented in PyTorch and trained on a cluster with 8 NVIDIA A100 GPUs. The network is involved in two parts, one of which is liver segmentation. In this phase, we resampled the image aspect size to 512×512 and processed their spacing counterparts into iso-voxels. Then we performed image up–down restriction according to the distribution of MRI intensity and normalized all input images. During the training period, we used $512 \times 512 \times 5$ multi-channel input patches (equivalent to the form of 2.5D) and $512 \times 512 \times 1$ outputs. We performed online augmentation of the images of the input network by applying random axis mirror flips with probability 0.5 in all 3 axes and random clockwise and counterclockwise rotations of $20°$. In addition to this, all images were scaled with random intensity in the range (0.9, 1.1). The batch size of each GPU was set to 16, the learning rate was set to 0.001, and a cosine annealing learning rate scheduler and five-fold cross-validation were used. On this server, after the adaptive network parameters module and experimental verification, the loss reduction effect under these hyperparameters was the best. The epoch was 300 and the total training time was 3 days. The other part is the fine segmentation of small tumors, which differs from the former only in that the input images were boxes detected by multilayer nnDetection and portioned into 64×64 sizes, and the other preprocessing and augmentation methods were the same. The total time spent on this part of training was 16 h.

3. Results

To evaluate the effectiveness of the multi-network fusion segmentation method for small objects segmentation, we compared the proposed method with nnU-Net and several other networks. All comparison methods are listed in Table 1, including single 3D U-Net, single nnU-Net, nnDetection plus nnU-Net, and nnU-Net segmentation plus nnDetection detection with fine segmentation by CSR-UNet (ours). The results were compared from multiple perspectives for each tumor occupancy, including overall segmentation and detection metrics, and metrics grouped by different size distribution. In addition, the number distribution by long-diameter size, tumor types, and tumor benignity or malignancy are also analyzed.

Table 1. Overall segmentation performance of liver tumors by different methods.

Method	Dice	IOU	F1-Score	VS	Recall
3D U-Net	0.801	0.740	0.816	0.851	0.733
nnU-Net	0.847	0.750	0.823	0.859	0.776
nnDetection + nnU-Net	0.856	0.762	0.891	0.904	0.858
nnDetection + nnU-Net + CSR-UNet	0.859	0.771	0.895	0.904	0.858
Proposed	**0.869**	**0.778**	**0.897**	**0.910**	**0.867**

"VS" means "volumetric similarity"; "IOU" means "intersection over union".

The metrics we evaluated for liver tumor segmentation include segmentation metrics: Dice, IOU, volumetric similarity (VS), F1-score, and detection metric recall. Table 1 presents the mean inference metrics of fusion models trained by three randomly selected test sets. The test set comprised 44 MRI data. The table summarizes the performance results of five experiments, namely CSR-UNet fusion network (ours), 3D U-Net segmentation alone, nnU-Net segmentation alone, nnU-Net segmentation plus nnDetection detection, and nnU-Net segmentation plus nnDetection detection plus CSR-UNet fine segmentation. All five experiments used the same MRI data preprocessing methodology as the proposed method and utilized their respective segmentation networks to isolate the liver and apply the same preprocessing on the liver region. And, all experiments test the same 44 test data. Our proposed multi-network fusion approach outperformed all other methods with the best overall segmentation metrics across all test sets.

We also conducted a tumor count analysis in the three randomly sampled test sets, categorized by long diameter and benign or malignant classification, as presented in Table 2. The table illustrates that the majority of liver tumors in the test sets were smaller than 30 mm, which is the primary focus of our study. In addition, we provide detailed information regarding tumor categories in the three test sets. While benign and malignant categories were relatively balanced, hepatic cysts constituted the largest tumor category. Our experimental investigation and quantitative metric calculations yielded segmentation and detection results for tumors of varying size distributions, which are summarized in Table 3. The presented table reveals that the detection and segmentation performance of liver tumors with long diameters of 5–10 mm yielded the lowest indexes, with Dice coefficients ranging between 0.418 and 0.532; however, for tumors with long diameters of 10–30 mm, all related indicators improved significantly, with a recall rate of one achieved for tumors larger than 30 mm across all five methods. All results metrics for our proposed method here were also the highest for liver tumors in the less than 30 mm range. Notably, the end-to-end segmentation technique, nnU-Net, demonstrated only marginal improvements over 3D UNet. In contrast, the multi-network fusion method, specifically CSR-UNet, yielded substantial improvements when compared to nnU-Net. Lastly, our proposed method demonstrated optimal performance across all metrics related to long-diameter detection and segmentation.

Table 2. Number (average) of size and type of liver tumors in the test set.

Diameter (mm)	Benign Tumor			Malignant Tumor	
	HCC	Metastases of Liver	ICC	Hepatic Cyst	Liver Hemangioma
5–10	24	83	60	105	31
10–30	84	85	74	130	78
>30	11	13	8	22	9

Table 3. Segmentation and detection metrics for tumor inference of different long diameters in our method and the comparison method.

Method	Diameter (mm)	Dice	IOU	F1-Score	Recall
3D U-Net	5–10	0.418	0.302	0.594	0.537
	10–30	0.520	0.382	0.829	0.847
	>30	0.821	0.749	1.000	1.000
nnU-Net	5–10	0.438	0.327	0.614	0.597
	10–30	0.521	0.430	0.869	0.857
	>30	0.842	0.791	1.000	1.000
nnDetection + nnU-Net	5–10	0.487	0.363	0.758	0.736
	10–30	0.531	0.398	0.910	0.905
	>30	0.857	0.807	1.000	1.000
nnDetection + nnU-Net + CSR-UNet	5–10	0.521	0.387	0.768	0.760
	10–30	0.552	0.448	0.910	0.760
	>30	0.873	0.829	1.000	1.000
Proposed	5–10	**0.532**	**0.409**	**0.785**	**0.761**
	10–30	**0.561**	**0.464**	**0.912**	**0.909**
	>30	**0.889**	**0.831**	1.000	1.000

Upon scrutinizing the inference result graph and the ground truth, our proposed method exhibits a relatively comprehensive efficacy in detecting small hepatocellular carcinoma. Nonetheless, certain small or poorly defined tumors are characterized by suboptimal boundary conformity, thereby resulting in diminished Dice and VS (volumetric similarity) scores. Moreover, the inadequacy of contrast and visualization in some tumors during the delayed phase impeded their accurate detection, leading to a proportion of false negatives.

To provide a rigorous elucidation, we posit that the suboptimal conformity of boundaries in certain smaller or indistinct tumors reduces the concurrence of the Dice and VS metrics. Additionally, the suboptimal contrast and visualization of some tumors during the delayed phase engendered erroneous classifications, resulting in an appreciable number of false negatives.

4. Discussion

In this paper, we proposed a method for small liver tumor detection and segmentation. Raw data from hospital screenings were collected and annotated to analyze the DCE images through expert annotation of additional information during the delay period. To maximize tumor ground segmentation results, we integrated detection and coarse and fine segmentation modules into our multi-network fusion method. The detection network employed nnDetection, which is a versatile adaptive detection network capable of detecting small targets comprehensively. Meanwhile, for the segmentation network, we developed a CSR-UNet network architecture that achieves more precise segmentation results for small liver cancers through preprocessing and training tumors at different scales. The detection and segmentation of small liver tumors through medical imaging is a crucial aspect of early disease diagnosis and treatment in the clinical setting. By comparing the results obtained from the test set, it can be inferred that the proposed model has the potential to assist in the early diagnosis of small liver tumors by providing valuable reference values; thus, this model holds promise for clinical applications in the detection and segmentation of small liver tumors.

Upon scrutinizing the inference result graph and the ground truth, our proposed method exhibits a relatively comprehensive efficacy in detecting small hepatocellular carcinoma. Nonetheless, certain small or poorly defined tumors are characterized by suboptimal boundary conformity, thereby resulting in diminished Dice and VS scores. Moreover, the inadequacy of contrast and visualization in some tumors during the delayed phase impeded their accurate detection, leading to a proportion of false negatives. To provide a rigorous elucidation, we posit that the suboptimal conformity of boundaries in certain smaller or indistinct tumors reduces the concurrence of the Dice and VS metrics. Additionally, the suboptimal contrast and visualization of some tumors during the delayed phase engendered erroneous classifications, resulting in an appreciable number of false negatives. Figure 5 presents the outcomes of our proposed method for detecting small hepatocellular carcinoma (HCC) with a diameter of less than 30 mm. Notably, the edges of these small HCCs appear indistinct in the images, rendering it challenging to determine whether they are tumors; however, our method can identify the majority of these small tumors. The comparison between the predicted results and the ground truth indicates that the accuracy of the segmentation is suboptimal. The small size of the HCCs leads to a limited number of pixels, resulting in relatively low values of segmentation-related metrics.

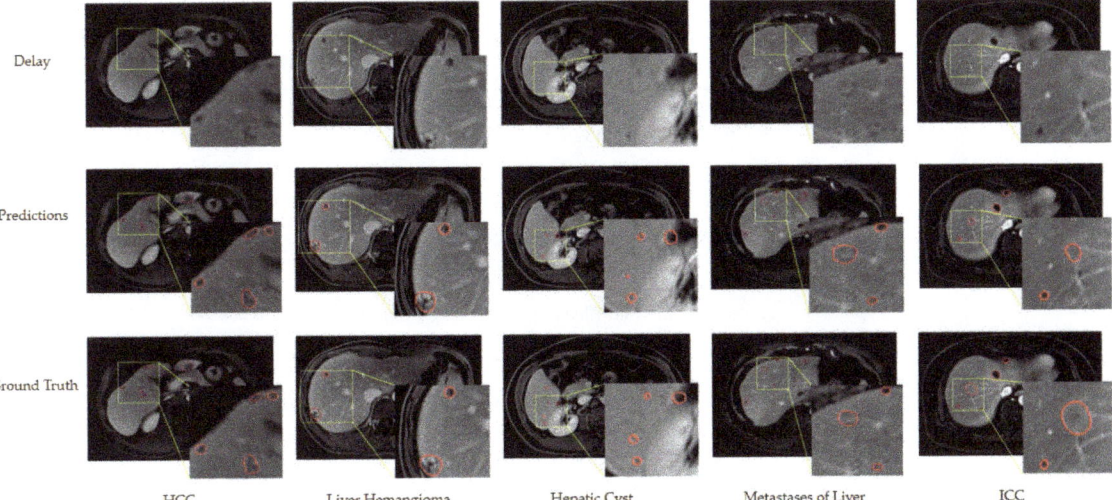

Figure 5. Typical results of our method on the test set. The MRIs are all delayed phases of DCE series. The predicted results and ground truth are circled with red edges in the figure.

Despite the promising results, there are limitations to our current method that require further improvements. Firstly, the proposed model was only tested on a specific MRI dataset. To validate its generality, multicenter external test sets containing enhanced CT images and other small objects need to be collected. Furthermore, since the distribution of different liver tumor types in the dataset is not well-balanced, collecting more varied tumor types is necessary for deeper evaluation. Secondly, although we identified that the delayed phase provides more pronounced visual effects for the five liver tumor types we studied, there is a possibility that more prominent tumor types in other phases were missed. Future research may involve analyzing MRI multimodal data to further examine these tumors. Thirdly, due to the multi-network fusion method's use of inference results from four neural networks, obtaining final segmentation results may take longer. Therefore, this method may be more suitable for patients with liver disease who do not require immediate surgery or require long-term follow-up. Fourthly, we did not model the classification for tumor type by single-class segmentation, and the method's sensitivity or specificity can only be statistically derived for certain species. Finally, there is some room for optimization in the three network frameworks we used. For example, CSR-UNet can enhance the fineness of some patch segmentation, and UHRNet [32] can optimize the decoder. Future research will explore various method combinations to improve small object segmentation accuracy and efficiency.

5. Conclusions

This research presents a highly effective method for segmenting liver tumors by fusing multiple networks. Even for small tumors, this approach achieves outstanding segmentation and detection performance, thanks to the complementary information provided by the different networks. The fusion network increases the performance of network training through adaptive network parameters. The loss function combines Focal loss and Tversky loss, enabling network learning to focus on and learn more detailed tumor feature information. Moreover, the segmentation results enable precise quantification of each tumor's long diameter and volume, providing valuable information for hepatologists and surgeons to monitor the progression and response to the treatment of patients with liver tumors. Ultimately, this novel approach maximizes the potential of liver tumor segmentation to inform clinical decision-making and improve patient outcomes.

Author Contributions: Conceptualization, S.W. and H.Y.; methodology, S.W.; software, S.W. and H.Y.; validation, S.W., H.Y. and C.L.; formal analysis, S.W. and C.L.; investigation, S.W. and H.Y.; resources, S.W. and C.L.; data curation, H.Y.; writing—original draft preparation, S.W.; writing—review and editing, S.W., R.Z., X.X. and H.Y.; visualization, S.W. and H.Y.; supervision, C.W. and H.W.; project administration, C.W. and H.W.; funding acquisition, H.W. All authors have read and agreed to the published version of the manuscript.

Funding: This work was supported by the National Natural Science Foundation of China (No. 82271956), Shanghai Municipal Science and Technology Major Project (No. 2018SHZDZX01).

Institutional Review Board Statement: Not applicable.

Informed Consent Statement: Not applicable.

Data Availability Statement: Data from this study were not provided in any public places. The code repository link https://github.com/wushu526/small_liver_tumor_segmentation (accessed on 14 June 2023).

Conflicts of Interest: Shu Wu and Cuiping Li are employed at the company Zhiyu Software Information Co., Ltd., Shanghai, China. Shu Wu and Cuiping Li have no economic or commercial interests to disclaim. The other authors declare no conflict of interest.

References

1. Bray, F.; Ferlay, J.; Soerjomataram, I.; Siegel, R.L.; Torre, L.A.; Jemal, A. Global cancer statistics 2018: GLOBOCAN estimates of incidence and mortality worldwide for 36 cancers in 185 countries. *CA Cancer J. Clin.* **2018**, *68*, 394–424. [CrossRef] [PubMed]
2. Li, W. Automatic segmentation of liver tumor in CT images with deep convolutional neural networks. *J. Comput. Commun.* **2015**, *3*, 146. [CrossRef]
3. Bilic, P.; Christ, P.; Li, H.B.; Vorontsov, E.; Ben-Cohen, A.; Kaissis, G.; Szeskin, A.; Jacobs, C.; Mamani, G.E.H.; Chartrand, G.; et al. The liver tumor segmentation benchmark (lits). *Med. Image Anal.* **2023**, *84*, 102680. [CrossRef] [PubMed]
4. Ringelhan, M.; O'Connor, T.; Protzer, U.; Heikenwalder, M. The direct and indirect roles of HBV in liver cancer: Prospective markers for HCC screening and potential therapeutic targets. *J. Pathol.* **2015**, *235*, 355–367. [CrossRef] [PubMed]
5. Christ, P.F.; Elshaer, M.E.A.; Ettlinger, F.; Bakshi, S. Automatic liver and lesion segmentation in CT using cascaded fully convolutional neural networks and 3D conditional random fields. In Proceedings of the International Conference on Medical Image Computing and Computer-Assisted Intervention 2016, Athens, Greece, 17–21 October 2016; Springer: Berlin/Heidelberg, Germany, 2016.
6. Zheng, H.; Gu, Y.; Qin, Y.; Huang, X.; Yang, J.; Yang, G.-Z. Small lesion classification in dynamic contrast enhancement MRI for breast cancer early detection. In Proceedings of the Medical Image Computing and Computer Assisted Intervention–MICCAI 2018, Granada, Spain, 16–20 September 2018; Springer: Berlin/Heidelberg, Germany, 2018.
7. Waqas, M.; Tu, S.; Halim, Z.; Rehman, S.U.; Abbas, G.; Abbas, Z.H. The role of artificial intelligence and machine learning in wireless networks security: Principle, practice and challenges. *Artif. Intell. Rev.* **2022**, *55*, 5215–5261. [CrossRef]
8. Lo, S.-C.; Lou, S.-L.; Lin, J.-S.; Freedman, M.; Chien, M.; Mun, S. Artificial convolution neural network techniques and applications for lung nodule detection. *IEEE Trans. Med. Imaging* **1995**, *14*, 711–718. [CrossRef] [PubMed]
9. Pavan, A.L.; Benabdallah, M.; Lebre, M.-A.; de Pina, D.R.; Jaziri, F.; Vacavant, A.; Mtibaa, A.; Ali, H.M.; Grand-Brochier, M.; Rositi, H.; et al. A parallel framework for HCC detection in DCE-MRI sequences with wavelet-based description and SVM classification. In Proceedings of the 33rd Annual ACM Symposium on Applied Computing, Pau, France, 9–13 April 2018.
10. Jin, Q.; Meng, Z.; Sun, C.; Cui, H.; Su, R. RA-UNet: A hybrid deep attention-aware network to extract liver and tumor in CT scans. *Front. Bioeng. Biotechnol.* **2020**, *8*, 1471. [CrossRef] [PubMed]

11. Tang, Y.; Tang, Y.; Zhu, Y.; Xiao, J.; Summers, R.M. E 2 Net: An edge enhanced network for accurate liver and tumor segmentation on CT scans. In Proceedings of the Medical Image Computing and Computer Assisted Intervention–MICCAI 2020: 23rd International Conference, Lima, Peru, 4–8 October 2020; Springer: Berlin/Heidelberg, Germany, 2018.
12. Umer, J.; Irtaza, A.; Nida, N. MACCAI LiTS17 liver tumor segmentation using RetinaNet. In Proceedings of the 2020 IEEE 23rd International Multitopic Conference (INMIC), Bahawalpur, Pakistan, 5–7 November 2020; IEEE: New York, NY, USA, 2020.
13. Ayalew, Y.A.; Fante, K.A.; Mohammed, M.A. Modified U-Net for liver cancer segmentation from computed tomography images with a new class balancing method. *BMC Biomed. Eng.* **2021**, *3*, 4. [CrossRef] [PubMed]
14. Wong, K.C.; Moradi, M.; Tang, H.; Syeda-Mahmood, T. 3D segmentation with exponential logarithmic loss for highly unbalanced object sizes. In Proceedings of the Medical Image Computing and Computer Assisted Intervention–MICCAI 2018, Granada, Spain, 16–20 September 2018; Springer: Berlin/Heidelberg, Germany, 2018.
15. Kofler, F.; Shit, S.; Ezhov, I.; Fidon, L.; Horvath, I.; Al-Maskari, R.; Li, H.B.; Bhatia, H.; Loehr, T.; Piraud, M.; et al. blob loss: Instance imbalance aware loss functions for semantic segmentation. *arXiv* **2022**, arXiv:2205.08209.
16. Isensee, F.; Jaeger, P.F.; Kohl, S.A.; Petersen, J.; Maier-Hein, K.H. nnU-Net: A self-configuring method for deep learning-based biomedical image segmentation. *Nat. Methods* **2021**, *18*, 203–211. [CrossRef] [PubMed]
17. Li, H.; Liu, X.; Boumaraf, S.; Liu, W.; Gong, X.; Ma, X. A new three-stage curriculum learning approach for deep network based liver tumor segmentation. In Proceedings of the 2020 International Joint Conference on Neural Networks (IJCNN), Glasgow, UK, 19–24 July 2020; IEEE: New York, NY, USA, 2020.
18. Li, X.; Zhu, S.; Song, L.; Wang, S.; Liang, Q. Algorithm for Segmentation of Liver Tumor Based on Improved U-Net Model. In Proceedings of the 2021 International Conference on Electronic Information Engineering and Computer Science (EIECS), Changchun, China, 23–25 September 2021; IEEE: New York, NY, USA, 2021.
19. Luan, S.; Xue, X.; Ding, Y.; Wei, W.; Zhu, B. Adaptive attention convolutional neural network for liver tumor segmentation. *Front. Oncol.* **2021**, *11*, 680807. [CrossRef] [PubMed]
20. Li, J.; Huang, G.; He, J.; Chen, Z.; Pun, C.; Yu, Z.; Ling, W.; Liu, L.; Zhou, J.; Huang, J. Shift-channel attention and weighted-region loss function for liver and dense tumor segmentation. *Med. Phys.* **2022**, *49*, 7193–7206. [CrossRef] [PubMed]
21. Yang, Z.; Li, S. Dual-path network for liver and tumor segmentation in CT images using Swin Transformer encoding approach. *Curr. Med. Imaging* **2022**, *19*, 1114–1123.
22. Fan, T.; Wang, G.; Wang, X.; Li, Y.; Wang, H. MSN-Net: A multi-scale context nested U-Net for liver segmentation. *Image Video Process.* **2021**, *15*, 1089–1097. [CrossRef]
23. Tang, W.; Zou, D.; Yang, S.; Shi, J.; Dan, J.; Song, G. A two-stage approach for automatic liver segmentation with Faster R-CNN and DeepLab. *Neural Comput. Appl.* **2020**, *32*, 6769–6778. [CrossRef]
24. Han, L.; Chen, Y.; Li, J.; Zhong, B.; Lei, Y.; Sun, M. Liver segmentation with 2.5 D perpendicular UNets. *Comput. Electr. Eng.* **2021**, *91*, 107118. [CrossRef]
25. Kota, N.S.; Reddy, G.U. Fusion based Gaussian noise removal in the images using curvelets and wavelets with Gaussian filter. *Int. J. Image Process* **2011**, *5*, 456–468.
26. Chartrand, G.; Cresson, T.; Chav, R.; Gotra, A.; Tang, A.; De Guise, J.A. Liver segmentation on CT and MR using Laplacian mesh optimization. *IEEE Trans. Biomed. Eng.* **2016**, *64*, 2110–2121. [CrossRef] [PubMed]
27. Baumgartner, M.; Jäger, P.F.; Isensee, F.; Maier-Hein, K.H. nnDetection: A self-configuring method for medical object detection. In Proceedings of the Medical Image Computing and Computer Assisted Intervention–MICCAI 2021, Strasbourg, France, 27 September–1 October 2021; Springer: Berlin/Heidelberg, Germany, 2021.
28. Jaeger, P.F.; Kohl, S.A.; Bickelhaupt, S.; Isensee, F.; Kuder, T.A.; Schlemmer, H.P.; Maier-Hein, K.H. Retina U-Net: Embarrassingly simple exploitation of segmentation supervision for medical object detection. In *Machine Learning for Health Workshop*; PLMR: Westminster, UK, 2020.
29. Jiang, Y.; Chen, L.; Zhang, H.; Xiao, X. Breast cancer histopathological image classification using convolutional neural networks with small SE-ResNet module. *PLoS ONE* **2019**, *14*, e0214587. [CrossRef] [PubMed]
30. Salehi, S.S.M.; Erdogmus, D.; Gholipour, A. Tversky loss function for image segmentation using 3D fully convolutional deep networks. In Proceedings of the Machine Learning in Medical Imaging: 8th International Workshop, MLMI 2017, Quebec City, QC, Canada, 10 September 2017; Springer: Berlin/Heidelberg, Germany, 2017.
31. Abraham, N.; Khan, N.M. A novel focal tversky loss function with improved attention u-net for lesion segmentation. In Proceedings of the 2019 IEEE 16th International Symposium on Biomedical Imaging (ISBI 2019), Venice, Italy, 8–11 April 2019; IEEE: New York, NY, USA, 2019.
32. Huang, R.; Wang, C.; Li, J.; Sui, Y. DF-UHRNet: A Modified CNN-Based Deep Learning Method for Automatic Sea Ice Classification from Sentinel-1A/B SAR Images. *Remote Sens.* **2023**, *15*, 2448. [CrossRef]

Disclaimer/Publisher's Note: The statements, opinions and data contained in all publications are solely those of the individual author(s) and contributor(s) and not of MDPI and/or the editor(s). MDPI and/or the editor(s) disclaim responsibility for any injury to people or property resulting from any ideas, methods, instructions or products referred to in the content.

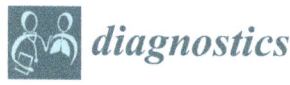

Comment

AI-Enabled Fusion of Medical Imaging, Behavioral Analysis and Other Systems for Enhanced Autism Spectrum Disorder. Comment on Jönemo et al. Evaluation of Augmentation Methods in Classifying Autism Spectrum Disorders from fMRI Data with 3D Convolutional Neural Networks. *Diagnostics* 2023, *13*, 2773

Daniele Giansanti

Centre Tisp, The Italian National Institute of Health, 00161 Rome, Italy; daniele.giansanti@iss.it; Tel.: +39-06-49902701

Citation: Giansanti, D. AI-Enabled Fusion of Medical Imaging, Behavioral Analysis and Other Systems for Enhanced Autism Spectrum Disorder. Comment on Jönemo, J.; Abramian, D.; Eklund, A. Evaluation of Augmentation Methods in Classifying Autism Spectrum Disorders from fMRI Data with 3D Convolutional Neural Networks. *Diagnostics* 2023, *13*, 2773. *Diagnostics* **2023**, *13*, 3545. https://doi.org/10.3390/diagnostics13233545

Academic Editor: Zhuhuang Zhou

Received: 12 October 2023
Accepted: 21 November 2023
Published: 28 November 2023

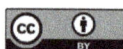

Copyright: © 2023 by the author. Licensee MDPI, Basel, Switzerland. This article is an open access article distributed under the terms and conditions of the Creative Commons Attribution (CC BY) license (https://creativecommons.org/licenses/by/4.0/).

I am writing to you in regard to the *research article "Johan Jönemo, David Abramian, and Anders Eklund*—Evaluation of Augmentation Methods in Classifying Autism Spectrum Disorders from fMRI Data with 3D Convolutional Neural Networks" [1].

In the Special Issues (SIs) that I coordinate, I always try to identify an article that stimulates a discussion with scholars for wide-ranging future development. In this SI [2], I identified your article. Autism, as a neurodevelopmental disorder, affects social behavior, communication and interaction. It manifests as difficulties in understanding other people's emotions, as verbal and non-verbal communication, as restricted interest in certain topics and as the repetitiveness of behaviors and routines. Each autistic individual is unique in his or her characteristics and level of functioning [3]. The therapeutic approach varies depending on individual needs and often involves multidisciplinary interventions.

This uniqueness is reflected in the *difficulty of diagnosis* [4,5], which requires a multifaceted approach from different medical disciplines, and in treatment that increasingly highlights the need for *personalized medicine* dedicated to autism [6,7].

Among the important activities in diagnosis are the following [4,5]:

- Observation and interviews;
- Physical exams and medical history;
- Developmental assessment and screening;
- Psychological and psychomotor evaluation;
- Assessment of social behavior and social interactions;
- Language and communication assessment;
- Sensory assessment;
- Functional behavior assessment;
- Genetic, metabolic, biochemical, immunological and neurobiological assessments;
- Assessments of environmental factors;
- Medical imaging assessment.

Functional Magnetic Resonance Imaging (fMRI) has played and is playing a significant role in advancing our understanding of autism spectrum disorder (ASD) by allowing researchers to investigate brain activity and connectivity in individuals with ASD. A search on PubMed with the composite key "Search: (fmri [Title/Abstract]) AND (autism [Title/Abstract]) Filters: Systematic Review Sort by: Publication Date" identified 14 systematic reviews starting from 2011, clearly identifying the potential of fMRI applied to autism, and also highlighting the need of an umbrella review [7–21]. fMRI allows, for example, for functional connectivity studies, Resting State fMRI (rs-fMRI), Task-Based fMRI, the neural correlation of social and communication impairments, and sensory processing and sensory integration investigation. Furthermore longitudinal fMRI studies can track brain development and changes in connectivity patterns over time in individuals with autism, which is very useful for understanding how the brain develops in those with ASD and how this leads to behavioral and cognitive changes. In fMRI, Machine Learning and Predictive Modeling have shown potential in earlier and more precise diagnosis and also in identifying specific biomarkers. Progress due to personalized interventions and therapies can be monitored just by means of fMRI, a useful tool to assess effectiveness in this filed.

I found your study very interesting and attractive.

I believe that, as you have highlighted, 3D augmentation techniques together with artificial intelligence (AI) applied to fMRI are promising.

I believe that this is a line of research that should be insisted upon.

I would also like to discuss with you the evolution prospects.

It is clear that autism requires a multidisciplinary approach and represents an area in which personalized medicine (PM) can undergo important development.

Multiple diagnostic approaches also play an important role in PM as in autism.

fMRI certainly has a key role and 3D augmentation and can represent a further boost in diagnosis and classification. AI is increasingly helping us in all of this, allowing for the classification of increasingly important volumes of data.

Personally, among the development directions of your study, I see potential in the application of AI tools to data reservoirs that, in the future, could include both the 3D-augmentation-based imaging method proposed by you and data coming from the many other multifaceted diagnostic activities not based on imaging.

I would like this comment open a scientific discussion with scholars as I am increasingly convinced that fMRI has been instrumental in uncovering the neural underpinnings of autism, shedding light on altered brain connectivity, social and sensory processing differences, and potential biomarkers; therefore, all the tools (and therefore, also the AI-based tools) integrating fMRI findings with other research approaches could contribute to a comprehensive understanding of autism and open the door to targeted interventions and treatments.

Conflicts of Interest: The author declares no conflict of interest.

References

1. Jönemo, J.; Abramian, D.; Eklund, A. Evaluation of Augmentation Methods in Classifying Autism Spectrum Disorders from fMRI Data with 3D Convolutional Neural Networks. *Diagnostics* **2023**, *13*, 2773. [CrossRef] [PubMed]
2. Available online: https://www.mdpi.com/journal/diagnostics/special_issues/3FXN9682V0 (accessed on 15 November 2023).
3. Available online: https://www.cdc.gov/ncbddd/autism/screening.html#:~:text=Diagnosing%20autism%20spectrum%20disorder%20(ASD,months%20of%20age%20or%20younger (accessed on 15 November 2023).
4. Available online: https://www.cdc.gov/ncbddd/autism/hcp-dsm.html (accessed on 15 November 2023).
5. Lord, C.; Elsabbagh, M.; Baird, G.; Veenstra-Vanderweele, J. Autism spectrum disorder. *Lancet* **2018**, *392*, 508–520. [CrossRef] [PubMed]
6. National Institute of Mental Health. A Parent's Guide to Autism Spectrum Disorder. 2011. Available online: http://www.nimh.nih.gov/health/publications/a-parents-guide-to-autism-spectrum-disorder/index.shtml (accessed on 8 March 2012).
7. Kotte, A.; Joshi, G.; Fried, R.; Uchida, M.; Spencer, A.; Woodworth, K.Y.; Kenworthy, T.; Faraone, S.V.; Biederman, J. Autistic traits in children with and without ADHD. *Pediatrics* **2013**, *132*, e612–e622. [CrossRef] [PubMed]
8. Morrel, J.; Singapuri, K.; Landa, R.J.; Reetzke, R. Neural correlates and predictors of speech and language development in infants at elevated likelihood for autism: A systematic review. *Front. Hum. Neurosci.* **2023**, *17*, 1211676. [CrossRef] [PubMed]
9. Xiao, J.; Wu, J. Effectiveness of the Neuroimaging Techniques in the Recognition of Psychiatric Disorders: A Systematic Review and Meta-analysis of RCTs. *Curr. Med. Imaging* **2023**, *20*, e260523217379. [CrossRef]
10. Kangarani-Farahani, M.; Izadi-Najafabadi, S.; Zwicker, J.G. How does brain structure and function on MRI differ in children with autism spectrum disorder, developmental coordination disorder, and/or attention deficit hyperactivity disorder? *Int. J. Dev. Neurosci.* **2022**, *82*, 681–715. [CrossRef] [PubMed]
11. Fathabadipour, S.; Mohammadi, Z.; Roshani, F.; Goharbakhsh, N.; Alizadeh, H.; Palizgar, F.; Cumming, P.; Michel, T.M.; Vafaee, M.S. The neural effects of oxytocin administration in autism spectrum disorders studied by fMRI: A systematic review. *J. Psychiatr. Res.* **2022**, *154*, 80–90. [CrossRef] [PubMed]

12. Santana, C.P.; de Carvalho, E.A.; Rodrigues, I.D.; Bastos, G.S.; de Souza, A.D.; de Brito, L.L. rs-fMRI and machine learning for ASD diagnosis: A systematic review and meta-analysis. *Sci. Rep.* **2022**, *12*, 6030. [CrossRef] [PubMed]
13. Miranda, L.; Paul, R.; Pütz, B.; Koutsouleris, N.; Müller-Myhsok, B. Systematic Review of Functional MRI Applications for Psychiatric Disease Subtyping. *Front. Psychiatry* **2021**, *12*, 665536. [CrossRef] [PubMed]
14. Walsh, M.J.M.; Wallace, G.L.; Gallegos, S.M.; Braden, B.B. Brain-based sex differences in autism spectrum disorder across the lifespan: A systematic review of structural MRI, fMRI, and DTI findings. *Neuroimage Clin.* **2021**, *31*, 102719. [CrossRef] [PubMed]
15. Kohl, S.H.; Mehler, D.M.A.; Lührs, M.; Thibault, R.T.; Konrad, K.; Sorger, B. The Potential of Functional Near-Infrared Spectroscopy-Based Neurofeedback-A Systematic Review and Recommendations for Best Practice. *Front. Neurosci.* **2020**, *14*, 594, Erratum in *Front. Neurosci.* **2022**, *16*, 907941. [CrossRef] [PubMed]
16. Lukito, S.; Norman, L.; Carlisi, C.; Radua, J.; Hart, H.; Simonoff, E.; Rubia, K. Comparative meta-analyses of brain structural and functional abnormalities during cognitive control in attention-deficit/hyperactivity disorder and autism spectrum disorder. *Psychol. Med.* **2020**, *50*, 894–919. [CrossRef] [PubMed]
17. Clements, C.C.; Zoltowski, A.R.; Yankowitz, L.D.; Yerys, B.E.; Schultz, R.T.; Herrington, J.D. Evaluation of the Social Motivation Hypothesis of Autism: A Systematic Review and Meta-analysis. *JAMA Psychiatry* **2018**, *75*, 797–808. [CrossRef] [PubMed]
18. Wigton, R.; Radua, J.; Allen, P.; Averbeck, B.; Meyer-Lindenberg, A.; McGuire, P.; Shergill, S.S.; Fusar-Poli, P. Neurophysiological effects of acute oxytocin administration: Systematic review and meta-analysis of placebo-controlled imaging studies. *J. Psychiatry Neurosci.* **2015**, *40*, E1–E22. [CrossRef] [PubMed]
19. Hamilton, A.F. Reflecting on the mirror neuron system in autism: A systematic review of current theories. *Dev. Cogn. Neurosci.* **2013**, *3*, 91–105. [CrossRef] [PubMed]
20. Philip, R.C.; Dauvermann, M.R.; Whalley, H.C.; Baynham, K.; Lawrie, S.M.; Stanfield, A.C. A systematic review and meta-analysis of the fMRI investigation of autism spectrum disorders. *Neurosci. Biobehav. Rev.* **2012**, *36*, 901–942. [CrossRef] [PubMed]
21. Sugranyes, G.; Kyriakopoulos, M.; Corrigall, R.; Taylor, E.; Frangou, S. Autism spectrum disorders and schizophrenia: Meta-analysis of the neural correlates of social cognition. *PLoS ONE* **2011**, *6*, e25322. [CrossRef] [PubMed]

Disclaimer/Publisher's Note: The statements, opinions and data contained in all publications are solely those of the individual author(s) and contributor(s) and not of MDPI and/or the editor(s). MDPI and/or the editor(s) disclaim responsibility for any injury to people or property resulting from any ideas, methods, instructions or products referred to in the content.

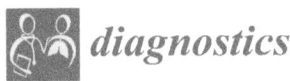

Review

An Umbrella Review of the Fusion of fMRI and AI in Autism

Daniele Giansanti

Centro Nazionale TISP, Istituto Superiore di Sanità, Viale Regina Elena 299, 00161 Roma, Italy; daniele.giansanti@iss.it; Tel.: +39-0649902701

Abstract: The role of functional magnetic resonance imaging (fMRI) is assuming an increasingly central role in autism diagnosis. The integration of Artificial Intelligence (AI) into the realm of applications further contributes to its development. This study's objective is to analyze emerging themes in this domain through an umbrella review, encompassing systematic reviews. The research methodology was based on a structured process for conducting a literature narrative review, using an umbrella review in PubMed and Scopus. Rigorous criteria, a standard checklist, and a qualification process were meticulously applied. The findings include 20 systematic reviews that underscore key themes in autism research, particularly emphasizing the significance of technological integration, including the pivotal roles of fMRI and AI. This study also highlights the enigmatic role of oxytocin. While acknowledging the immense potential in this field, the outcome does not evade acknowledging the significant challenges and limitations. Intriguingly, there is a growing emphasis on research and innovation in AI, whereas aspects related to the integration of healthcare processes, such as regulation, acceptance, informed consent, and data security, receive comparatively less attention. Additionally, the integration of these findings into Personalized Medicine (PM) represents a promising yet relatively unexplored area within autism research. This study concludes by encouraging scholars to focus on the critical themes of health domain integration, vital for the routine implementation of these applications.

Keywords: autism; artificial intelligence; autism spectrum disorders; fMRI

Citation: Giansanti, D. An Umbrella Review of the Fusion of fMRI and AI in Autism. *Diagnostics* **2023**, *13*, 3552. https://doi.org/10.3390/diagnostics13233552

Academic Editor: Malek Makki

Received: 21 October 2023
Revised: 22 November 2023
Accepted: 25 November 2023
Published: 28 November 2023

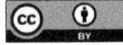

Copyright: © 2023 by the author. Licensee MDPI, Basel, Switzerland. This article is an open access article distributed under the terms and conditions of the Creative Commons Attribution (CC BY) license (https://creativecommons.org/licenses/by/4.0/).

1. Introduction

1.1. fMRI: The Functioning and the Integration with AI

1.1.1. An Introduction to fMRI

The advanced technology of functional magnetic resonance imaging, abbreviated to fMRI, has revolutionized the landscape of neuroscience and brain research [1–10]. Born around the 1990s from the fusion of sophisticated magnetic resonance imaging techniques and the understanding of brain activity, fMRI offers an extraordinary window into the functioning of the human brain [2,6]. This non-invasive methodology allows scientists to peer deeply into the brain as it engages in a wide range of cognitive activities, providing detailed pictures of neural activity in real time from complex elaborations [7–9]. Unlike other neuroimaging techniques [4,11], fMRI does not require the insertion of electrodes or the use of ionizing radiation, making it safe and suitable for a wide spectrum of applications, from scientific research to diagnosis and condition monitoring neurologically. The basis of fMRI lies in the idea that neural activity is related to changes in cerebral blood flow, and this principle is exploited to map brain regions involved in specific cognitive functions or behavioral responses [1,3,10]. Over the years, fMRI has made significant contributions to our understanding of the brain, unlocking secrets of how different parts of the brain work together to influence behavior, sensory perception, language processing, and many other complex functions [1,4,5]. This progress has been further catalyzed by the integration of artificial intelligence, enabling advanced analysis of complex data and the identification of subtle patterns, opening new perspectives for research and the diagnosis of brain conditions [12–14].

1.1.2. Integrating fMRI and AI for the Brain Study

Artificial intelligence (AI) plays a fundamental role in the interpretation and processing of data from fMRI, providing sophisticated tools to analyze in depth the functioning of the human brain [12–25]. One high-impact area is advanced data analytics, where AI can identify complex patterns and correlations that would be difficult or impossible to identify manually [13,17,22]. This means that AI can help reveal subtle relationships between brain activity and certain stimuli or conditions, leading to a deeper understanding of cognitive and neural functions [16,20]. Furthermore, AI is essential for automating critical processes such as brain segmentation and mapping of brain regions [14,15]. This automation significantly speeds up the analysis process and ensures greater accuracy, allowing scientists to focus more on interpreting results rather than manipulating raw data [18,19,21]. Another powerful application is the prediction of brain responses to certain stimuli or tasks based on historical fMRI data [23]. AI can create predictive models that indicate how the brain might react in different situations, offering valuable insights for understanding the neural basis of different cognitive and behavioral activities [13,15,20]. Integrating multi-omics data are another important frontier where AI can contribute. By combining fMRI data with genetic, proteomic, or other biological information, AI can help create a comprehensive view of the relationship between brain functioning and biological factors, paving the way for new discoveries and personalized therapeutic approaches. In synthesis, it is possible to affirm that AI amplifies the human ability to analyze and interpret fMRI data, enabling a deeper understanding of brain dynamics [24,25]. This synergy between fMRI and AI promises to radically transform neuroscientific research and open new ways to diagnose and treat brain disorders more accurately and effectively.

1.2. Diagnosis in Autism

The diagnosis of autism spectrum disorders (ASD) is a nuanced process shaped by the disorder's inherent complexity [26–31]. Central to this complexity is the spectrum nature of autism, which encompasses a diverse range of symptoms and severity levels [32]. From social and communication challenges to variable behaviors, each individual's experience is unique, necessitating personalized approaches to diagnosis and intervention. Adding to the intricacy is the variability in symptom manifestation, making the diagnostic journey a challenging one. The developmental trajectory introduces another layer of complexity, as symptoms may not fully emerge until a child encounters new social and cognitive demands. Overlap with other developmental disorders and mental health conditions further complicates the diagnostic landscape. Clinicians must carefully distinguish between autism and conditions like ADHD or intellectual disabilities through meticulous evaluations. Social communication challenges form a core feature of autism, ranging from a lack of interest in socializing to nuanced struggles in interpreting nonverbal cues. Navigating these subtleties is crucial for accurate diagnoses. Cultural sensitivity is paramount, acknowledging that the presentation of autism symptoms can be influenced by cultural norms. Comorbidity, the co-occurrence of autism with other conditions, adds complexity, necessitating comprehensive evaluations. The evolving nature of diagnostic criteria, from DSM-IV to DSM-5, highlights the importance of staying current in the field.

One of the problems of diagnosis is that the manifestations of autism vary widely [26], giving rise to the yet-cited concept of the "spectrum" [32], which includes individuals with mild to severe symptoms. Signs of autism can emerge from early childhood but are often identified in preschool or school age, when they become more evident. Symptoms include difficulty with verbal and nonverbal communication, difficulty interacting with others, repetitive and restricted interests and activities, and increased or decreased sensory sensitivity. To diagnose autism, a multidisciplinary approach is used [32–34]. Specialists, such as psychologists, child psychiatrists, and pediatricians, conduct interviews and observations to evaluate the individual's behavior, language, social skills, and cognitive abilities. Diagnosis is often completed through structured questionnaires, developmental assessments, and assessments of communication skills. In addition to behavioral assessments and questionnaires, genetic analysis can be an integral part of the diagnosis of autism, since there is a genetic component to its etiology. Blood tests and genetic tests can identify genetic abnormalities associated with autism. Innovation in autism diagnostics comes through the integration of cutting-edge technologies such as fMRI [35].

1.3. Integrating fMRI in Autism Diagnosis

fMRI may serve as an invaluable tool in unraveling the mysteries of the autistic brain, providing a detailed exploration of neural activity and connectivity unique to individuals on the autism spectrum [35]. In the initial phases of an fMRI study, special attention is given to participant preparation, recognizing the potential sensory sensitivities often associated with autism [34,35]. Beyond the standard procedure briefing, efforts are made to ensure the comfort of individuals with autism in the MRI environment, acknowledging their heightened sensitivity to sensory stimuli. During the scanning process, individuals with autism engage in tasks designed to activate specific cognitive processes relevant to the challenges associated with autism spectrum disorders. Tasks may be tailored to investigate social cognition, communication, or sensory processing—core aspects often affected by individuals with autism. Alternatively, resting-state fMRI provides a unique avenue to explore intrinsic brain connectivity patterns without the imposition of specific tasks, allowing researchers to uncover spontaneous neural activity associated with autism. Structural imaging captures high-resolution images of the autistic brain's anatomy, laying the groundwork for a comprehensive understanding of the structural nuances associated with the condition [35]. As the participant's brain responds to tasks or conditions, the fMRI scanner detects changes in blood oxygenation levels, offering insights into the neural correlates of various cognitive processes. This dynamic data acquisition is particularly relevant when investigating how the autistic brain processes and responds to social cues, sensory stimuli, and other stimuli that may be challenging for individuals on the autism spectrum. In the subsequent analysis phase, researchers delve into the intricacies of the data, applying sophisticated statistical methods to identify significant changes in brain activity specific to autism. Connectivity analyses play a pivotal role in examining how different brain regions communicate in individuals with autism. Short-range and long-range connectivity patterns are scrutinized, shedding light on the unique neural networks associated with the condition. Interpreting fMRI results within the context of autism research requires a nuanced understanding of the specific challenges and strengths of individuals on the spectrum. The integration of fMRI findings with other data sources, such as behavioral assessments and clinical measures, provides a holistic perspective on the neural basis of autism spectrum disorders. In essence, fMRI serves as a powerful ally in the ongoing quest to deepen our understanding of the autistic brain, contributing valuable insights into the complexities of this neurodevelopmental condition. In the context of autism, fMRI can help visualize brain activity patterns and specific neural connections that may be different compared to neurotypical individuals. fMRI allows us to examine brain activity during social, communication, or specific tasks, providing insights into neurofunctional differences in people with autism.

1.4. Integrating AI in Autism

1.4.1. A Brief Recall of the Artificial Intelligence in the Health Domain

AI is a multidisciplinary field focused on developing intelligent machines capable of performing tasks that typically require human intelligence. It encompasses a range of techniques, including machine learning, natural language processing, and computer vision. Machine learning, a subset of AI, involves training algorithms on data to enable them to learn patterns and make predictions or decisions without explicit programming.

There is an increasing interest in investigating the impact of AI in the healthcare domain. For example, the four recent systematic reviews [36–39] offer a holistic and nuanced understanding of the multifaceted landscape of AI in healthcare. From identifying barriers to implementation and acknowledging diverse stakeholder preferences to delving into the role of AI in chronic care and evaluating its economic implications, these inquiries collectively contribute to shaping a comprehensive narrative on the present and future of AI in healthcare. The intersection of these diverse perspectives provides valuable guidance for researchers, practitioners, and policymakers aiming to harness the potential of AI to enhance healthcare delivery. In the study proposed in [36], the authors scrutinize the barriers obstructing the seamless integration of AI into healthcare practices. This inquiry into challenges offers a valuable starting point for understanding the practical impediments that need addressing to realize the full potential of AI technologies in healthcare delivery. The systematic review reported in [37] takes a broader perspective by examining the preferences of multiple stakeholders regarding the use of AI in healthcare. This systematic review not only acknowledges the diverse perspectives of stakeholders but also recognizes the significance of aligning AI solutions with the preferences and needs of various actors within the complex healthcare ecosystem. The inclusivity of stakeholder preferences becomes pivotal in designing and implementing AI technologies that are both effective and accepted across different healthcare contexts. The overview reported in [38] focuses on a specific dimension—AIs role in managing chronic medical conditions. This targeted exploration reveals how AI interventions contribute to the ongoing care of individuals with persistent health issues. Understanding the nuances of AI applications in chronic care is critical for envisioning comprehensive healthcare strategies that leverage technological advancements for improved patient outcomes.

The last work [39] contributes a unique perspective by conducting a systematic literature review on the economic evaluations of AI-based healthcare interventions. This inquiry into the economic dimensions of AI implementation sheds light on the cost-effectiveness and efficiency of integrating AI technologies. Such insights are indispensable for policymakers and healthcare providers as they navigate the complex landscape of healthcare financing and resource allocation.

1.4.2. The Application of AI with the Focus on Autism

AI is playing a particularly impactful role in autism research [40,41].

Research trends indicate an increasing interest in the applications of AI within this domain [42], encompassing a spectrum from diagnostic tools to seamless integrations with IoT technologies [43,44]. This surge underscores the transformative impact of AI, showcasing its versatile utilization and integration across various facets of the field. From advancing diagnostic capabilities to forging synergies with cutting-edge IoT technologies, the trajectory of AI applications within this realm is marked by a remarkable and expansive evolution, signifying its pivotal role in shaping the landscape of healthcare.

AI, particularly machine learning (ML) and deep learning, plays a pivotal role in addressing ASD challenges. ML excels in pattern recognition, aiding in early ASD detection through behavioral and physiological data analysis [40,41]. Predictive modeling tailors support strategies, while naturalistic behavioral analysis, powered by computer vision and ML, informs interventions by decoding subtle cues [44]. Deep learning, especially in neural networks, unveils intricate neural mechanisms through fMRI data analysis, contributes to understanding communication challenges, and identifies genetic markers associated with autism [40]. Overall, AI stands as a dynamic force, promising transformative potential in ASD research, from early detection to personalized interventions and a profound understanding of complexities. The intersection of AI and autism exemplifies technology's capacity for improving the lives of individuals on the spectrum, unlocking new possibilities and insights.

A fast search in Pubmed using the composite key

"("artificial intelligence"[Title/Abstract] AND ("autism s"[All Fields] OR "autisms"[All Fields] OR "autistic disorder"[MeSH Terms] OR ("autistic"[All Fields] AND "disorder"[All Fields]) OR "autistic disorder"[All Fields] OR "autism"[All Fields])) AND (systematicreview[Filter])" identify 11 systematic reviews [45–55] focused on the impact of AI on autism.

Collectively, these explorations narrate a compelling story of how AI is becoming a powerful ally in the realm of autism research. From precision interventions to immersive technologies and advanced diagnostics, each theme contributes to the evolving narrative of leveraging technology for a deeper understanding and improved support for individuals on the autism spectrum.

Each one of the systematic reviews helps us to identify how, in the dynamic exploration of AI within the realm of autism research, a multitude of themes have emerged, each shedding light on the nuanced intersections of technology and neurodevelopmental disorders.

1. *Precision Psychiatry and Pharmacogenomics*

The first systematic review [45] ushers us into a realm where machine learning converges with pharmacogenomics, envisioning a future of precision psychiatry. This integration holds promise for tailoring psychiatric interventions to individual genetic profiles, potentially revolutionizing the treatment landscape for individuals on the autism spectrum.

2. *Virtual Reality-Based Techniques for Health Improvement*

The systematic review reported in [46] offers insights into the potential of virtual reality for human exercise and health enhancement. This systematic review prompts contemplation on how immersive technologies could be harnessed to address specific health challenges faced by individuals with autism, fostering holistic well-being.

3. *Bibliometric Analysis of AI in Autism Treatment*

The study available in [47] provides a meta-analysis, exploring the bibliometric landscape of AI in the treatment of autism spectrum disorders. This comprehensive overview not only reveals current research trends but also emphasizes the evolving priorities within the broader AI and autism research community, with potential implications for future interventions.

4. *Hybridization of Medical Tests and Sociodemographic Characteristics*

The authors of the overview reported in [48] delve into a systematic review, investigating the hybridization of medical tests and sociodemographic characteristics in the context of autism. This approach underscores a comprehensive diagnostic strategy, acknowledging the multifaceted factors influencing autism spectrum disorder diagnosis.

5. *Triage and Priority-Based Healthcare Diagnosis*

The study proposed in [49] brings practical applications to the forefront, focusing on triage and priority-based healthcare diagnosis. This prompts reflection on how AI can streamline diagnostic processes, potentially ensuring timely interventions tailored to the specific needs of individuals with autism.

6. *Mobile and Wearable AI in Child and Adolescent Psychiatry*

The contribution reported in [50] shifts the discourse towards mobile and wearable AI, conducting a scoping review in child and adolescent psychiatry. This exploration signifies a paradigm shift towards technology-driven mental health interventions for younger populations, including those on the autism spectrum.

7. *Robot-Assisted Therapy for Children with Autism*

A systematic review reported in [51] introduces robotics into the conversation through a systematic review of robot-assisted therapy for children with autism. The exploration of robotics as a therapeutic tool sparks contemplation on how technology could enhance therapeutic interventions and support individuals on the spectrum.

8. *Machine-Learning Models in Behavioral Assessment*

A navigation on the application of machine-learning models in behavioral assessment for autism spectrum disorder is reported in [52]. This suggests a shift towards more sophisticated computational methods, offering the potential for a deeper understanding of behavioral patterns and individualized interventions.

9. *Deep Learning in Psychiatric Disorders Classification*

The authors of [53] guide the discussion towards the integration of deep learning in classifying psychiatric disorders, particularly in the context of autism. This prompts consideration of how advanced computational techniques can refine the classification and understanding of psychiatric conditions associated with autism.

10. *Impact of Technology on Autism Spectrum Disorder*

The work proposed in [54] contributes a systematic literature review on the broader impact of technology, also integrated with AI, on individuals with autism spectrum disorder. This holistic overview underscores the transformative role of technology in enhancing the lives of individuals on the spectrum, opening avenues for support and intervention.

11. *Deep Learning in Neurology*

The authors of the overview available in [55] delve into the application of deep learning in neurology, with a focus also on autism, signaling a systematic exploration of advanced computational techniques in understanding neurological disorders, including those that may co-occur with autism. This offers insights into the potential for technology-driven advancements in neurology for individuals on the spectrum.

1.5. Integrating the Two Tools of AI and fMRI in Autism

AI and fMRI serve as two essential arms in autism research, offering complementary strengths. fMRI, as described above, provides detailed insights into neural mechanisms, capturing changes in brain activity related to social behavior and cognition, especially with interventions like oxytocin. On the other hand, AI, as also described above, particularly machine learning, enables sophisticated analysis of vast and complex datasets, identifying subtle patterns in individual responses. Together, these arms create a powerful synergy, enhancing our understanding of autism's neural underpinnings, personalizing interventions, and guiding the development of effective treatments [56,57].

Integrating fMRI with AI [56,57] can help identify complex patterns in brain activity in autism and predict individual behavior, providing valuable information for more precise diagnosis and personalized intervention strategies. In summary, autism is a complex neurodevelopmental disorder with a wide variety of manifestations. The diagnosis is multidisciplinary and involves behavioral assessments, structured questionnaires, and genetic analyses [32–34]. fMRI, also integrated with AI, may offer [35,56,57] significant potential to deepen the understanding of autism by visualizing patterns of brain activity, providing valuable insights for diagnosis, understanding the neural basis, and developing personalized therapies.

1.6. Rising Questions and Purpose of the Umbrella Review

Building on the preceding discussion, it becomes evident that there is a noteworthy importance attributed to both fMRI and AI within the context of autism. On one hand, the role of fMRI offers insights into neural activities and connectivity unique to individuals on the autism spectrum, providing a detailed exploration of the autistic brain. Simultaneously, AI brings its transformative capabilities, contributing to areas such as early detection, diagnostic precision, and personalized interventions for individuals with autism.

However, it is equally noteworthy to underscore that the potential synergies arising from the integration of AI and fMRI have not undergone a dedicated thematic analysis. The intricate interplay between these two powerful tools remains relatively unexplored territory. Understanding and harnessing the collaborative potential of AI and fMRI could unveil novel perspectives in unraveling the complexities of autism, offering a more comprehensive understanding of the neural underpinnings of this neurodevelopmental condition. Further exploration into this uncharted territory could pave the way for innovative approaches and interventions, presenting new avenues for advancing autism research and care.

The objective of this study was to perform an *umbrella review* [58,59] to summarize and critically evaluate the scientific evidence emerging from the systematic reviews regarding the application of artificial AI in the analysis of fMRI data in subjects with autism spectrum disorder (ASD). The overall goal is to achieve a thorough understanding of the contribution made by this technological integration in enhancing.

2. Methods

This review used a standardized checklist designed for the narrative category of reviews (see [60]). The narrative review, designed as an *umbrella review* (a review that considers the produced systematic reviews [58,59]), was performed based on targeted searches using specific composite keys on PubMed and Scopus.

The overview literature accompanying the main survey was conducted using both a qualification checklist and a qualification methodology based on proposed quality parameters described in [61] to decide the inclusion of the study in the overview.

See Algorithm 1 used in the literature overview.

Algorithm 1 The proposed algorithm for the umbrella review.

1. Set the search query to:
   "fMRI"[Title/Abstract] OR "functional magnetic resonance"[Title/Abstract]) AND ("autism"[Title/Abstract] OR "ASD"[Title/Abstract] OR "autistic"[Title/Abstract])) AND (systematicreview[Filter])"
2. Conduct a targeted search on Pubmed and Scopus using the search query from step 1.
3. Select studies published in peer-reviewed journals that focus on the field
4. For each study, evaluate the following parameters:
   - N1: Is the rationale for the study in the introduction clear?
   - N2: Is the design of the work appropriate?
   - N3: Are the methods described clearly?
   - N4: Are the results presented clearly?
   - N5: Are the conclusions based and justified by results?
   - N6: Did the authors disclose all the conflicts of interests?
5. Assign a graded score to parameters N1–N5, ranging from 1 (minimum) to 5 (maximum).
6. For parameter N6, assign a binary assessment of "Yes" or "No" to indicate if the authors disclosed all the conflicts of interest.
7. Preselect studies that meet the following criteria:
   - Parameter N6 must be "Yes".
   - Parameters N1–N5 must have a score greater than 3.
8. Include the preselected studies in the overview.

From the studies sourced from PubMed, 100% were included, while from Scopus, 96% were considered [62–81]. It is noteworthy that those selected from Scopus were also available on PubMed, indicating an overlapping inclusion. The reviewers, who were three in number, hold a Master's degree in diagnostic healthcare professions, with a strong focus on diagnostic imaging. Their training at the University involved comprehensive courses and specialized training in Artificial Intelligence.

3. Results

During the review process, a comprehensive examination of the literature revealed a total of 20 systematic reviews [62–81]. These systematic reviews collectively delve into the pivotal theme concerning the criticality of fMRI. This exploration often includes a comparative analysis with other diagnostic instruments, such as the devices for whole-brain voxel-based morphometry [64], EEG, MEG, TMS, eyetracking, EMG [68], and near infrared spectroscopy [62,63], shedding light on the evolving landscape of diagnostic tools and emphasizing the significance of fMRI in this context. Among these systematic reviews, only one [69] specifically focuses on evaluating the potential of fMRI as a catalyst for personalized medicine (PM) in the realm of autism. This focus could be particularly strategic, given the unique nature of this condition, as extensively emphasized [65]. The research highlights fMRIs indispensable role in analyzing the discussed impact of oxytocin [66,77].

In a broader context, these systematic reviews unearth potentialities and opportunities in various analytical domains. This encompasses both the modeling of brain structures and understanding brain responses to an array of stimuli—be they behavioral; social; or of other psychological/psychiatric origins [62,63,76,79]. Additionally, the utility of fMRI extends to motor activities [68], further underscoring its versatility and applicability.

Moreover, fMRI emerges as an invaluable tool, not only for deciphering influencing factors in brain patterns and responses but also for offering promising prospects in the field of predictive medicine, as showcased in [71]. The integration of fMRI with artificial intelligence (AI) amplifies this potential significantly [64,67,69,71,75].

While these studies reiterate the paramount importance of fMRI, they also interlace moments of enthusiasm [63,71] and caution [62,64,67]—an observation particularly relevant in the context of navigating this integration with AI. This integration holds immense potential, offering a substantial contribution to the realms of classification and guidance [71]. The delicate balance between enthusiasm and prudence is accentuated, especially in the context of carefully considering the implications and impact of integrating fMRI with AI.

The profound influence and indispensable presence of technology resonate throughout practically every study subjected to analysis [62–81]. A meticulous scrutiny and in-depth examination unveil a discernible bifurcation into the subsequent thematic domains arranged into subparagraphs. Here, systematic reviews stand as the bedrock, offering a preeminent and guiding influence in delineating the paramount thematic contributions.

Theme 1: Investigating the potential of the fMRI along with other Medical Imaging Devices (Section 3.1): At the forefront stands the awe-inspiring potential of fMRI technology, transcending conventional boundaries in diagnostic capabilities. This extends beyond fMRI to encompass an array of groundbreaking technological contributions, collectively propelling our understanding of diagnostics to unprecedented heights.

Theme 2: Integrating fMRI with Artificial Intelligence (Section 3.2): A pivotal discussion point centers on the seamless integration of fMRI technology with the immense potential of AI. This convergence represents a monumental stride forward, a union of cutting-edge advancements in fMRI and AI, promising a future where the whole is truly greater than the sum of its parts.

Theme 3: Personalized Medicine Through AI and fMRI (Section 3.3): Emerging as a beacon of promise, AI is steering us towards an era of personalized medicine. This transformative shift signifies a departure from the one-size-fits-all approach, embracing a model of healthcare that is finely attuned to the unique needs and characteristics of each individual.

Theme 4: The Role of Oxytocin (Section 3.4): Within the realm of scientific inquiry, a captivating enigma revolves around oxytocin. Here, fMRI technology emerges as an indispensable tool, shedding light on the intricacies of oxytocin's functions and effects.

3.1. Theme 1: Investigating the Potential of the fMRI along with Other Medical Imaging Devicses

The major theme that was identified by the reviewer is related to the analysis of the impact and potential of fMRI technologies in comparison with other methodologies. [62,63,65,68,70,72–74,76,79–81]. The reviewed studies collectively explore various aspects of neuroimaging in the context of psychiatric and neurodevelopmental disorders, particularly focusing on ASD. The research encompasses investigations into the neural correlates of speech and language development in infants at elevated risk for autism, the effectiveness of neuroimaging techniques in recognizing psychiatric disorders, and technologies supporting the diagnosis and treatment of neurodevelopmental disorders [62–70]. Scholars demonstrate interest in brain structure and function differences in children with ASD, developmental coordination disorder, and attention deficit hyperactivity disorder (ADHD) [74]. Furthermore, the studies touch on the neural effects of physical activity and movement interventions in individuals with developmental disabilities [68], systematic reviews of functional MRI applications for psychiatric disease subtyping, and brain-based sex differences in ASD across the lifespan [70]. Areas of investigation include functional near-infrared spectroscopy (fNIRS) [72,73] in speech and language impairment, the potential of fNIRS-based neurofeedback, comparative meta-analyses of brain structural and functional abnormalities in ADHD and ASD, and the accuracy of machine learning algorithms for ASD diagnosis based on brain FMRI studies. The exploration of the social motivation hypothesis in ASD [76] is also addressed. The studies extend to neuroimaging's role in supporting the DSM-5 proposed symptom dyad in ASD [74] and meta-analyses of fMRI investigations in ASD [79].

Overall, the comprehensive body of research reflects a multidimensional approach to understanding the neural underpinnings of various psychiatric and neurodevelopmental conditions, with a prominent focus on ASD.

Table 1 reports the key elements of interest gleaned from systematic reviews pertinent to this emerging theme.

Table 1. Key elements emerging from the studies in theme 1.

Systematic Review	Highlights
[62]	The study emphasizes speech and language delays in young autistic children, utilizing neuroimaging, especially fMRI, to explore early neurobiological indicators. Key findings encompass atypical neural lateralization, connectivity alterations, and varied neural sensitivities, with an early detection potential of as early as 6 weeks. These results underscore fMRIs ability to reveal early signs of delays before behavioral manifestations, highlighting the importance of standardized paradigms.
[63]	The study reported different neuroimaging techniques to identify brain abnormalities associated with psychiatric conditions, emphasizing the intricate interplay of physiology and anatomy in these disorders. The meta-analysis strongly advocates for the utilization of neuroimaging techniques, particularly emphasizing the physiological and anatomical insights provided by fMRI, in the accurate detection of psychiatric disorders, including autism.
[65]	The study delves into the neural intricacies of brain structure and function in children with co-occurring neurodevelopmental disorders, using structural MRI, diffusion tensor imaging, and resting-state fMRI. It emphasizes the uniqueness of neural correlates for each disorder, shedding light on their distinct characteristics despite common co-occurrence.
[68]	The study highlights significant neural effects and behavioral improvements resulting from interventions based on motion activity, with chronic interventions showing greater efficacy. The review calls for more extensive research with larger sample sizes and standardized neuroimaging tools to better comprehend the underlying neural mechanisms that benefit individuals with developmental disabilities, emphasizing the crucial interplay of anatomy and physiology in this context.
[70]	The study stresses the need to prioritize females in ASD research due to their distinct phenotypic trajectories and age-related brain differences. It underscores the influence of sex-related biological factors, proposing a comprehensive approach to understanding brain-based sex differences in ASD, focusing on anatomy and physiology. The review of neuroimaging studies identifies consistent sex differences in brain regions, suggesting unique neurodevelopmental patterns in females with ASD. The concept of a 'female protective effect' gains support, emphasizing genetic and endocrine influences on brain development.

Table 1. Cont.

Systematic Review	Highlights
[72]	The study focused on near-infrared spectroscopy (fNIRS), highlighting its potential advantages in exploring the neural connections to speech and language issues across diverse conditions, including autism spectrum disorders. The findings suggest that fNIRS holds promise for early diagnosis, assessment of treatment responses, and applications in neuroprosthetics and neurofeedback.
[73]	The study identifies practicality, portability, and reduced sensitivity to movement artifacts as advantages of fNIRS as a functional neuroimaging technique. However, it notes variations in study quality and a lack of large, randomized controlled trials. Although some studies suggest the feasibility of modulating brain function in autism, conclusions remain premature. The study highlights the potential for clinical translation and emphasizes the need for improved research practices and reporting for further methodological advancements in fNIRS-neurofeedback.
[74]	The study reveals distinct structural and functional brain irregularities in attention-deficit/hyperactivity disorder (ADHD) and ASD during cognitive control tasks. Specifically, ADHD is associated with reduced gray matter volume in the ventromedial orbitofrontal area, whereas ASD is characterized by increased gray matter volume in regions like the bilateral temporal and right dorsolateral prefrontal areas. Functional differences emerge as underactivation in the medial prefrontal region and overactivation in the bilateral ventrolateral prefrontal cortices and precuneus in ASD. Conversely, individuals with ADHD demonstrate right inferior fronto-striatal underactivation, particularly during motor response inhibition.
[76]	The study investigates how individuals with ASD process rewarding stimuli, particularly if these differences extend beyond social rewards. Utilizing fMRI, the research uncovers distinct patterns of reward processing in ASD individuals, encompassing both social and nonsocial rewards, with atypical brain activation in specific striatal regions. Notably, heightened brain activation occurs when individuals with ASD are exposed to their restricted interests, challenging traditional notions of the social motivation hypothesis.
[78]	The study in [58] revisits the attention-grabbing potential link between dysfunction in the mirror neuron system and challenges in social interaction and communication in individuals with ASD. Various neuroscience methods, including EEG, MEG, TMS, eyetracking, EMG, and fMRI, were used to assess the integrity of the mirror system in autism. Notably, fMRI emerges as the most effective measure of mirror system function. In fMRI studies, those using emotional stimuli reveal group differences, while those employing non-emotional hand action stimuli do not show similar distinctions.
[79]	The work analyzes studies using functional fMRI and diffusion tensor imaging (DTI) data to evaluate their alignment with the proposed social communication and behavioral symptom dyad in individuals diagnosed with ASD according to the DSM-5. The results reveal abnormalities in brain function and structure within various networks, such as fronto-temporal and limbic networks linked to social and pragmatic language deficits, temporo-parieto-occipital networks associated with syntactic-semantic language deficits, and fronto-striato-cerebellar networks related to repetitive behaviors and restricted interests in individuals with ASD.

Table 1. Cont.

Systematic Review	Highlights
[80]	In the study, one of the most consistently observed findings is a disruption in the function of brain regions associated with social interactions in ASD. These differences in activation within the social brain may stem from a diminished preference for social stimuli rather than a fundamental malfunction of these brain areas. Accumulating evidence suggests challenges in effectively integrating various functional brain regions and difficulties in finely adjusting brain function based on changing task demands in individuals with ASD.
[81]	The study investigates the brain regions associated with social cognition deficits in ASD and Schizophrenia (SZ). The results show that both ASD and SZ exhibit reduced activation in certain brain areas linked to social cognition, particularly in the medial prefrontal region. However, there are specific differences in brain activation patterns and engagement with stimuli between the two disorders. These findings offer valuable insights for future research and understanding of these conditions.

The study proposed in [62] remarked that speech and language delays are common in young autistic children and are often a concern for parents before their child's second birthday; therefore, understanding the neural mechanisms behind these delays could improve early detection and intervention. The work aimed to consolidate evidence on early neurobiological indicators and predictors of speech and language development using various neuroimaging techniques, with particular reference to fMRI in infants with and without a family history of autism. Three main themes emerged from the systematic review: (1) atypical neural lateralization related to language in infants at a higher likelihood of autism (EL infants) compared to those at lower likelihood (LL infants); (2) structural and functional connectivity alterations; and (3) varied neural sensitivities to speech and non-speech stimuli, detectable as early as 6 weeks of age. These findings suggest that neuroimaging techniques may detect early signs of speech and language delays before behavioral delays become evident. Future research should standardize experimental paradigms and address practical implementation in non-academic, community-based settings.

According to [63], neuroimaging plays a crucial role in understanding brain development, diagnosing mental illnesses, including autism, and distinguishing between conditions. This study conducted a systematic review and meta-analysis of randomized controlled trials to assess the efficacy of using neuroimaging for detecting psychiatric disorders, particularly autism. The trials included in this study used various neuroimaging techniques to detect brain abnormalities associated with psychiatric disorders, including autism. The meta-analysis strongly recommends the use of neuroimaging techniques, in particular fMRI, for detecting psychiatric disorders, including autism.

The study proposed in [65] aimed to systematically review and analyze the neural similarities and differences in brain structure and function, assessed by neuroimaging, in children with commonly co-occurring neurodevelopmental disorders, including autism. The applied technologies were structural MRI, diffusion tensor imaging, and resting-state fMRI. The interpretation of the results revealed that the neural correlates of co-occurring conditions were distinct and more widespread compared to a single diagnosis. The majority of findings (77%) indicated distinct neural correlates for each neurodevelopmental disorder rather than shared features, suggesting the distinctiveness of each disorder despite their common co-occurrence. However, the limited number of studies and the lack of correction for multiple comparisons necessitate a cautious interpretation of these results.

The systematic review proposed in [68] addresses developmental disabilities, including autism, and highlights the potential of physical activity interventions to enhance behavior, applicable to both those with and without these disabilities. It emphasizes a scarcity of reviews on how such interventions affect individuals with developmental disabilities, including autism. Synthesizing evidence from 32 papers, it underscores substantial neural effects and behavioral improvements resulting from these interventions. Chronic interventions show more significant effects compared to single sessions. The review explores neural changes induced by these interventions using various neuroimaging techniques, revealing promising alterations in neural activity. Despite promising results, this study calls for further research with larger sample sizes and standardized neuroimaging tools to deepen our understanding of the neural mechanisms benefiting individuals with developmental disabilities, including autism.

The need to focus on females with ASD in neuroscience research, recognizing their unique phenotypic trajectories and age-related brain differences, was underscored in [70]. Sex-related biological factors, such as hormones and genes, likely play a crucial role in ASD development and neurodevelopmental pathways. A comprehensive lifespan approach is advocated to fully grasp brain-based sex differences in ASD. The study synthesizes neuroimaging research, revealing consistent sex differences in brain regions across neurotypical and ASD cohorts. Age-related brain differences point to distinctive neurodevelopmental patterns in females with ASD. The concept of a 'female protective effect' in ASD gains support, emphasizing genetic and endocrine influences on brain development. The interplay of sex-related biology with peripheral processes, especially the stress axis and brain arousal system, shapes unique neurodevelopmental patterns in males and females with ASD. This study calls for further research integrating behavior, sex hormones, and brain development to deepen our understanding of ASD.

Two studies examine the usefulness of Functional Near-Infrared Spectroscopy in the Study of Speech and Language in autism [72,73].

In the first study [72], a systematic review of functional near-infrared spectroscopy (fNIRS) studies revealed its potential benefits in investigating the neural correlates of speech and language impairment across various conditions, such as autism spectrum disorders, developmental speech and language disorders, cochlear implantation, deafness, and more. fNIRS could aid in early diagnosis, treatment response assessment, neuroprosthetic functioning, and neurofeedback.

In the second study [73], a systematic review focused on fNIRS-based neurofeedback studies. It found that fNIRS, as a functional neuroimaging technique, offers practicality, portability, and reduced sensitivity to movement artifacts. However, the quality of the studies varied, and large randomized controlled trials were lacking. While some studies indicated the feasibility of modulating brain functioning, especially in clinical populations like stroke, ADHD, autism, and social anxiety, specific clinical utility conclusions remain premature. With improved research and reporting practices, fNIRS-neurofeedback holds potential for clinical translation and further methodological advancements.

These studies collectively demonstrate the potential of fNIRS (which can represent a valid complementary tool for the fMRI) in understanding and addressing communication disorders and brain functioning, especially in populations with speech or language impairment. The technology holds promise for improved diagnosis, treatment, and neurofeedback applications.

The systematic review reported in [74] also proposed a comparative meta-analysis. The focus was on unraveling the unique and shared structural and functional brain irregularities in individuals with attention-deficit/hyperactivity disorder (ADHD) and autism spectrum disorder (ASD) during cognitive control tasks. When it comes to structural abnormalities, the analysis highlighted that ADHD is associated with a reduction in gray matter volume in the ventromedial orbitofrontal area. In contrast, individuals with ASD tend to exhibit an increase in gray matter volume in certain brain regions, particularly the bilateral temporal and right dorsolateral prefrontal areas. In terms of functional abnormalities during cognitive control tasks, the findings were intriguing. For ASD, there was a notable pattern of underactivation in the medial prefrontal region. Additionally, there was overactivation observed in the bilateral ventrolateral prefrontal cortices and precuneus. On the other hand, individuals with ADHD demonstrated right inferior fronto-striatal underactivation, especially during motor response inhibition. This underactivation was distinct from ASD and was accompanied by shared underactivation in the right anterior insula. In essence, this analysis illuminated the distinct structural and functional brain differences between ADHD and ASD, providing valuable insights into the unique neural mechanisms underlying these neurodevelopmental disorders.

The study, along with a meta-analysis reported in [76], delved into how individuals with ASD process rewarding stimuli, investigating whether these differences are limited to social rewards. Utilizing fMRI, the study aimed to reconcile conflicting findings in existing research. The key findings were:-The study uncovers distinct patterns of reward processing in individuals with ASD, encompassing both social and nonsocial rewards. -It highlights atypical brain activation in specific striatal regions.-Intriguingly, heightened brain activation is observed in individuals with ASD when exposed to their restricted interests, challenging traditional notions from the social motivation hypothesis.

These insights propose a broader interpretation of the social motivation hypothesis, indicating that atypical reward processing in ASD extends beyond social stimuli to include nonsocial rewards and fixations on restricted interests.

The meta-analysis hints at a potential explanation for the discrepancies in previous studies—a variation in the age composition of the study samples. This underscores the need for further research to comprehend the developmental trajectory of reward processing in ASD. In essence, this meta-analysis offers a nuanced understanding of how individuals with ASD process rewards, expanding beyond the conventional focus on social motivations. It sheds light on the intricate nature of reward processing in this population and advocates for considering age-related aspects to gain a comprehensive perspective.

The study reported in [78] recalled how the potential link between dysfunction in the mirror neuron system and challenges in social interaction and communication among individuals with autism spectrum conditions has garnered significant attention. Studies utilizing various neuroscience methods (EEG/MEG/TMS/eyetracking/EMG/fMRI) to assess the integrity of the mirror system in autism were analyzed. A thorough review of the selected papers revealed a diverse array of current data, particularly emphasizing the challenge of interpreting studies employing weakly localized measures of mirror system integrity. Notably, fMRI emerged as the most effectively localized measure of mirror system function. Within fMRI studies, those employing emotional stimuli have reported group differences, while those utilizing non-emotional hand action stimuli have not shown similar distinctions. In sum, the evidence for a comprehensive dysfunction of the mirror system in autism remained limited. An alternative model was proposed, emphasizing abnormal social top-down response modulation in autism and providing valuable insights into current data. The paper concluded by discussing the implications of this model and suggesting future research directions.

In [59], the authors conducted a thorough review of studies utilizing functional fMRI and diffusion tensor imaging (DTI) data to assess if these findings align with the proposed social communication and behavioral symptom dyad in individuals diagnosed with ASD according to the DSM-5. The consistent findings across these studies revealed abnormalities in brain function and structure within various networks, such as fronto-temporal and limbic networks linked to social and pragmatic language deficits, temporo-parieto-occipital networks associated with syntactic-semantic language deficits, and fronto-striato-cerebellar networks related to repetitive behaviors and restricted interests in individuals with ASD. As a result, this comprehensive review offers partial support for the proposed ASD dyad outlined in DSM-5.

A systematic review and meta-analysis of fMRI studies on ASD were conducted in [80]. One of the most consistently observed findings was a disruption in the function of brain regions associated with social interactions. These differences in activation within the social brain might stem from a diminished preference for social stimuli rather than a fundamental malfunction of these brain areas. Accumulating evidence suggests challenges in effectively integrating various functional brain regions and difficulties in finely adjusting brain function based on changing task demands in individuals with ASD. However, the authors conclude that existing research is limited by small sample sizes and a predominant focus on high-functioning males with autism.

This study proposed in [81] aimed to understand the brain regions associated with social cognition deficits in ASD and Schizophrenia (SZ). They conducted a systematic review of relevant studies and analyzed the data. The results showed that both ASD and SZ exhibit reduced activation in certain brain areas linked to social cognition, particularly in the medial prefrontal region. However, there were specific differences in brain activation patterns and engagement with stimuli between the two disorders. The findings offer valuable insights for future research and understanding of these conditions.

3.2. Theme 2: Integrating fMRI with Artificial Intelligence

Five systematic reviews have focused on analyzing the integration of AI with fMRI, highlighting opportunities, challenges, and bottlenecks [64,67,69,71,75]

In summary, these studies collectively explore the application of technology, including machine learning and neuroimaging techniques like fMRI, EEG, MRI, and neurofeedback, in the context of mental health research and specifically Neurodevelopmental Disorders (NDDs), with a focus on ASD. The findings suggest promise in technology-based diagnosis and intervention for NDDs, highlighting the potential of machine learning classifiers, resting-state fMRI (rs-fMRI) data, and the concept of "predictome" for predicting mental illness, including ASD. However, they emphasize the need for more high-quality research and well-designed studies to address potential biases, enhance sensitivity, and fully realize the clinical potential of these technological approaches. Table 2 reports the key elements emerging for this theme.

The review reported in [64] explored the increasing interest in utilizing technology in mental health research, particularly for Neurodevelopmental Disorders (NDDs). The focus was on summarizing studies that utilized technologies such as machine learning, fMRI, EEG, MRI, and neurofeedback for diagnosing and treating disorders, notably Autism Spectrum Disorder. The results suggest promise in technology-based diagnosis and intervention for NDDs, with a significant emphasis on ASD. However, the need for more high-quality research due to potential biases in existing studies is highlighted.

The study conducted in [67] addressed the challenges in ASD diagnosis through behavioral criteria and emphasized the need for brain imaging biomarkers to facilitate diagnosis. The focus was on using machine learning classifiers based on resting-state fMRI (rs-fMRI) data to achieve this. The meta-analysis indicates promising accuracy using rs-fMRI data but suggests that combining other brain imaging or phenotypic data could further enhance sensitivity. However, further, well-designed studies are essential to fully realizing the potential of this approach.

An investigation proposed in [71] discussed the extensive application of neuroimaging-based approaches, particularly machine learning, to study autism. It introduced the concept of "predictome," which involves using brain network features from neuroimaging modalities to predict mental illness. The systematic review covered various psychiatric disorders, including schizophrenia, major depression, bipolar disorder, and autism spectrum disorder (ASD), and emphasized the potential for individualized prediction and characterization. It also identifies the need for more research in this domain.

The study reported in [75] faced the increasing application of machine learning algorithms in diagnosing ASD and their potential clinical implications. A systematic review and meta-analysis were conducted to summarize the available evidence on the accuracy of machine learning algorithms in diagnosing ASD. The results suggest acceptable accuracy, particularly when utilizing structural magnetic resonance imaging (sMRI). However, the study emphasized the necessity for further well-designed studies to enhance the potential use of machine learning algorithms in clinical settings.

Table 2. Key elements emerging from the studies in theme 2.

Systematic Review	Highlights
[64]	The study explores the growing interest in employing technology for mental health research, specifically in Neurodevelopmental Disorders (NDDs). It summarizes studies using various technologies like machine learning, fMRI, EEG, MRI, and neurofeedback for diagnosing and treating ASD disorders. While the results suggest promise in technology-based diagnosis and intervention for NDDs, with a focus on ASD, the need for more high-quality research is emphasized due to potential biases in existing studies.
[67]	The study addresses challenges in ASD diagnosis based on behavioral criteria and emphasizes the need for brain imaging biomarkers to facilitate diagnosis. It focuses on using machine learning classifiers based on resting-state fMRI (rs-fMRI) data, indicating promising accuracy. However, the study suggests that combining other brain imaging or phenotypic data could further enhance sensitivity, emphasizing the necessity for further well-designed studies.
[71]	The review discusses the extensive application of neuroimaging-based approaches, particularly machine learning, to study autism. It introduces the concept of "predictome," using brain network features to predict mental illness. The contribution covers various psychiatric disorders, including ASD, emphasizing the potential for individualized prediction and characterization while identifying the need for more research in this domain.
[75]	The study reviews the increasing use of machine learning algorithms in diagnosing ASD and their clinical implications. A systematic review and meta-analysis summarize evidence on the accuracy of machine learning algorithms, particularly those using structural magnetic resonance imaging (sMRI). While acceptable accuracy is suggested, the study underscores the necessity for further well-designed studies to enhance the potential use of machine learning algorithms in clinical settings.

The study reported in [69], discussed in Section 3.3, focused on the potential of using AI and fMRI to empower personalized medicine in autism.

In summary, these articles collectively highlighted the significant role of technology, particularly fMRI and AI, in understanding and diagnosing ASD and other neurodevelopmental disorders. While there is promise and potential in utilizing these technologies for diagnosis and intervention, according to the studies, further high-quality research is essential to realizing their full clinical potential.

3.3. Theme 3: The Personalized Medicine through AI and fMRI

The analysis underscores, particularly in [65], that each patient with autism possesses a unique profile, highlighting the distinctiveness of this disorder. This characteristic uniqueness renders autism a promising domain for delving into personalized medicine (PM), wherein fMRI, owing to its potent diagnostic capabilities, could play a pivotal role. Currently, only one review study has delved into this aspect of fMRI [69]. The study underscored that PM is leading a profound shift in psychiatric disorder research, notably within the realm of autism. Traditionally, psychiatric disorders relied on symptom-based classifications; however, there is now a notable surge in efforts to unravel the fundamental mechanisms and etiology of these conditions. PM is actively seeking data-driven approaches to enhance diagnosis, prognosis, and treatment selection tailored to the individual needs of patients. The review thoroughly examined the burgeoning field of fMRI, focusing on unsupervised machine learning applications for disease subtyping while considering the unique characteristics of autism. Among the studies meeting inclusion criteria, several effectively utilized fMRI data to interpret disease clusters derived from both symptoms and biomarkers, shedding light on the psychiatric symptoms present in autism. This underscored the imperative to customize treatment approaches. The study emphasized that, despite being in an early exploratory stage, the field of PM for psychiatric disorders, particularly autism, is gaining significant momentum. However, conclusive results necessitate further validation and larger sample sizes. "The review strongly stressed the need to explore more accessible and clinically viable functional proxies, complementing fMRI technology in the pursuit of effective personalized psychiatric care, particularly in the context of autism".

3.4. Theme 4: The Role of Oxytocin

The combination of fMRI and AI offers a potent approach to dissecting the intricate role of oxytocin (OXT) in the brain. fMRI enables the visualization of neural responses influenced by oxytocin, particularly in social and emotional processing. AI, with its analytical prowess, delves into complex fMRI datasets, identifying subtle patterns and correlations. When these two technologies synergize, researchers gain a holistic view of OXTs impact, incorporating genetic, behavioral, and other neuroimaging data for personalized insights. AIs predictive modeling holds promise for anticipating individual responses to oxytocin but presents challenges in navigating the complexity of real-world social scenarios. OXT has a notable impact on neural activity, particularly during the processing of social stimuli. fMRI was shown to be crucial to this understanding in two systematic reviews [66,77].

In the context of both systematic reviews, there remains a conspicuous absence of a substantial contribution from Artificial Intelligence (AI). This observation, while indicative of the current state, presents an opportunity and impetus for researchers to embark on a more extensive exploration and incorporation of AI methodologies. Recognizing this gap underscores the potential for researchers to further unlock the capabilities of AI in enhancing the depth and breadth of future scientific investigations.

The first study [77] remarked how the OXT influenced the brain regions, including the temporal lobes and insula. Notably, the left insula showed significant hyperactivation following OXT administration, suggesting a modulation of neural circuits associated with emotional processing. These effects appeared to vary depending on factors such as sex and specific tasks. The authors were also invited to interpret the conclusions cautiously due to the limited number of studies and the limited sample size, which prevented a more detailed exploration of potential confounding factors.

The review reported in [66] remarked that studies involving intranasal oxytocin (IN-OXT) administration in individuals with autism spectrum disorder (ASD) suggested that OXT does alter brain activation in this population. fMRI has played a critical role in investigating these effects. The effects of OXT administration interacted with the type of task performed during fMRI studies. However, the overall results did not conclusively indicate a full restoration of normal brain activation in regions typically associated with ASD. Therefore, while there is a consistent body of evidence indicating that OXT affects brain activation in individuals with ASD, the exact implications for addressing their social deficits remain uncertain.

In summary, both articles underscore the critical role of fMRI in understanding how oxytocin affects neural activity, especially in the context of social and emotional processing. The use of fMRI has been instrumental in unraveling the effects of oxytocin and its potential implications for disorders like autism spectrum disorder. However, based on these two studies, further research is needed to fully comprehend the extent and nuances of these effects, and the use of AI could make an important contribution in this regard.

4. Discussion

4.1. The Trends in the Studies on Autism Focused on AI and fMRI

fMRI emerged as a powerful brain imaging technology in the 1990s. This tool has revolutionized our understanding of the human brain and its functions. Much of the initial fMRI research was focused on understanding the general mechanisms of the brain.

Furthermore, a more limited but equally important portion of fMRI research has been devoted to autism. This approach has opened new perspectives on understanding brain functioning in autism spectrum disorders, providing valuable information for the development of therapeutic and support approaches. Brain images generated by fMRI have made it possible to identify some peculiarities in the brain activity patterns associated with autism, thus contributing to the growing understanding of this complex neurological condition. A search was conducted on Pubmed with the keys shown in Box 1 to analyze the trends. This research has reported a total of 71,184 studies to date on the application of fMRI in the *health domain* since the 1990s. Figure 1 highlights how an important part of these studies focused on the application of fMRI to the brain (93.2%). Figure 2 provides a sketch of the number of fMRI studies focused on autism (2.1%).

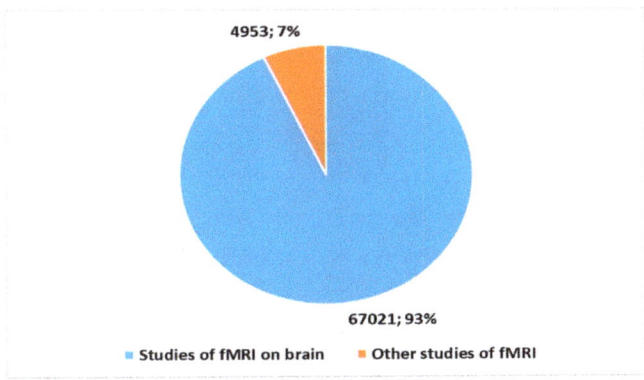

Figure 1. Studies focusing on fMRI.

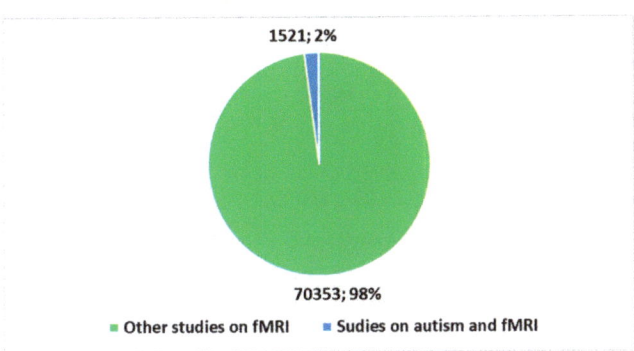

Figure 2. Studies on autism focusing fMRI.

Subsequently, integrating fMRI research with artificial intelligence (AI) has produced significant results. The use of advanced algorithms and neural networks trained on fMRI data has made it possible to identify complex patterns and correlations within brain images. Figure 3 shows the evolution of fMRI studies on integration with AI since the end of the 1990s (through research conducted using the keys in Box 1). There have been two important accelerations. The first acceleration was recorded in the last decade, when 87.1% of the total works were produced. The latest acceleration occurred starting with the COVID-19 pandemic, in which 49.3% of all works on this topic were produced in a period of approximately three years. The AI application has expanded our understanding of the neurological changes associated with autism, helping to identify distinctive biomarkers and improve early diagnosis. Furthermore, AI applied to the analysis of fMRI data has made it possible to predict behavior and individual responses to treatments, allowing for personalized and targeted intervention for those living with autism. This development has opened promising perspectives for the optimization of therapies and the adaptation of intervention strategies according to the specific needs of everyone. Figure 4 shows the total number of works produced in the context of the integration of AI and fMRI in autism, starting in 2010 (always using the keys in Box 1). Also, in this case, there was an important acceleration in the last decade (with 95.8% of the total works produced) and with the explosion of the pandemic (with 45.4% of the total works produced).

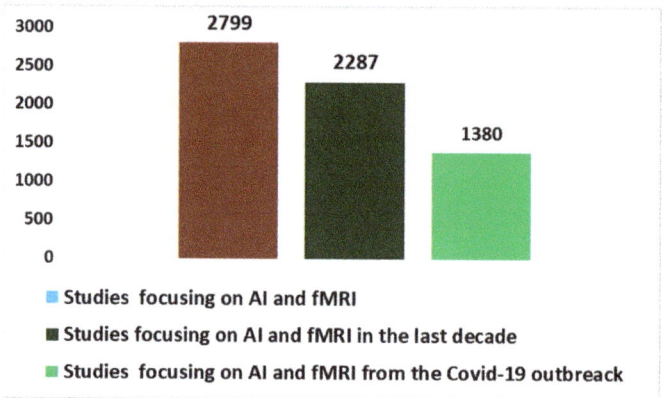

Figure 3. Studies focusing on AI and fMRI.

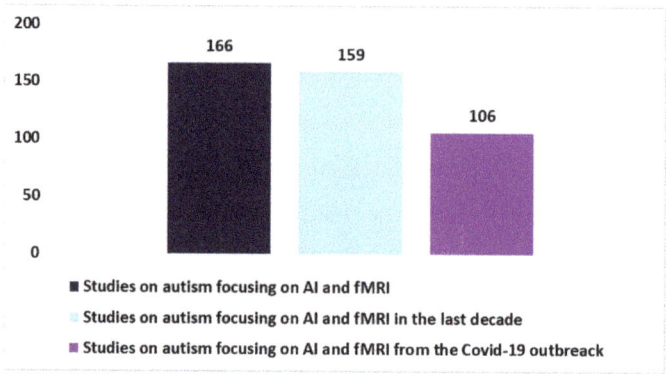

Figure 4. Studies on autism focusing on AI and fMRI.

4.2. Interpretation of Results

4.2.1. Interpretation of Results: Highlights

The importance of conducting an *umbrella review* of the applications of fMRI and AI integration in autism lies in the need to obtain an in-depth and accurate understanding of the current state of research. In light of the trends highlighted in Figures 1–4, studies on fMRI in autism (Figure 2) and fMRI and AI on autism are growing and represent a non-trivial part of the percentage of studies on fMRI in general (Figure 1) and with an increasing amount of AI integration (Figure 3). Therefore, an *umbrella review* of existing systematic reviews offers an in-depth and critical analysis with several advantages [58,59]. An integrated review of systematic reviews provides a holistic perspective on existing evidence, reducing information fragmentation and promoting a comprehensive understanding of discoveries. This facilitates the recognition of areas needing further research or methodological improvements. Additionally, it highlights emerging trends and best practices in the integration of fMRI and AI in autism, guiding future research efforts. Ultimately, this global review supports clinical decision-making, enhancing evidence-based practice for autism patients.

Box 1. The proposed composite key.

> *((fMRI[Title/Abstract]) OR (Functional Magnetic Resonance[Title/Abstract]))*
>
> *((fMRI[Title/Abstract]) OR (functional magnetic resonance[Title/Abstract])) AND (Brain)*
>
> *((fMRI[Title/Abstract]) OR (functional magnetic resonance[Title/Abstract])) AND ((autism[Title/Abstract]) OR (ASD[Title/Abstract]) OR (autistic[Title/Abstract]))*
>
> *((fMRI[Title/Abstract]) OR (functional magnetic resonance[Title/Abstract])) AND ((artificial intelligence[Title/Abstract]) OR (machine learning[Title/Abstract]) OR (deep learning[Title/Abstract]) OR (neural network[Title/Abstract])*
>
> *((fMRI[Title/Abstract]) OR (functional magnetic resonance[Title/Abstract])) AND ((autism[Title/Abstract]) OR (ASD[Title/Abstract]) OR (autistic[Title/Abstract])) AND ((artificial intelligence[Title/Abstract]) OR (machine learning[Title/Abstract]) OR (deep learning[Title/Abstract]) OR (neural network[Title/Abstract]))*

From this overview of systematic reviews, important themes have clearly emerged, receiving varying degrees of attention. Technology garnered widespread interest across the systematic reviews, particularly in the context where fMRI played a prominent role. The analysis led to the organization of the results into themes based on the dominance of content. Beyond the theme where technology took center stage (including studies involving fMRI in comparison with other technological solutions) [62,63,65,68,70,72–74,76,79–81], other themes have also surfaced. The extensively explored theme is that of AI integrated with fMRI. Here, systematic reviews have demonstrated a polarization around [64,67,71,75] the promising applications for technology-based diagnosis and intervention in NDDs, highlighting the potential of machine learning classifiers, resting-state fMRI (rs-fMRI) data, and the "predictome" concept for predicting mental illness, including ASD. Nevertheless, they underscore the imperative for additional high-quality research and well-designed studies to mitigate potential biases, enhance sensitivity, and fully unlock the clinical potential of these technological approaches. Another related theme that has been identified is that of personalized medicine. Only one specific study delved into the potential of combining AI and fMRI to enable PM for autism, tailoring treatments to the unique needs of individuals with ASD [69]. Another important theme that emerged regarding the prominent role of fMRI is that of analyzing the role of oxytocin [66,77], highlighting the need to foster research in the integration of AI as a specific tool in this field.

An overview of the most recent production of articles between 2022/2023 in Pubmed (last composite *key in* Box 1) is useful for comparing the themes that emerged in the systematic reviews as well as those that emerged in the umbrella review.

The dominant themes of technologies and AI emerge from the literature based on scientific articles [82–114]. This is in line with the *umbrella review*.

A brief examination identifies the following among the dominant concerns of technology and AI:

1. *Genetic and Sensory Factors in ASD Prediction*

The study reported in [82] explored the sensory signature of unaffected biological parents and how it can be used to predict the risk of autism in their offspring. This research delves into the genetic and sensory factors that may play a role in the development of autism. It highlights the importance of studying familiar connections and sensory characteristics for early prediction and intervention.

2. *Machine Learning and Graph Analysis for ASD Classification*

A cluster of articles [83,85,88,90,93,95,99,101,104,106,111,113,114] focuses on using advanced computational techniques, including machine learning, deep learning, and graph analysis, to classify and diagnose autism. These articles represent the growing interest in leveraging data-driven approaches to understand and categorize individuals with ASD. They investigate various data sources, from fMRI data to multi-site datasets, and aim to enhance accuracy and efficiency in ASD diagnosis.

3. *Functional Connectivity and Resting State Analysis*

Articles such as [82,84,86,108,110] emphasized the significance of studying functional connectivity and resting state fMRI data in the context of autism. These articles investigate how patterns of brain activity at rest can reveal insights into ASD. They explored methods to analyze and interpret these patterns, providing valuable information for understanding the disorder.

4. *AI and Technology in ASD Diagnosis*

Articles [91,114] looked in general at the role of artificial intelligence (AI) and technology in diagnosing autism. They considered the integration of AI in analyzing imaging data such as DTI, MRI, and fMRI scans. Additionally, article [91] provided a survey perspective on the current state of AI technology in autism diagnosis, highlighting the potential for technology to assist in this area.

5. *Neural Network and Deep Learning Approaches*

Several articles [93,104,108,114] examined the use of neural networks, including convolutional neural networks (CNNs), in the context of ASD diagnosis. These deep learning methods were employed to process and interpret complex brain imaging data, with the goal of improving diagnostic accuracy.

6. *Graph Neural Networks and Connectivity Analysis*

Articles [90,95,99,111] delved into the application of graph neural networks and connectivity analysis for diagnosing autism. These methods considered the interrelationships and patterns within functional brain networks, offering insights into the brain's role in autism.

7. *Multi-Site Data and Site-Dependent Analysis*

Articles [99,112,113] addressed the challenges associated with using data from multiple sites for autism diagnosis. They explore techniques to minimize site-dependent variations and improve the reliability of classification models. These articles highlighted the importance of standardization and robustness in multi-site studies.

8. *Interpretable and Explainable AI in ASD Diagnosis*

Articles [101,108] focused on the interpretability of AI methods and the importance of understanding how AI arrives at its conclusions in the context of ASD diagnosis. This theme is crucial for gaining insights into the decision-making processes of AI models in clinical applications.

These detected patterns of interest can certainly be a starting point for scholars to identify possible lines of study and address them towards specific systematic reviews in the future.

4.2.2. Interpretation of Results: Problems, Limits, Perspectives, and Final Reflections
Problems, Limits, and Perspectives

The *umbrella review* shows that the integration of fMRI in autism research comes with several notable challenges and limitations, as indicated in the provided analysis conducted in the umbrella review. Firstly [62], there is a call for greater harmonization of experimental paradigms both within and across neuroimaging modalities. This is crucial because variability in the design of experiments can make it difficult to draw meaningful comparisons and generalizations across different studies. Without standardized protocols and paradigms, the results obtained from various fMRI studies may not be directly comparable, which can hinder progress in the field. Another significant issue [64] highlighted is the high risk of bias in many studies. Research quality is of paramount importance, and studies with a high risk of bias can undermine the credibility and reliability of their findings. To advance our understanding of the relationship between fMRI data and autism, it is essential to conduct research with rigorous methodology and transparent reporting. Moreover, the limited sample sizes and a lack of corrections for multiple comparisons in many studies are significant challenges [65]. Small sample sizes can result in limited statistical power, making it challenging to detect meaningful effects. Additionally, the absence of corrections for multiple comparisons can lead to spurious or false-positive findings, which can have serious implications for the accuracy and validity of results. The outcome [66] also raises questions about the implications of findings related to OXT alterations in the fMRI brain networks of individuals with autism. While there is evidence of such alterations, it remains unclear how these changes in brain activation relate to the alleviation of social deficits in individuals with autism. Understanding the clinical significance of these fMRI findings is vital for informing potential treatments and interventions. The cost and signal-to-noise ratio limitations of fMRI may also present an obstacle [67]. Despite being a valuable tool for measuring brain function, fMRI is associated with high costs and a relatively low signal-to-noise ratio. As a result, some authors [67] suggest that it may not be the most practical and cost-effective option for clinical applications. This limitation prompts researchers to explore more accessible and clinically-ready functional proxies for assessing brain function in the context of autism. Research on sex differences in autism using fMRI is another area that demands attention [70]. The outcome points out that a more comprehensive and lifespan-oriented approach is needed in this regard. Understanding the relationships between behavior, sex hormones, and brain development in autism could provide valuable insights, but this area remains underexplored. Even if machine learning algorithms for diagnosing autism based on fMRI data have shown promise, in some cases, the accuracy varies. The limitations highlighted in the outcome of the analysis [75] suggest the need for further well-designed studies to enhance the potential use of these algorithms in clinical settings. Machine learning may offer a valuable diagnostic tool, but its full potential is yet to be realized. Finally, the limitations of the existing literature, such as the use of small sample sizes and a focus on high-functioning males with autism, suggest the need for a broader and more inclusive approach to research [60]. This will help ensure that the findings are more representative of the entire spectrum of individuals with autism and can be more readily generalized to diverse populations. In summary, integrating fMRI with autism research faces challenges related to standardization, bias, sample sizes, data correction, clinical relevance, cost, sex differences, machine learning, and the representativeness of the studied populations. Addressing these challenges is vital for improving the quality and applicability of fMRI-based research in the context of autism.

Several missing or underexplored yet intriguing themes have also surfaced in this context. Within the systematic reviews scrutinized regarding the application of fMRI in autism, as analyzed in the *umbrella review*, we encounter the following absent themes:

1. The regulatory aspect concerns the integration of Medical Devices.
2. The issues of cybersecurity and privacy.
3. Acceptance and consent.

Furthermore, this observation, which is corroborated by a comparison with recent literature [82–104], highlights a current trend leaning more towards the development of innovative, specialized Artificial Intelligence tools than their routine integration into the healthcare domain.

This suggests a distinctive direction in research, emphasizing the creation of novel AI solutions tailored to the specific needs of autism research and diagnosis rather than immediate integration into standard healthcare practices.

The *umbrella review* therefore indirectly suggests focusing on the themes reported in (1–3). Among the underexplored themes, we find the one of the PM, which analyzes only a systematic review [69].

PM, also known as precision medicine or personalized medicine, could represent an innovative approach in the field of autism [115]. This approach would carefully consider individual differences, including genetics, lifestyle, and environment, with the aim of personalizing disease prevention, diagnosis, and treatment with the aim of maximizing therapeutic efficacy and minimizing side effects [115–117], while also integrating with AI [118,119]. In the specific context of autism, personalized medicine could seek to adapt treatments based on the specific genetic and biological characteristics of each individual suffering from autism spectrum disorder (ASD) [120]. This could mean identifying specific subtypes of autism based on genetic, biochemical, and neurophysiological markers. This customization would allow for a more accurate diagnosis and personalized assessment of each patient's clinical picture, helping to identify the most suitable and effective treatments [121,122]. Furthermore, PM could revolutionize the development of new drugs, guiding research towards the creation of more targeted therapies, considering the genetic and biological variations that influence autism. This could lead to the development of more effective drugs with fewer side effects. In essence, the integration of PM in the field of autism could lead to a more targeted and effective therapeutic approach, considering the specific needs of each individual [123,124]. This could translate into a significant improvement in the quality of life of autism patients and their families, opening new perspectives in the treatment and management of the condition. The *umbrella review* highlighted the integration of fMRI and AI in autism [69] as an articulated path due to the need for a contemporary multidomain and heterogeneous approach in several multifaced fields.

Final Reflections

We are currently witnessing a significant impact resulting from the introduction of Artificial Intelligence (AI) in the health domain. This impact is notably observed in the focused efforts to improve the accuracy and efficiency of diagnoses and assessments within specific medical contexts, achieved through the implementation of advanced AI methodologies [125,126]. The significance of AI utilization also becomes evident in the thematic exploration undertaken in this umbrella review, specifically regarding the integration of functional Magnetic Resonance Imaging (fMRI) with AI in the context of autism. By delving into the problems, limitations, and emerging perspectives revealed through this umbrella review, we gain valuable insights. It allows us to not only pinpoint areas of concern (Table 3) but also identify themes that remain underexplored (Table 4) and recognize emerging trends (Table 5). This comprehensive understanding serves as a guide, offering directions for both scholars and stakeholders in the healthcare domain. These directions, informed by the current state of AI integration in medical research, lay the foundation for future developments that can potentially transform the landscape of healthcare practices.

Table 3 outlines key areas of concern and suggests actions to enhance the integration of functional Magnetic Resonance Imaging (fMRI) in autism research. Each issue is identified, accompanied by recommended steps for improvement.

Table 4 reports the underexplored themes: It focuses on critical regulatory, cybersecurity, and ethical aspects associated with the integration of medical devices in autism research, particularly in the context of functional Magnetic Resonance Imaging (fMRI). The table highlights key issues and suggests areas for investigation and improvement.

Table 5 reports the emerging trends: It clearly invites researchers and stakeholders to understand and explore the potential benefits of integrating precision medicine into autism research. It underscores the importance of personalized approaches to enhance therapeutic efficacy and minimize side effects, ultimately contributing to an improved quality of life for individuals with autism and their families.

Table 3. Areas of concern and improvement.

Issue	Needed/Suggested Action
Harmonization of Experimental Paradigms	Investigate methods for greater harmonization of experimental paradigms within and across neuroimaging modalities to enhance comparability between studies.
Bias in Studies	Explore strategies to minimize bias in fMRI studies, emphasizing rigorous methodology and transparent reporting to improve the credibility and reliability of findings.
Sample Sizes and Statistical Power	Conduct studies with larger sample sizes and appropriate corrections for multiple comparisons to increase statistical power and reduce the likelihood of spurious or false-positive findings.
Clinical Relevance of Findings	Investigate the clinical significance of fMRI findings, particularly regarding alterations in brain networks, to better understand their implications for the development of treatments and interventions.
Cost and Signal-to-Noise Ratio Limitations	Explore alternative, more cost-effective functional proxies for assessing brain function in the context of autism, considering the high costs and signal-to-noise ratio limitations associated with fMRI.
Sex Differences in Autism	Conduct research on sex differences in autism using fMRI, adopting a comprehensive and lifespan-oriented approach to understand the relationships between behavior, sex hormones, and brain development.
Machine learning algoritms	Further refine and validate machine learning algorithms for diagnosing autism based on fMRI data, addressing the limitations highlighted in existing studies, to enhance their potential use in clinical settings.
Inclusive Research Approach	Advocate for a broader and more inclusive approach to research by expanding the focus beyond high-functioning males and small sample sizes, ensuring findings are representative of the entire spectrum of individuals with autism.

Table 4. Underexplored themes.

Issue	Needed/Suggested Action
Regulatory Aspect of Medical Devices	Investigate the regulatory aspects concerning the integration of medical devices in autism research, addressing potential challenges and opportunities.
Cybersecurity and Privacy	Explore the issues of cybersecurity and privacy in the context of fMRI data and autism research, ensuring the ethical handling and protection of sensitive information.
Acceptance and Consent	Examine the themes of acceptance and consent in fMRI-based autism research, considering the perspectives of individuals participating in studies and ensuring ethical practices.

4.3. Limitations

The methodology employed for this review was grounded in an umbrella review, a comprehensive approach that scrutinizes systematic reviews sourced from two prominent databases, namely Scopus and PubMed. Umbrella reviews [58,59] serve as powerful tools for distilling key themes prevalent in studies within a specific domain, leveraging the analysis of high-caliber research, particularly systematic reviews. It is crucial to acknowledge, however, that delving into more nuanced and specific aspects necessitates a broader exploration, encompassing studies of diverse types, including articles and communications.

Table 5. Emerging trends.

Issue	Needed/Suggested Action
Precision Medicine in Autism	Explore the potential of precision medicine in autism research, considering individual differences in genetics, lifestyle, and environment for personalized disease prevention, diagnosis, and treatment.
Improving the quality of life	Investigate how the integration of precision medicine in autism research could lead to a more targeted and effective therapeutic approach, ultimately improving the quality of life for individuals with autism and their families.

5. Conclusions

In conclusion, this study, conducted through the umbrella review, strongly underscores the predominant themes addressed in systematic reviews, focusing on technological integration (with fMRI playing a pivotal role) and the utilization of AI. Equally deserving of attention is the mysterious role of oxytocin. The study not only highlights the immense potential but also the formidable challenges and limitations in this domain. It is worth noting that there is a growing and fervent interest in advancing research and innovation in AI within this context, contrasting with the comparatively lesser emphasis on themes related to the integration of processes in the health domain, such as regulation, acceptance, consent, and data security. Furthermore, the integration into PM stands out as an exceptionally vital and relatively uncharted territory, which, intriguingly, holds remarkable promise for autism research.

Funding: This research received no external funding.

Conflicts of Interest: The author declares no conflict of interest.

References

1. Uğurbil, K. Development of functional imaging in the human brain (fMRI); the University of Minnesota experience. *Neuroimage* **2012**, *62*, 613–619. [CrossRef] [PubMed]
2. Bandettini, P.A. fMRI. In *Special Collection: CogNet*; The MIT Press: Cambridge, MA, USA, 2020; ISBN 9780262356770. [CrossRef]
3. Krueger, G.; Granziera, C. The history and role of long duration stimulation in fMRI. *NeuroImage* **2012**, *62*, 1051–1055. [CrossRef] [PubMed]
4. Raichle, M.E. A brief history of human brain mapping. *Trends Neurosci.* **2009**, *32*, 118–126. [CrossRef] [PubMed]
5. Jardetzky, O. fMRI in Brain Research in Its Historical Context. *Am. J. Bioeth.* **2008**, *8*, 43–45. [CrossRef] [PubMed]
6. Icon Group International: FMRI: Webster's Timeline History, 1970–2007; Icon Group International: Las Vegas, NV, USA, 2010.
7. Practice Parameter, fMRI Brain. Available online: https://www.acr.org/-/media/ACR/Files/Practice-Parameters/fmr-brain.pdf (accessed on 23 November 2023).
8. Ashburner, J. *Preparing fMRI Data for Statistical Analysis Functional MRI Techniques*; Filippi, M., Ed.; Humana Press: Totowa, NJ, USA, 2009.
9. Henson, R.N.A. Analysis of fMRI time series. In *Human Brain Function*, 2nd ed.; Frackowiak, R.S.J., Friston, K.J., Frith, C., Dolan, R., Friston, K.J., Price, C.J., Zeki, S., Ashburner, J., Penny, W.D., Eds.; Academic Press: Cambridge, MA, USA, 2003.
10. Leong, A.T.L.; Wu, E.X. Functional MRI: Making connections in the brain. *eLife* **2017**, *6*, e32064. [CrossRef]
11. Scrivener, C.L.; Reader, A.T. Variability of EEG electrode positions and their underlying brain regions: Visualizing gel artifacts from a simultaneous EEG-fMRI dataset. *Brain Behav.* **2022**, *12*, e2476. [CrossRef] [PubMed]
12. FDA Authorizes Marketing of Diagnostic Aid for Autism Spectrum Disorder. Available online: https://www.fda.gov/news-events/press-announcements/fda-authorizes-marketing-diagnostic-aid-autism-spectrum-disorder (accessed on 20 November 2023).
13. Zhang, Z.; Li, G.; Xu, Y.; Tang, X. Application of Artificial Intelligence in the MRI Classification Task of Human Brain Neurological and Psychiatric Diseases: A Scoping Review. *Diagnostics* **2021**, *11*, 1402. [CrossRef] [PubMed]
14. Yin, W.; Li, L.; Wu, F.-X. Deep learning for brain disorder diagnosis based on fMRI images. *Neurocomputing* **2022**, *469*, 332–345. [CrossRef]
15. Nenning, K.H.; Langs, G. Machine learning in neuroimaging: From research to clinical practice. *Radiologie* **2022**, *62* (Suppl. S1), 1–10. [CrossRef]

16. Macpherson, T.; Churchland, A.; Sejnowski, T.; DiCarlo, J.; Kamitani, Y.; Takahashi, H.; Hikida, T. Natural and Artificial Intelligence: A brief introduction to the interplay between AI and neuroscience research. *Neural Netw.* **2021**, *144*, 603–613. [CrossRef]
17. Kocak, B. Artificial intelligence to predict task activation from resting state fMRI. *Eur. Radiol.* **2021**, *31*, 5251–5252. [CrossRef]
18. Bajaj, V.; Sinha, G.R. *Artificial Intelligence-Based Brain-Computer Interface*, 1st ed.; Academic Press: Cambridge, MA, USA, 2022.
19. Zhao, Y.; Chen, Y.; Cheng, K.; Huang, W. Artificial intelligence based multimodal language decoding from brain activity: A review. *Brain Res. Bull.* **2023**, *201*, 110713. [CrossRef] [PubMed]
20. Stephan, K.E.; Friston, K.J. Analyzing effective connectivity with functional magnetic resonance imaging. *Wiley Interdiscip. Rev. Cogn. Sci.* **2010**, *1*, 446–459. [CrossRef] [PubMed]
21. Qian, J.; Li, H.; Wang, J.; He, L. Recent Advances in Explainable Artificial Intelligence for Magnetic Resonance Imaging. *Diagnostics* **2023**, *13*, 1571. [CrossRef] [PubMed]
22. Rezaei, S.; Gharepapagh, E.; Rashidi, F.; Cattarinussi, G.; Sanjari Moghaddam, H.; Di Camillo, F.; Schiena, G.; Sambataro, F.; Brambilla, P.; Delvecchio, G. Machine learning applied to functional magnetic resonance imaging in anxiety disorders. *J. Affect. Disord.* **2023**, *342*, 54–62. [CrossRef] [PubMed]
23. Rashid, M.; Singh, H.; Goyal, V. The use of machine learning and deep learning algorithms in functional magneticresonance imaging—A systematic review. *Expert Syst.* **2020**, *37*, e12644. [CrossRef]
24. Chan, Y.H.; Wang, C.; Soh, W.K.; Rajapakse, J.C. Combining Neuroimaging and Omics Datasets for Disease Classification Using Graph Neural Networks. *Front Neurosci.* **2022**, *16*, 866666. [CrossRef] [PubMed]
25. Uddin, M.; Wang, Y.; Woodbury-Smith, M. Artificial intelligence for precision medicine in neurodevelopmental disorders. *NPJ Digit. Med.* **2019**, *2*, 112. [CrossRef]
26. CDC. Autism Spectrum Disorders. Available online: https://www.cdc.gov/ncbddd/autism/facts.html (accessed on 23 November 2023).
27. Autism Speak, What Is Autism? Available online: https://www.autismspeaks.org/what-autism (accessed on 23 November 2023).
28. NHS. What Is Autism? Available online: https://www.nhs.uk/conditions/autism/what-is-autism/ (accessed on 23 November 2023).
29. NIH. Autism Spectrum Disorders. Available online: https://www.nimh.nih.gov/health/topics/autism-spectrum-disorders-asd (accessed on 23 November 2023).
30. WHO. Autism. Available online: https://www.who.int/news-room/fact-sheets/detail/autism-spectrum-disorders (accessed on 23 November 2023).
31. APS. What Is Autism Spectrum Disorder? Available online: https://www.psychiatry.org/patients-families/autism/what-is-autism-spectrum-disorder (accessed on 23 November 2023).
32. Mughal, S.; Faizy, R.M.; Saadabadi, A. *Autism Spectrum Disorder*; StatPearls Publishing: Treasure Island, FL, USA, 2023.
33. Grabrucker, A.M. (Ed.) *Autims Spectrum Disordes*; Exon Publications: Brisbane, QLD, Australia, 2021.
34. Matson, J.L. *Handbook of Assessment and Diagnosis of Autism Spectrum Disorder*; Springer: Berlin/Heidelberg, Germany, 2016.
35. Casanova, F.M. *Imaging the Brain in Autism*; Springer: Berlin/Heidelberg, Germany, 2013.
36. Ahmed, M.I.; Spooner, B.; Isherwood, J.; Lane, M.; Orrock, E.; Dennison, A. A Systematic Review of the Barriers to the Implementation of Artificial Intelligence in Healthcare. *Cureus* **2023**, *15*, e46454. [CrossRef]
37. Vo, V.; Chen, G.; Aquino, Y.S.J.; Carter, S.M.; Do, Q.N.; Woode, M.E. Multi-stakeholder preferences for the use of artificial intelligence in healthcare: A systematic review and thematic analysis. *Soc. Sci. Med.* **2023**, *338*, 116357. [CrossRef]
38. Singareddy, S.; Sn, V.P.; Jaramillo, A.P.; Yasir, M.; Iyer, N.; Hussein, S.; Nath, T.S. Artificial Intelligence and Its Role in the Management of Chronic Medical Conditions: A Systematic Review. *Cureus* **2023**, *15*, e46066. [CrossRef]
39. Vithlani, J.; Hawksworth, C.; Elvidge, J.; Ayiku, L.; Dawoud, D. Economic evaluations of artificial intelligence-based healthcare interventions: A systematic literature review of best practices in their conduct and reporting. *Front. Pharmacol.* **2023**, *14*, 1220950. [CrossRef] [PubMed]
40. Kautish, S.; Dhiman, G. (Eds.) *Artificial Intelligence for Accurate Analysis and Detection of Autism Spectrum Disorder (Advances in Medical Diagnosis, Treatment, and Care)*; IGI Global Publisher: Hershey, PA, USA, 2021.
41. Mintz, J.; Gyori, M.; Aagaard, M. (Eds.) *Touching the Future Technology for Autism? Lessons from the HANDS Project*; IOS Press: Amsterdam, The Netherlands, 2012.
42. Wu, X.; Deng, H.; Jian, S.; Chen, H.; Li, Q.; Gong, R.; Wu, J. Global trends and hotspots in the digital therapeutics of autism spectrum disorders: A bibliometric analysis from 2002 to 2022. *Front. Psychiatry* **2023**, *14*, 1126404. [CrossRef] [PubMed]
43. Marciano, F.; Venutolo, G.; Ingenito, C.M.; Verbeni, A.; Terracciano, C.; Plunk, E.; Garaci, F.; Cavallo, A.; Fasano, A. Artificial Intelligence: The "Trait D'Union" in Different Analysis Approaches of Autism Spectrum Disorder Studies. *Curr. Med. Chem.* **2021**, *28*, 6591–6618. [CrossRef] [PubMed]
44. Abdel Hameed, M.; Hassaballah, M.; Hosney, M.E.; Alqahtani, A. An AI-Enabled Internet of Things Based Autism Care System for Improving Cognitive Ability of Children with Autism Spectrum Disorders. *Comput. Intell. Neurosci.* **2022**, *2022*, 2247675, Retraction in: *Comput. Intell. Neurosci.* **2023**, *2023*, 9878709. [CrossRef] [PubMed]

45. Del Casale, A.; Sarli, G.; Bargagna, P.; Polidori, L.; Alcibiade, A.; Zoppi, T.; Borro, M.; Gentile, G.; Zocchi, C.; Ferracuti, S.; et al. Machine Learning and Pharmacogenomics at the Time of Precision Psychiatry. *Curr. Neuropharmacol.* **2023**, *21*, 2395–2408. [CrossRef] [PubMed]
46. Ali, S.G.; Wang, X.; Li, P.; Jung, Y.; Bi, L.; Kim, J.; Chen, Y.; Feng, D.D.; Magnenat Thalmann, N.; Wang, J.; et al. A systematic review: Virtual-reality-based techniques for human exercises and health improvement. *Front. Public Health* **2023**, *11*, 1143947. [CrossRef] [PubMed]
47. Zhang, S.; Wang, S.; Liu, R.; Dong, H.; Zhang, X.; Tai, X. A bibliometric analysis of research trends of artificial intelligence in the treatment of autistic spectrum disorders. *Front. Psychiatry* **2022**, *13*, 967074. [CrossRef]
48. Alqaysi, M.E.; Albahri, A.S.; Hamid, R.A. Diagnosis-Based Hybridization of Multimedical Tests and Sociodemographic Characteristics of Autism Spectrum Disorder Using Artificial Intelligence and Machine Learning Techniques: A Systematic Review. *Int. J. Telemed. Appl.* **2022**, *2022*, 3551528. [CrossRef]
49. Joudar, S.S.; Albahri, A.S.; Hamid, R.A. Triage and priority-based healthcare diagnosis using artificial intelligence for autism spectrum disorder and gene contribution: A systematic review. *Comput. Biol. Med.* **2022**, *146*, 105553. [CrossRef]
50. Welch, V.; Wy, T.J.; Ligezka, A.; Hassett, L.C.; Croarkin, P.E.; Athreya, A.P.; Romanowicz, M. Use of Mobile and Wearable Artificial Intelligence in Child and Adolescent Psychiatry: Scoping Review. *J. Med. Internet Res.* **2022**, *24*, e33560. [CrossRef] [PubMed]
51. Alabdulkareem, A.; Alhakbani, N.; Al-Nafjan, A. A Systematic Review of Research on Robot-Assisted Therapy for Children with Autism. *Sensors* **2022**, *22*, 944. [CrossRef] [PubMed]
52. Cavus, N.; Lawan, A.A.; Ibrahim, Z.; Dahiru, A.; Tahir, S.; Abdulrazak, U.I.; Hussaini, A. A Systematic Literature Review on the Application of Machine-Learning Models in Behavioral Assessment of Autism Spectrum Disorder. *J. Pers. Med.* **2021**, *11*, 299. [CrossRef] [PubMed]
53. Quaak, M.; van de Mortel, L.; Thomas, R.M.; van Wingen, G. Deep learning applications for the classification of psychiatric disorders using neuroimaging data: Systematic review and meta-analysis. *Neuroimage Clin.* **2021**, *30*, 102584. [CrossRef] [PubMed]
54. Valencia, K.; Rusu, C.; Quiñones, D.; Jamet, E. The Impact of Technology on People with Autism Spectrum Disorder: A Systematic Literature Review. *Sensors* **2019**, *19*, 4485. [CrossRef] [PubMed]
55. Valliani, A.A.; Ranti, D.; Oermann, E.K. Deep Learning and Neurology: A Systematic Review. *Neurol. Ther.* **2019**, *8*, 351–365. [CrossRef] [PubMed]
56. Liu, M.; Li, B.; Hu, D. Autism Spectrum Disorder Studies Using fMRI Data and Machine Learning: A Review. *Front. Neurosci.* **2021**, *15*, 697870. [CrossRef] [PubMed]
57. Feng, M.; Xu, J. Detection of ASD Children through Deep-Learning Application of fMRI. *Children* **2023**, *10*, 1654. [CrossRef]
58. The University of Melbourne Library. Library Guides, Umbrella Review. Available online: https://unimelb.libguides.com/whichreview/umbrellareview (accessed on 23 November 2023).
59. Choi, G.J.; Kang, H. The umbrella review: A useful strategy in the rain of evidence. *Korean J. Pain.* **2022**, *35*, 127–128. [CrossRef]
60. ANDJ Narrative Checklist. Available online: https://it.scribd.com/document/434616519/ANDJ-Narrative-Review-Checklist (accessed on 23 November 2023).
61. Giansanti, D. The Regulation of Artificial Intelligence in Digital Radiology in the Scientific Literature: A Narrative Review of Reviews. *Healthcare* **2022**, *10*, 1824. [CrossRef]
62. Morrel, J.; Singapuri, K.; Landa, R.J.; Reetzke, R. Neural correlates and predictors of speech and language development in infants at elevated likelihood for autism: A systematic review. *Front. Hum. Neurosci.* **2023**, *17*, 1211676. [CrossRef] [PubMed]
63. Xiao, J.; Wu, J. Effectiveness of the Neuroimaging Techniques in the Recognition of Psychiatric Disorders: A Systematic Review and Meta-analysis of RCTs. *Curr. Med. Imaging* **2023**, *20*, e260523217379. [CrossRef]
64. Ribas, M.O.; Micai, M.; Caruso, A.; Fulceri, F.; Fazio, M.; Scattoni, M.L. Technologies to support the diagnosis and/or treatment of neurodevelopmental disorders: A systematic review. *Neurosci. Biobehav. Rev.* **2023**, *145*, 105021. [CrossRef]
65. Kangarani-Farahani, M.; Izadi-Najafabadi, S.; Zwicker, J.G. How does brain structure and function on MRI differ in children with autism spectrum disorder, developmental coordination disorder, and/or attention deficit hyperactivity disorder? *Int. J. Dev. Neurosci.* **2022**, *82*, 681–715. [CrossRef] [PubMed]
66. Fathabadipour, S.; Mohammadi, Z.; Roshani, F.; Goharbakhsh, N.; Alizadeh, H.; Palizgar, F.; Cumming, P.; Michel, T.M.; Vafaee, M.S. The neural effects of oxytocin administration in autism spectrum disorders studied by fMRI: A systematic review. *J. Psychiatr. Res.* **2022**, *154*, 80–90. [CrossRef] [PubMed]
67. Santana, C.P.; de Carvalho, E.A.; Rodrigues, I.D.; Bastos, G.S.; de Souza, A.D.; de Brito, L.L. rs-fMRI and machine learning for ASD diagnosis: A systematic review and meta-analysis. *Sci. Rep.* **2022**, *12*, 6030. [CrossRef] [PubMed]
68. Su, W.C.; Amonkar, N.; Cleffi, C.; Srinivasan, S.; Bhat, A. Neural Effects of Physical Activity and Movement Interventions in Individuals with Developmental Disabilities—A Systematic Review. *Front. Psychiatry* **2022**, *13*, 794652. [CrossRef]
69. Miranda, L.; Paul, R.; Pütz, B.; Koutsouleris, N.; Müller-Myhsok, B. Systematic Review of Functional MRI Applications for Psychiatric Disease Subtyping. *Front. Psychiatry* **2021**, *12*, 665536. [CrossRef]
70. Walsh, M.J.M.; Wallace, G.L.; Gallegos, S.M.; Braden, B.B. Brain-based sex differences in autism spectrum disorder across the lifespan: A systematic review of structural MRI, fMRI, and DTI findings. *Neuroimage Clin.* **2021**, *31*, 102719. [CrossRef]
71. Rashid, B.; Calhoun, V. Towards a brain-based predictome of mental illness. *Hum. Brain Mapp.* **2020**, *41*, 3468–3535. [CrossRef]
72. Butler, L.K.; Kiran, S.; Tager-Flusberg, H. Functional Near-Infrared Spectroscopy in the Study of Speech and Language Impairment Across the Life Span: A Systematic Review. *Am. J. Speech Lang. Pathol.* **2020**, *29*, 1674–1701. [CrossRef] [PubMed]

73. Kohl, S.H.; Mehler, D.M.A.; Lührs, M.; Thibault, R.T.; Konrad, K.; Sorger, B. The Potential of Functional Near-Infrared Spectroscopy-Based Neurofeedback–A Systematic Review and Recommendations for Best Practice. *Front. Neurosci.* **2020**, *14*, 594, Erratum in *Front. Neurosci.* **2022**, *16*, 907941. [CrossRef] [PubMed]
74. Lukito, S.; Norman, L.; Carlisi, C.; Radua, J.; Hart, H.; Simonoff, E.; Rubia, K. Comparative meta-analyses of brain structural and functional abnormalities during cognitive control in attention-deficit/hyperactivity disorder and autism spectrum disorder. *Psychol. Med.* **2020**, *50*, 894–919. [CrossRef] [PubMed]
75. Moon, S.J.; Hwang, J.; Kana, R.; Torous, J.; Kim, J.W. Accuracy of Machine Learning Algorithms for the Diagnosis of Autism Spectrum Disorder: Systematic Review and Meta-Analysis of Brain Magnetic Resonance Imaging Studies. *JMIR Ment. Health* **2019**, *6*, e14108. [CrossRef] [PubMed]
76. Clements, C.C.; Zoltowski, A.R.; Yankowitz, L.D.; Yerys, B.E.; Schultz, R.T.; Herrington, J.D. Evaluation of the Social Motivation Hypothesis of Autism: A Systematic Review and Meta-analysis. *JAMA Psychiatry* **2018**, *75*, 797–808. [CrossRef] [PubMed]
77. Wigton, R.; Radua, J.; Allen, P.; Averbeck, B.; Meyer-Lindenberg, A.; McGuire, P.; Shergill, S.S.; Fusar-Poli, P. Neurophysiological effects of acute oxytocin administration: Systematic review and meta-analysis of placebo-controlled imaging studies. *J. Psychiatry Neurosci.* **2015**, *40*, E1–E22. [CrossRef] [PubMed]
78. Hamilton, A.F. Reflecting on the mirror neuron system in autism: A systematic review of current theories. *Dev. Cogn. Neurosci.* **2013**, *3*, 91–105. [CrossRef]
79. Pina-Camacho, L.; Villero, S.; Fraguas, D.; Boada, L.; Janssen, J.; Navas-Sánchez, F.J.; Mayoral, M.; Llorente, C.; Arango, C.; Parellada, M. Autism spectrum disorder: Does neuroimaging support the DSM-5 proposal for a symptom dyad? A systematic review of functional magnetic resonance imaging and diffusion tensor imaging studies. *J. Autism Dev. Disord.* **2012**, *42*, 1326–1341. [CrossRef]
80. Philip, R.C.; Dauvermann, M.R.; Whalley, H.C.; Baynham, K.; Lawrie, S.M.; Stanfield, A.C. A systematic review and meta-analysis of the fMRI investigation of autism spectrum disorders. *Neurosci. Biobehav. Rev.* **2012**, *36*, 901–942. [CrossRef]
81. Sugranyes, G.; Kyriakopoulos, M.; Corrigall, R.; Taylor, E.; Frangou, S. Autism spectrum disorders and schizophrenia: Meta-analysis of the neural correlates of social cognition. *PLoS ONE* **2011**, *6*, e25322. [CrossRef]
82. Chen, C.; Cheng, Y.; Wu, C.T.; Chiang, C.H.; Wong, C.C.; Huang, C.M.; Martínez, R.M.; Tzeng, O.J.L.; Fan, Y.T. A sensory signature of unaffected biological parents predicts the risk of autism in their offspring. *Psychiatry Clin. Neurosci.* **2023**. [CrossRef] [PubMed]
83. Shao, L.; Fu, C.; Chen, X. A heterogeneous graph convolutional attention network method for classification of autism spectrum disorder. *BMC Bioinform.* **2023**, *24*, 363. [CrossRef] [PubMed]
84. Kim, Y.G.; Ravid, O.; Zhang, X.; Kim, Y.; Neria, Y.; Lee, S.; He, X.; Zhu, X. Explaining Deep Learning-Based Representations of Resting State Functional Connectivity Data: Focusing on Interpreting Nonlinear Patterns in Autism Spectrum Disorder. *bioRxiv* **2023**. [CrossRef]
85. Jönemo, J.; Abramian, D.; Eklund, A. Evaluation of Augmentation Methods in Classifying Autism Spectrum Disorders from fMRI Data with 3D Convolutional Neural Networks. *Diagnostics* **2023**, *13*, 2773. [CrossRef]
86. Wang, X.; Chu, Y.; Wang, Q.; Cao, L.; Qiao, L.; Zhang, L.; Liu, M. Unsupervised contrastive graph learning for resting-state functional MRI analysis and brain disorder detection. *Hum. Brain Mapp.* **2023**, *44*, 5672–5692. [CrossRef] [PubMed]
87. Zhang, S.; Chen, X.; Shen, X.; Ren, B.; Yu, Y.; Yang, H.; Jiang, X.; Shen, D.; Zhou, Y.; Zhang, X.Y. A-GCL: Adversarial graph contrastive learning for fMRI analysis to diagnose neurodevelopmental disorders. *Med. Image Anal.* **2023**, *90*, 102932. [CrossRef] [PubMed]
88. Ma, Y.; Wang, Q.; Cao, L.; Li, L.; Zhang, C.; Qiao, L.; Liu, M. Multi-Scale Dynamic Graph Learning for Brain Disorder Detection with Functional MRI. *IEEE Trans. Neural Syst. Rehabil. Eng.* **2023**, *31*, 3501–3512. [CrossRef]
89. Artiles, O.; Al Masry, Z.; Saeed, F. Confounding Effects on the Performance of Machine Learning Analysis of Static Functional Connectivity Computed from rs-fMRI Multi-site Data. *Neuroinformatics* **2023**, *21*, 651–668. [CrossRef]
90. Qiang, N.; Gao, J.; Dong, Q.; Li, J.; Zhang, S.; Liang, H.; Sun, Y.; Ge, B.; Liu, Z.; Wu, Z.; et al. A deep learning method for autism spectrum disorder identification based on interactions of hierarchical brain networks. *Behav. Brain Res.* **2023**, *452*, 114603. [CrossRef]
91. Helmy, E.; Elnakib, A.; ElNakieb, Y.; Khudri, M.; Abdelrahim, M.; Yousaf, J.; Ghazal, M.; Contractor, S.; Barnes, G.N.; El-Baz, A. Role of Artificial Intelligence for Autism Diagnosis Using DTI and fMRI: A Survey. *Biomedicines* **2023**, *11*, 1858. [CrossRef]
92. Lei, D.; Zhang, T.; Wu, Y.; Li, W.; Li, X. Autism spectrum disorder diagnosis based on deep unrolling-based spatial constraint representation. *Med. Biol. Eng. Comput.* **2023**, *61*, 2829–2842. [CrossRef]
93. Benabdallah, F.Z.; Drissi El Maliani, A.; Lotfi, D.; El Hassouni, M. A Convolutional Neural Network-Based Connectivity Enhancement Approach for Autism Spectrum Disorder Detection. *J. Imaging* **2023**, *9*, 110. [CrossRef] [PubMed]
94. Liu, M.; Zhang, H.; Shi, F.; Shen, D. Hierarchical Graph Convolutional Network Built by Multiscale Atlases for Brain Disorder Diagnosis Using Functional Connectivity. *IEEE Trans. Neural Netw. Learn. Syst.* **2023**. [CrossRef]
95. Alves, C.L.; Toutain, T.G.L.O.; de Carvalho Aguiar, P.; Pineda, A.M.; Roster, K.; Thielemann, C.; Porto, J.A.M.; Rodrigues, F.A. Diagnosis of autism spectrum disorder based on functional brain networks and machine learning. *Sci. Rep.* **2023**, *13*, 8072. [CrossRef] [PubMed]
96. Saha, P. Eigenvector Centrality Characterization on fMRI Data: Gender and Node Differences in Normal and ASD Subjects. *J. Autism Dev. Disord.* **2023**. [CrossRef] [PubMed]

97. Ren, P.; Bi, Q.; Pang, W.; Wang, M.; Zhou, Q.; Ye, X.; Li, L.; Xiao, L. Stratifying ASD and characterizing the functional connectivity of subtypes in resting-state fMRI. *Behav. Brain Res.* **2023**, *449*, 114458. [CrossRef] [PubMed]
98. D'Souza, N.S.; Venkataraman, A. mSPD-NN: A Geometrically Aware Neural Framework for Biomarker Discovery from Functional Connectomics Manifolds. *arXiv* **2023**, arXiv:2303.14986v1.
99. Kang, L.; Chen, J.; Huang, J.; Jiang, J. Autism spectrum disorder recognition based on multi-view ensemble learning with multi-site fMRI. *Cogn. Neurodyn.* **2023**, *17*, 345–355. [CrossRef]
100. Manikantan, K.; Jaganathan, S. A Model for Diagnosing Autism Patients Using Spatial and Statistical Measures Using rs-fMRI and sMRI by Adopting Graphical Neural Networks. *Diagnostics* **2023**, *13*, 1143. [CrossRef]
101. Yousefian, A.; Shayegh, F.; Maleki, Z. Detection of autism spectrum disorder using graph representation learning algorithms and deep neural network, based on fMRI signals. *Front. Syst. Neurosci.* **2023**, *16*, 904770. [CrossRef]
102. Song, I.; Lee, T.H. Considering dynamic nature of the brain: The clinical importance of connectivity variability in machine learning classification and prediction. *bioRxiv* **2023**. [CrossRef]
103. Abbas, S.Q.; Chi, L.; Chen, Y.P. DeepMNF: Deep Multimodal Neuroimaging Framework for Diagnosing Autism Spectrum Disorder. *Artif. Intell. Med.* **2023**, *136*, 102475. [CrossRef] [PubMed]
104. ElNakieb, Y.; Ali, M.T.; Elnakib, A.; Shalaby, A.; Mahmoud, A.; Soliman, A.; Barnes, G.N.; El-Baz, A. Understanding the Role of Connectivity Dynamics of Resting-State Functional MRI in the Diagnosis of Autism Spectrum Disorder: A Comprehensive Study. *Bioengineering* **2023**, *10*, 56. [CrossRef] [PubMed]
105. Wang, Z.; Xu, Y.; Peng, D.; Gao, J.; Lu, F. Brain functional activity-based classification of autism spectrum disorder using an attention-based graph neural network combined with gene expression. *Cereb. Cortex* **2023**, *33*, 6407–6419. [CrossRef] [PubMed]
106. Hao, X.; An, Q.; Li, J.; Min, H.; Guo, Y.; Yu, M.; Qin, J. Exploring high-order correlations with deep-broad learning for autism spectrum disorder diagnosis. *Front. Neurosci.* **2022**, *16*, 1046268. [CrossRef] [PubMed]
107. Jiang, X.; Yan, J.; Zhao, Y.; Jiang, M.; Chen, Y.; Zhou, J.; Xiao, Z.; Wang, Z.; Zhang, R.; Becker, B.; et al. Characterizing functional brain networks via Spatio-Temporal Attention 4D Convolutional Neural Networks (STA-4DCNNs). *Neural Netw.* **2023**, *158*, 99–110. [CrossRef] [PubMed]
108. Deng, X.; Zhang, J.; Liu, R.; Liu, K. Classifying ASD based on time-series fMR using spatial-temporal transformer. *Comput. Biol. Med.* **2022**, *151 Pt B*, 106320. [CrossRef]
109. Mahmood, U.; Fu, Z.; Ghosh, S.; Calhoun, V.; Plis, S. Through the looking glass: Deep interpretable dynamic directed connectivity in resting fMRI. *Neuroimage* **2022**, *264*, 119737. [CrossRef]
110. Ma, H.; Cao, Y.; Li, M.; Zhan, L.; Xie, Z.; Huang, L.; Gao, Y.; Jia, X. Abnormal amygdala functional connectivity and deep learning classification in multifrequency bands in autism spectrum disorder: A multisite functional magnetic resonance imaging study. *Hum. Brain Mapp.* **2023**, *44*, 1094–1104. [CrossRef]
111. Zhang, H.; Song, R.; Wang, L.; Zhang, L.; Wang, D.; Wang, C.; Zhang, W. Classification of Brain Disorders in rs-fMRI via Local-to-Global Graph Neural Networks. *IEEE Trans. Med. Imaging* **2023**, *42*, 444–455. [CrossRef]
112. Huang, Z.A.; Hu, Y.; Liu, R.; Xue, X.; Zhu, Z.; Song, L.; Tan, K.C. Federated Multi-Task Learning for Joint Diagnosis of Multiple Mental Disorders on MRI Scans. *IEEE Trans. Biomed. Eng.* **2023**, *70*, 1137–1149. [CrossRef] [PubMed]
113. Kunda, M.; Zhou, S.; Gong, G.; Lu, H. Improving Multi-Site Autism Classification via Site-Dependence Minimization and Second-Order Functional Connectivity. *IEEE Trans. Med. Imaging* **2023**, *42*, 55–65. [CrossRef] [PubMed]
114. Han, T.; Gong, X.; Feng, F.; Zhang, J.; Sun, Z.; Zhang, Y. Privacy-Preserving Multi-Source Domain Adaptation for Medical Data. *IEEE J. Biomed. Health Inform.* **2023**, *27*, 842–853. [CrossRef] [PubMed]
115. Goetz, L.H.; Schork, N.J. Personalized medicine: Motivation, challenges, and progress. *Fertil. Steril.* **2018**, *109*, 952–963. [CrossRef] [PubMed]
116. Delpierre, C.; Lefèvre, T. Precision and personalized medicine: What their current definition says and silences about the model of health they promote. Implication for the development of personalized health. *Front. Sociol.* **2023**, *8*, 1112159. [CrossRef] [PubMed]
117. Shlyakhto, E.V. Scientific Basics of Personalized Medicine: Realities and Opportunities. *Her. Russ. Acad. Sci.* **2022**, *92*, 671–682. [CrossRef] [PubMed]
118. Evers, A.W.; Rovers, M.M.; Kremer, J.A.; Veltman, J.A.; Schalken, J.A.; Bloem, B.R.; van Gool, A.J. An integrated framework of personalized medicine: From individual genomes to participatory health care. *Croat. Med. J.* **2012**, *53*, 301–303. [CrossRef] [PubMed]
119. Schork, N.J. Artificial Intelligence and Personalized Medicine. *Cancer Treat. Res.* **2019**, *178*, 265–283. [CrossRef] [PubMed]
120. Johnson, K.B.; Wei, W.Q.; Weeraratne, D.; Frisse, M.E.; Misulis, K.; Rhee, K.; Zhao, J.; Snowdon, J.L. Precision Medicine, AI, and the Future of Personalized Health Care. *Clin. Transl. Sci.* **2021**, *14*, 86–93. [CrossRef] [PubMed]
121. Loth, E.; Murphy, D.G.; Spooren, W. Defining Precision Medicine Approaches to Autism Spectrum Disorders: Concepts and Challenges. *Front. Psychiatry* **2016**, *7*, 188. [CrossRef]
122. Kostic, A.; Buxbaum, J.D. The promise of precision medicine in autism. *Neuron* **2021**, *109*, 2212–2215. [CrossRef]
123. Gabis, L.V.; Gross, R.; Barbaro, J. Editorial: Personalized Precision Medicine in Autism Spectrum-Related Disorders. *Front Neurol.* **2021**, *12*, 730852. [CrossRef]
124. Frye, R.E.; Boles, R.; Rose, S.; Rossignol, D. *A Personalized Medicine Approach to the Diagnosis and Management of Autism Spectrum Disorder*; MDPI: Basel, Switzerland, 2022.

125. Savas, S.; Damar, Ç. Transfer-learning-based classification of pathological brain magnetic resonance images. *ETRI J.* **2023**, 1–14. [CrossRef]
126. Savaş, S.; Topaloğlu, N.; Kazcı, Ö.; Koşar, P.N. Performance Comparison of Carotid Artery Intima Media Thickness Classification by Deep Learning Methods. In Proceedings of the HORA2019, Nevsehir, Turkey, 5–7 July 2019.

Disclaimer/Publisher's Note: The statements, opinions and data contained in all publications are solely those of the individual author(s) and contributor(s) and not of MDPI and/or the editor(s). MDPI and/or the editor(s) disclaim responsibility for any injury to people or property resulting from any ideas, methods, instructions or products referred to in the content.

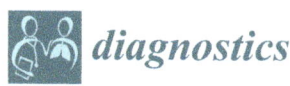

Article

Fractional Flow Reserve-Based Patient Risk Classification

Marijana Stanojević Pirković [1], Ognjen Pavić [2,3], Filip Filipović [3], Igor Saveljić [2,3], Tijana Geroski [3,4], Themis Exarchos [5] and Nenad Filipović [3,4,*]

1. Faculty of Medical Sciences, University of Kragujevac, 34000 Kragujevac, Serbia; marijanas14@gmail.com
2. Institute for Information Technologies, University of Kragujevac, 34000 Kragujevac, Serbia; opavic@kg.ac.rs (O.P.); isaveljic@kg.ac.rs (I.S.)
3. Bioengineering Research and Development Center (BioIRC), 34000 Kragujevac, Serbia; filipovicfilip1999@gmail.com (F.F.); tijanas@kg.ac.rs (T.G.)
4. Faculty of Engineering, University of Kragujevac, 34000 Kragujevac, Serbia
5. Department of Informatics, Ionian University, 49100 Corfu, Greece; themis.exarchos@gmail.com
* Correspondence: fica@kg.ac.rs; Tel.: +381-698449673

Abstract: Cardiovascular diseases (CVDs) are a leading cause of death. If not treated in a timely manner, cardiovascular diseases can cause a plethora of major life complications that can include disability and a loss of the ability to work. Globally, acute myocardial infarction (AMI) is responsible for about 3 million deaths a year. The development of strategies for prevention, but also the early detection of cardiovascular risks, is of great importance. The fractional flow reserve (FFR) is a measurement used for an assessment of the severity of coronary artery stenosis. The goal of this research was to develop a technique that can be used for patient fractional flow reserve evaluation, as well as for the assessment of the risk of death via gathered demographic and clinical data. A classification ensemble model was built using the random forest machine learning algorithm for the purposes of risk prediction. Referent patient classes were identified by the observed fractional flow reserve value, where patients with an FFR higher than 0.8 were viewed as low risk, while those with an FFR lower than 0.8 were identified as high risk. The final classification ensemble achieved a 76.21% value of estimated prediction accuracy, thus achieving a mean prediction accuracy of 74.1%, 77.3%, 78.1% and 83.6% over the models tested with 5%, 10%, 15% and 20% of the test samples, respectively. Along with the machine learning approach, a numerical approach was implemented through a 3D reconstruction of the coronary arteries for the purposes of stenosis monitoring. Even with a small number of available data points, the proposed methodology achieved satisfying results. However, these results can be improved in the future through the introduction of additional data, which will, in turn, allow for the utilization of different machine learning algorithms.

Keywords: cardiovascular diseases; acute myocardial infarction; fractional flow reserve; machine learning; ensemble; random forest; 3D reconstruction

Citation: Stanojević Pirković, M.; Pavić, O.; Filipović, F.; Saveljić, I.; Geroski, T.; Exarchos, T.; Filipović, N. Fractional Flow Reserve-Based Patient Risk Classification. *Diagnostics* **2023**, *13*, 3349. https://doi.org/10.3390/diagnostics13213349

Academic Editors: Daniele Giansanti and Dania Cioni

Received: 21 September 2023
Revised: 14 October 2023
Accepted: 19 October 2023
Published: 31 October 2023

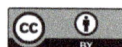

Copyright: © 2023 by the authors. Licensee MDPI, Basel, Switzerland. This article is an open access article distributed under the terms and conditions of the Creative Commons Attribution (CC BY) license (https://creativecommons.org/licenses/by/4.0/).

1. Introduction

The World Health Organization estimates that cardiovascular diseases are the leading cause of death in the world with 17.9 million fatal outcomes annually. Cardiovascular diseases are responsible for significant medical, social and economic consequences globally. They represent one of the leading causes of disability, a loss in the ability to work and premature mortality, as well as place high costs on health care systems. According to the literature data, CVDs result in 31.8% of all the reported deaths in the world, and half of these outcomes are as a result of ischemic heart diseases [1–3].

Acute myocardial infarction is manifested through the necrosis of the heart muscle, which occurs due to coronary artery occlusion and the insufficient oxygenation of cardiomyocytes. The prevalence of acute myocardial infarction is about three million people, with more than a million deaths per year occurring in the United States [4]. Considering the serious consequences of this disease, there is a need to develop strategies for the prevention and early detection of cardiovascular risks, as well as for the rapid diagnosis of AMI for the timely application of adequate therapy [5].

The rupture of unstable atherosclerotic plaque, thrombosis and the acute reduction in blood flow through the coronary artery, with its consequent occlusion, are some of the possible mechanisms of AMI development [6,7]. A study suggested that that the characterization of culprit lesions by optical coherence tomography supported the concept that plaque erosion is more common in cases of non-ST-segment-elevation myocardial infarction (NSTEMI), while plaque rupture is more prominent in cases of ST-segment-elevation myocardial infarction (STEMI) [8].

Dyslipidemia is one of the key proposed factors in the progression of atherosclerosis. It has also been shown that a decrease in the concentration of low-density lipoprotein cholesterol (LDL-C) in high-risk patients is one of the key strategies in the prevention of ischemic heart disease [9,10]. Namely, the reduction in LDL concentration by 1 mmol/L over five years in middle-aged people reduces the risk of developing CVD by 20% [11].

The laboratory measurement of cardiac biomarkers enables the rapid diagnosis and monitoring of patients with AMI, as well as the possibility of individualizing the therapy according to the characteristics and risks of the patient. A laboratory establishment of CKMB activity is used in diagnosis, the assessment of the severity of the clinical picture and in the prediction of the prognosis of AMI. This isoenzyme, due to myocardial necrosis, shows an increase in activity in the patient's serum after 4 to 8 h from the onset of chest pain; this then reaches a maximum within 18–24 h, and then returns back to a normal value after 24–48 h [12]. According to the data from the literature, the establishing of CKMB activity together with concentrations of myoglobin, troponin I and NT-proBNP, also have a—apart from diagnostic—prognostic significance [13].

The dominant biomarkers of myocardial damage today are certainly cardiac troponins (i.e., TnI and TnT). High-sensitivity troponins entered the clinical practice guidelines and were incorporated into the universal diagnostics definition of AMI [14]. The diagnosis of AMI is established by the detection of an increase or decrease in cardiac biomarkers, especially troponin, with at least one concentration that is larger than the 99th percentile of the healthy population and at least one symptom of ischemia [15,16].

The establishment of NT-proBNP is significant in the assessment of ventricular dysfunction and myocardial ischemia. This highly specific and sensitive cardiac biomarker is also a powerful predictor of the development of heart failure and mortality after AMI [17,18].

In current clinical guidelines, the most important diagnostic/therapeutic strategy in the management of patients with confirmed AMI is the invasive coronary angiography. By performing this procedure, the disease is indicated within 24 h in patients who meet at least one of the high-risk criteria for AMI (high cardiac troponins, dynamic changes in the electrocardiogram or a Global Registry of Acute Coronary Events risk score of >10). Percutaneous coronary intervention enables the establishment of a flow through the occluded coronary artery (which is the cause of AMI), as well as helps in gaining insights into the condition of other blood vessels.

Fractional flow reserve measurement is used to quantitatively assess the severity of the coronary artery stenosis identified during invasive coronary angiography. FFR is defined as the ratio between the maximum possible blood flow in the diseased coronary artery and the theoretically possible maximum blood flow in the normal coronary artery. During angiography, FFR is measured using a wire (catheter) for measuring coronary pressure, as well as by calculating the ratio between the coronary pressure distal to the coronary artery and the pressure in the aorta when under conditions of maximum myocardial hyperemia. This ratio shows the potential decrease in the flow distal to coronary stenosis. In healthy people, the FFR is 1, whereas an FFR lower than 0.75–080 indicates myocardial ischemia. FFR values less than 0.75 indicate the need for revascularization [19,20].

Multidetector computed tomography fractional flow reserve (MDC FFR) is used for a more elaborate assessment of the hemodynamic significance of coronary artery stenosis when compared to classic FFR. This quantitative technique is built on processing, based on a mathematical model of fluid dynamics, the obtained data.

A decision tree algorithm is a supervised classification algorithm that is based on a binary tree structure. This algorithm splits the ranges of input variables to create conditions with which the dataset can be split between two or more classes. Each condition represents a node of the binary tree. Each node branches into two other nodes, where each branch represents one of the two possible outcomes of the set condition. The leaves of the decision tree represent classes, which are then assigned to the samples of data.

A random forest classification algorithm is a supervised classification algorithm that is based on an ensemble of multiple decision tree models. Each decision tree model contained within the random forest has the same aforementioned way of making decisions, but it is trained with different, randomly selected subsets of data. Each decision tree is capable of making its own decisions, but the final output of the random forest is made by counting the number of times each class was chosen by the decision trees and by selecting the class that was chosen the highest number of times. The random forest approach reduces variance in classification with its voting process when compared to a single decision tree, and it achieves this while also reducing the overfitting of the model by feeding each tree with a smaller subset of the initial set of data.

In recent times, artificial intelligence has been gaining a strong foothold in medical science. Machine learning and deep learning models are gaining a widespread use in the automation of disease classification, disease development over time, as well as risk monitoring through the use of classification and regression analysis algorithms. Several studies have been conducted for the purposes of FFR patient risk classification [21–23]. All of these studies used data comprising computed tomography angiography (CTA) images for training convolutional neural networks. In this paper, we propose a methodology based on an ensemble of machine learning models for the purposes of patient risk classification through fractional flow reserve measurements using demographic and clinical data. The created system is meant to serve as a decision support tool for medical experts.

2. Materials and Methods

This section of the paper contains information on the available data, as well as the methodology used for the data preprocessing and the creation of the final classification model. The methodology used is depicted in Figure 1.

2.1. Dataset

Our dataset is composed of the clinical data gathered from patients in the form of biomarkers and the descriptive data points regarding primary and follow up diagnosis, as well as the descriptive data points that define the position and degree of stenosis and lesions in three defined arteries from the left and right coronary artery trees. Along with the aforementioned data collected directly from patients, our dataset contains simulated FFR values, which represent the target to be used in the classification of patients into high-risk or low-risk classes.

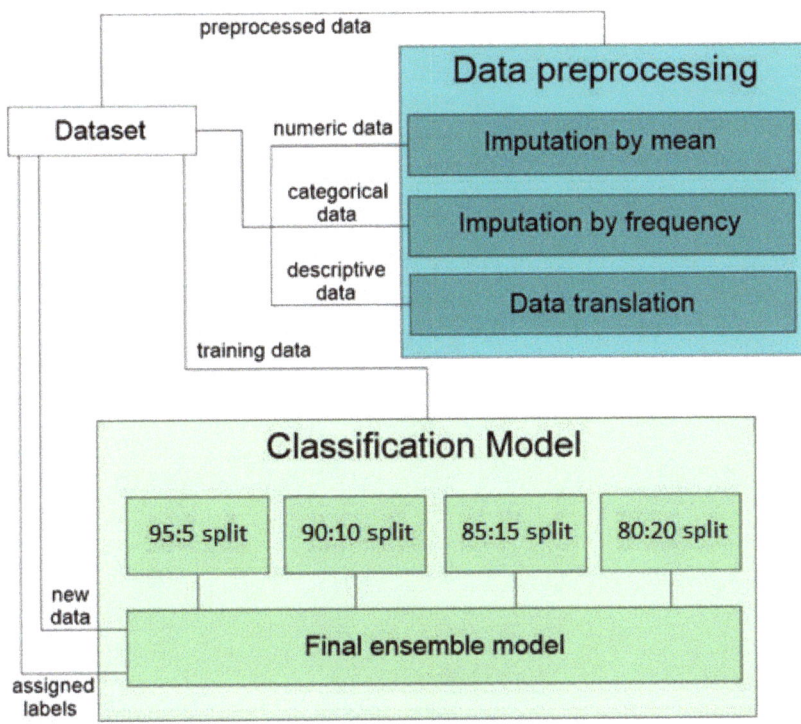

Figure 1. Graphical representation of the applied methodology.

During the visits, blood samples were taken from the patients according to the usual standards of clinical biochemistry. All biomarkers were determined in the Laboratory Diagnostic Service of the University Clinical Center Kragujevac. Standard laboratory methods were used in all the patients to establish the following values: hematological parameters (total number of leukocytes); concentrations of biochemical parameters (glucose, urea, creatinine, uric acid, cholesterol, triacylglycerols and LDL); the enzyme activity of cardiomyocyte damage markers (CK, CKMB, AST and LDH); and cardio-specific proteins (hs TNI and NT-proBNP). Hematological parameters were established on a DxH900 hematological counter, Beckman Coulter Analysers and biochemical parameters. The cardio-specific enzymes were established on an Oly AU 680 biochemical analyzer and on Beckman Coulter Analyzers. An Abbot Allinity immunochemical analyzer was used to establish the concentration of hsTNI, whereas the concentration of NT-proBNP was measured on a Cobas e411 immunochemical analyzer (Roche Diagnostics, Mannheim, Germany). All laboratory measurements included the implementation of regular internal and external quality controls in accordance with the recommendations of good laboratory practice. The study conduction was complied with the code of ethics of the World Medical Association (Declaration of Helsinki), and it was also approved by the Ethics Board of University Clinical Centre Kragujevac.

In our study, we have included patients suffering from coronary artery disease, where 80% had a history of AMI. Most of the patients had between 40% and 50% of stenosis, which meant that they belonged to the intermediate class of coronary artery stenosis; this was the reason virtual FFR was applied as a validation tool.

All the features used in the creation of a machine learning model, as well as their data types and ranges, are shown in Table 1.

Table 1. Dataset description.

Name	Type	Range
Numeric FFR	Numeric	0–1
Risk class	Binary	[0, 1]
Smoker	Binary	[0, 1]
Gender	Binary	[0, 1]
Age	Numeric	36–73
CK	Numeric	61–3353
CKMB	Numeric	11–324
AST	Numeric	12–348
LDH	Numeric	210–2557
Troponin	Numeric	0.0124–58.96
pBNP	Numeric	48.1–32,700.0
CRP	Numeric	3.3–122.6
Leukocyte	Numeric	7.1–18.61
Glucose	Numeric	4.7–16.3
Urea	Numeric	5.0–23.2
Creatinine	Numeric	59.0–1447.0
Ac. uricum	Numeric	204.0–532.0
Cholesterol	Numeric	3.33–7.4
Trig	Numeric	0.88–8.3
HDL	Numeric	0.7–2.07
LDL	Numeric	2.57–5.88
Atherosclerosis index	Numeric	3.23–6.17
Cholesterol/HDL	Numeric	3.28–9.43
LAD	Descriptive/Numeric	0–1
LCx	Descriptive/Numeric	0–1
RCA	Descriptive/Numeric	0–1

The dataset contained data on 276 patients, of which 181 had simulated FFR values. Of the 181 labeled patients, 123 belonged to the low-risk class and 58 belonged to the high-risk class. Our approach included the training of a machine learning model with 181 patients for which the simulated FFR values were available. The geometries for the numerical simulation of FFR for these 181 patients were taken from the invasive coronary angiography images. In addition, a 3D finite element model was built based on the methodology published in [24]. Details on the 3D reconstruction and analysis are given in Section 2.3. We have already published several papers related to the numerical simulations, and we have obtained a good match with the measurements of FFR [25,26]. Now, this methodology was used as a standard to compare with the results of ML model.

The remaining 95 patients were patients who had suffered an AMI in the past, as well as had clinical and demographic data available; however, these patients were unlabeled because their geometric coronary angiography data were not available. Because the 95 unlabeled patients still represented possible real world combinations of the feature values, these patients were used for missing data imputation. However, the labels could not be assigned to those patients, so they could not have been used for the validation of machine learning models in any way. The 95 unlabeled patients were fed into the final classification model in order to demonstrate the application of the proposed methodology on those patients with unknown FFR values. The main challenge was that the data of those 181 patients was a very low amount of data that was used for training. After this, the model was applied to predict the values for the new 95 patients (for which the FFR values were unknown). Nevertheless, since the final machine learning model was meant to classify the patients using non-geometric parameters, it was expected that the model would achieve similar classification results to the results obtained during the testing on labeled data. It is important to emphasize that the application of the proposed methodology to the unlabeled data cannot be viewed as a validation attempt. The application of the proposed methodology represents a transfer of the learned medical knowledge from the labeled subset of patients to the patients for whom the ground truth was unknown. The added value of the proposed methodology was that the numerical calculations with a combination of the real measurements of the FFR could help in the future to significantly increase the size of the dataset, as well as increase the accuracy of the proposed ML models.

The problem of missing data in a dataset was tackled using a conventional approach, whereby the missing samples were filled in depending on the type of data contained in the column in question. Namely, the numeric data were replaced by the mean value of the already present values in the examined column, and the categorical data were replaced by the most common value in the column. For the purposes of data imputation, there was an attempt at using a multiple imputation approach via chained equations, but the results were very poor because of the low correlation between the different features; as such, the aforementioned approach yielded far greater results.

As for the descriptive data regarding stenosis and the lesion values of the three arteries, they were required to be translated into numeric values so that they could be used during the training of the classification model. The problem arose with the formatting of the descriptive data, and this was because very similar situations were described in completely different ways; as such, there was no way of translating these data other than translating them directly by hand and approximating the meaning. The data were translated as follows:

- Data that contained percentile values for the narrowing of the observed artery were translated as a numeric sample corresponding to the percentage value.
- Data that contained an approximation of the narrowing in the form of a range of values were translated as a numeric sample that corresponded to the average value of the observed range.
- Data that did not contain percentage values of the narrowing but did have an indication that the narrowing was not substantial were translated as if they held information of a 10% narrowing.
- Data that did not contain percentage values of the narrowing but did have an indication that the narrowing was very minor were translated as if they held information of a 5% narrowing.
- Data that did not contain percentage values of the narrowing but indicated an orderly arterial lumen were translated as if there was no narrowing at all.
- Data that did not contain any indication of the size of the narrowing nor contained the previously mentioned phrases with which the narrowing was estimated were not translated at all. Instead, they were approximated as a mean value of all of the other translated values.

Lastly, the available simulated FFR values were written in the form of a floating-point notation between the values of 0 and 1. These values had to be transcribed into categorical values that represented the risk class of the patient so that they could be used as output values of the classification model.

With regard to FFR, the patients could be divided into 3 risk classes. The low-risk class was defined by an FFR greater than 0.8, while the high-risk class was defined by an FFR lower than 0.74. There also existed a class between the values of 0.74 and 0.8, which was defined as a border class because the patients in this range could be considered both high-risk and low-risk; the final classification was the doctor's prerogative [27]. When transcribing the data, this border class was viewed as a part of the high-risk class and was merged. This was performed because of the inherent risk of falsely putting high-risk patients as anything other than a high-risk class.

2.2. Data Correlation

After data preprocessing, we ran tests to find the correlations between the input values and the designated output FFR value. These correlations were calculated with the aim of expanding the dataset using high correlation features to create more labeled data. The correlation between the features and the patients' FFR is shown in Table 2.

Table 2. Feature correlations with the FFR.

Feature	Correlation with the FFR	Feature	Correlation with the FFR
Smoker	−0.39	Urea	0.15
Gender	−0.19	Creatinine	0.11
Age	0.21	Ac. Uricum	0.40
CK	−0.21	Cholesterol	−0.02
CKMB	−0.07	Trig	0.09
AST	−0.14	HDL	0.03
HDL	−0.33	LDL	0.06
Troponin	0.25	Atherosclerosis index	0.16
pBNP	0.33	Cholesterol/HDL	0.02
CRP	−0.18	LAD	0.50
Leukocyte	−0.23	LCx	0.25
Glucose	0.30	RCA	0.30

With the available data, it was not possible to expand the dataset because there were no features that had a high correlation with the FFR values. The classification model had to be created using only the initial data, which presented a challenge due to the small amount of labeled data.

2.3. 3D Reconstruction and Analysis

Three-dimensional models of the right and left coronary arteries were reconstructed from DICOM angiography images. An eight-node brick element was obtained as the final element. PAK-F software, version 2023 [28] was used for the numerical solution of the fluid flow problems. The three-dimensional flow of a viscous incompressible fluid that is considered here is governed by the Navier–Stokes equations [28], and its continuity equation can be written as follows:

$$\rho(u_i \cdot \nabla)u_i + \nabla p_i - \mu \Delta u_i = 0 \tag{1}$$

$$\nabla u_i = 0 \tag{2}$$

where u_i is velocity, p_i is pressure, μ is the dynamic viscosity and ρ is the density of blood. The first equation represents the balance of linear momentum, while Equation (2) expresses the incompressibility condition. By applying the Galerkin method on the previous two equations, we obtained the final form of the discretized Navier Stokes equations as follows:

$$\begin{bmatrix} \frac{1}{\Delta t}\mathbf{M} + {}^{n+1}\hat{\mathbf{K}}_{vv}^{i-1} & \mathbf{K}_{vp} \\ \mathbf{K}_{vp}^T & 0 \end{bmatrix} \begin{Bmatrix} \Delta \mathbf{V}^i \\ \Delta \mathbf{P}^i \end{Bmatrix} = \begin{Bmatrix} {}^{n+1}\mathbf{F}_{ext}^{i-1} \\ 0 \end{Bmatrix} - \begin{bmatrix} \frac{1}{\Delta t}\mathbf{M} + {}^{n+1}\mathbf{K}_{vv}^{i-1} & \mathbf{K}_{vp} \\ \mathbf{K}_{vp}^T & 0 \end{bmatrix} \begin{Bmatrix} {}^{n+1}\mathbf{V}^{i-1} \\ {}^{n+1}\mathbf{P}^{i-1} \end{Bmatrix} + \begin{Bmatrix} \frac{1}{\Delta t}\mathbf{M}^n \mathbf{V} \\ 0 \end{Bmatrix} \tag{3}$$

FFR is defined as the ratio of the maximum flow through a coronary artery in the presence of stenosis with the maximum flow through a normal coronary artery [29]:

$$FFR = \frac{Q^S}{Q^N} \quad (4)$$

where Q^S is the flow through an artery with stenosis, and Q^N is the flow through an artery without stenosis. The flow through an artery without stenosis can be calculated as follows:

$$Q^N = \frac{p_a - p_v}{R} \quad (5)$$

where p_a is the mean aortic pressure, p_v is the mean venous pressure and R is the resistance through the heart. The flow through the artery with stenosis is calculated in a similar way:

$$Q^S = \frac{p_d - p_v}{R} \quad (6)$$

where p_d is the mean distal pressure in coronary arteries with stenosis. When we substitute Equations (6) and (5) into Equation (4), we obtain the following:

$$FFR = \frac{p_d - p_v}{p_a - p_v} \approx \frac{p_d}{p_a} \quad (7)$$

In the case of healthy arteries, the FFR value is 1. Based on clinical trials, the critical value for stenting is any value that is ≤ 0.75.

Blood was considered as an incompressible Newtonian fluid with a dynamic viscosity of μ = 0.00365 Pas and a density of ρ = 1050 kg/m^3. In order to calculate the numerical FFR value, two separate simulations were performed for each case. A pressure of 100 mmHg was applied at the inlet, and the flow rates of 1 and 3 mL/s were applied at the outlet. Patient-specific microvascular resistance was considered a specific Windkessel boundary condition. This was algebraically coupled to calculate the outlet pressure and flow, which was informed in each time step of the 3D computational fluid dynamics simulation [26].

2.4. Classification Model

The main problem encountered in the development of our classification model was the inability to test the model's performance because of the small amount of data labeled with a risk class. More specifically, the data from 181 patients were not enough to build a comprehensive test set. To overcome this problem, we resorted to using an ensemble, which consists of a great number of less complex prediction models [30].

These less complex prediction models were also smaller ensemble models that were created using the random forest classification algorithm. First, we trained 19 random forest classification models that consisted of 50 decision trees and were without constraints in regard to the minimum samples required for creating branching nodes and leaves. The 181 labeled patients from the original dataset were split into 20 groups of data samples, each containing 5% of the data and including both high-risk and low-risk patients. Each of the models was trained using a different configuration of 19 groups of training samples, and they were tested with the one remaining group of samples. After that, we trained more models with every possible configuration of 18, 17 and 16 groups of training samples, as well as tested them with their respective combinations of 2, 3 and 4 remaining test sample groups.

The major drawback of the standard approach is that, when a model makes a wrong prediction with such a small test set, the final accuracy metric was severely impacted. To resolve this problem, we kept only the models that were deemed capable of predicting their respective test sets very precisely. In the case of models trained with a configuration of 19 training samples, only those models that predicted 6 out of 9 test samples correctly were kept. In the case of models that used bigger test sets, only those that achieved the set threshold for classification accuracy were kept. We achieved this by setting thresholds of 66%, 75%, 75% and 80% accuracy for the models being tested with 1, 2, 3 and 4 test sample groups, respectively. Only models above the given threshold were kept while the others were discarded. In the end, a total of 2785 classification models were obtained, and each model was trained with different configurations of the samples from our starting dataset.

The final model we created was an ensemble of these 2785 models. Each new sample from the original dataset was fed to every one of these models in succession. After new pieces of data were fed to all of the models in this ensemble, the final decision was made by counting up the outputs for each class and picking the one that was chosen most frequently.

3. Results

This section of the paper provides a review of the results acquired from the training and testing of the classification model, as well as presents the possible approaches through which to improve its performance in the future.

3.1. Classification Results

In the starting dataset, an imbalance can be noticed between the samples belonging to the high-risk class, of which there were 58 samples, and the low-risk class, of which there were 123 samples. Moreover, there was a risk of falsely classifying the patients into the low-risk class when they should be in the high-risk class. Hence, we first opted to evaluate our model using the F1 score metric on the high-risk class. However, we experienced some difficulties evaluating the final model in such a manner.

In the main, the F1 score metric was spoiled due to its tendency to evaluate the model through only using the results achieved from a single class. In this case specifically, there were multiple lower-level models that had been tested using only samples belonging to class 1, or, in this case, the low-risk class. In these situations, the F1 score was drastically lowered even though it was able to predict multiple test samples correctly. The problem was that the sizes of the test datasets were quite small and could not be increased in any way.

As a result, prediction accuracy was chosen as the main evaluation metric of our model's capabilities. The final model's accuracy was calculated as a mean of the accuracy of each of the lower-level models that were used in creating an ensemble for the final model. This accuracy metric is a simulated metric that evaluates the average performance of all the final model's pieces instead of the entire final model. The classification model achieved an estimated prediction accuracy of 76.21%. The average performances for the models trained with different configurations of training and test sets are shown in Table 3.

Table 3. Classification accuracy metrics.

Train: Test Split	Mean Prediction Accuracy
95%: 5% split	74.1%
90%: 10% split	77.3%
85%: 15% split	78.1%
80%: 20% split	83.6%
Final model	76.21%

3.2. Feature Importance

The importance of the features used during the training process of our classification model varied from one lower-level model to the next. This variation was caused by differences in the training data sample groups, which affected the model's ability to consolidate the concrete values for the importance of certain features.

However, some features varied less than others. Every training feature at our disposal was a crucial part of at least some of the classification models, but those features that did not vary much were the best features in a majority of the classification models and served as a backbone to the final classification ensemble. In the end, feature importance was calculated for the final model as a whole, and this was expressed as a mean value of the feature importance across all of the lower-level models. These feature importance values are shown in Table 4.

Table 4. The simulated feature importance of the final model.

Feature	Feature Importance	Feature	Feature Importance
Smoker	0.023	Glucose	0.058
Gender	0.014	Urea	0.048
Age	0.048	Creatinine	0.047
CK	0.042	Ac. Uricum	0.077
CKMB	0.045	Cholesterol	0.048
AST	0.047	Trig	0.037
LDH	0.048	HDL	0.043
Troponin	0.057	LDL	0.045
pBNP	0.074	Atherosclerosis index	0.009
CRP	0.041	Cholesterol/HDL	0.059
Leukocyte	0.058	Observed coronary artery	0.032

The feature importance of ac. uricum, pBNP, leukocyte, troponin and glucose varied very little between the different models. The feature importance of cholesterol/HDL, AST, urea and creatinine varied heavily between the models, ranging from being extremely important in some and mostly redundant in others. The feature importance of the atherosclerosis index, trig, smoker and gender was quite low across the board; however, the number of good models was slightly reduced every time one of these features was omitted from the training process.

These feature importance values, especially those that had very little variation between models, can be used to explain the learning and decision-making process—after the evaluation of the patient's state—of the final model to the patient.

3.3. Numerical Simulation Results

Figure 2 shows the results of four patients after a numerical simulation in the case of a flow rate of 3 mL/s. This flow rate was a standard maximum flow for the measurement of FFR when adenosine was intravenously administrated. A red circle can be seen in Figure 2, which marks the observed stenosis on the artery. As already mentioned, a good agreement between the numerical simulations and the measurements of FFR was obtained, and this was the reason we used numerical results to validate the ML model [25,26].

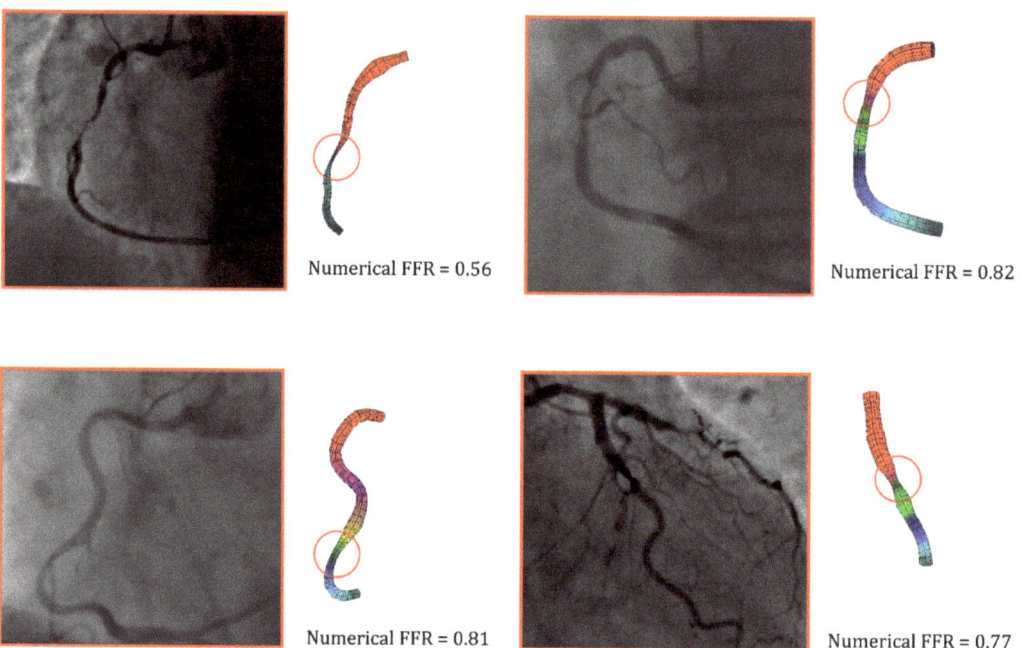

Figure 2. Pressure distribution, based on finite element analysis, in the coronary arteries. The FFR value was calculated based on numerical simulations.

4. Discussion

The main limiting factor during the creation of a classification model, for the purposes of classifying the patients based on their FFR, was the very low amount of available labeled data. The low amount of data severely limited the possibilities when choosing the base algorithm and tuning the parameters of the classification models. We hypothesized that the classification process could be drastically improved if there were more labeled data samples.

Also, the current model's prediction capabilities could be improved by adopting a different approach to building the ensemble. One of the ways through which to achieve this improvement is to fine tune the models by utilizing grid search during the training process. Fine tuning would exponentially increase the training time of the model, but it would also potentially increase its prediction performance in the end. Another approach that could be utilized was the creation of different types of classification models with the same configurations of training and testing datasets [31].

Furthermore, even though the imbalance between classes was not large, this imbalance, when paired with the size of the entire labeled dataset, rendered the use of traditionally good ensemble inclusions impossible. Namely, when working with small datasets, machine learning algorithms such as K-Nearest Neighbors and the Support Vector Machine achieve good classification results. However, each of these approaches had some drawbacks when used in this particular situation.

The Support Vector Machine algorithm is a kernel-based classifier, which divides the training data using multidimensional hyperplanes, the dimensionality of which is dependent on the dimensionality defined by the model input parameters. As an algorithm, it is capable of perfectly separating a dataset based on training data samples while keeping the Euclidean distance between the physical representations of the training data points in multidimensional space at the maximum. However, problems arise with the generalization capabilities of such models for newly introduced data. For this reason, a coefficient of error tolerance was introduced, which allows the algorithm to make minor mistakes during training but also increases the potential to better generalize when making decisions in the future. The problem in this particular situation arises when any high-risk patient is present in the test set as this reduces the number of available high-risk patients for training. Any value of allowed error tolerance renders the models incapable of predicting the high-risk class in an acceptable manner.

Similarly, the K-Nearest Neighbors algorithm, while not an algorithm that creates a mathematical model in the true meaning of those concepts, is still capable of splitting a multidimensional hyperspace into sections belonging to observed classes. The class separation of this algorithm is based on the proximity of similar training data points in the n-dimensional space. The high-risk patients defined two dense clusters within the aforementioned space, and this was achieved by clearly separating the zones within which the patient would be considered as under a high risk of AMI from those that could be considered to be under a low risk of suffering AMI. Introducing high-risk samples into the test set reduced the density of these clusters. This, consequently, greatly reduces the area inside the n-dimensional hyperspace within which the patient could be classified as high-risk, or, as in some situations, where those zones would be eliminated.

With the increase in the size and diversity of the dataset that was available for model training, the inclusion of a classification model other than the random forest model in the final ensemble became a possibility. While the introduction of new models would increase the time needed for training and parameter optimization, as well as slightly increase the time needed for prediction, the introduction of these models would, on the other hand, further reduce the output variance and greatly increase the versatility of the final ensemble.

High-quality data are seldom available in large amounts in fields of research like medicine due to ethical guidelines and patient privacy protection. Furthermore, medical data that are tied to specific diseases are, in some cases, region-specific, and they are also much sparser in some locations compared to others. In order to address these challenges, the proposed methodology serves as a proof of concept for a way in which to improve the automatic diagnosis approach when using a small amount of available data.

The main limiting factor of this study was the small amount of real data available as input to the ML model. Commonly used techniques for dataset enhancement that include the generation of new data through oversampling and the estimation of labels for unlabeled samples when using multiple imputations through chained equations are not always applicable to certain datasets and they do not always yield satisfying results.

Therefore, the added value of this paper primarily lies in the fact that we have proposed a methodology that deals with datasets that have a small amount of data. In fact, high amounts of data are hard to obtain in the medical field due to requiring ethical approvals and the need to ensure data privacy protection. As a result, this paper focuses on the novel methods that could be used on small datasets and can thus surpass traditional data enhancement methods. Although applied on a specific dataset regarding the assessment of the risk of suffering an acute myocardial infarction, the proposed methodology can be translated to other medical datasets as well. In addition, the novelty of the paper lies in the validation of the proposed methodology with simulated FFRs via the finite element method (FEM). The proposed approach would reduce the time needed for diagnosis and works to eliminate invasive coronography, as the data used in this paper were faster and easier to obtain than the real measurements of FFR.

In future research, numerical calculations combined with real measurements of FFR could be used to significantly increase the size of the dataset and achieve better accuracy in the proposed ML models. In addition to the improvement of the proposed machine learning approach to assessing the risk of AMI, an additional increase in the amount of available data would enable the transfer from machine learning algorithms to creating a specialized neural network for patient classification.

5. Conclusions

Cardiovascular diseases are the leading cause of death globally and a major contributor to life-altering complications such as a loss in the ability to work and physical disabilities. Acute myocardial infarction occurs due to coronary artery occlusion and the insufficient oxygenation of cardiomyocytes.

The main goal of this study was to create a decision support system that is capable of classifying patients into risk classes based on their calculated fractional flow reserve. The risk classes within the final ensemble model were defined by the observed FFR value of patients, where 0.8 was chosen as a threshold value. Patients with an FFR value higher than 0.8 were viewed as belonging to the low-risk class, while those with an FFR lower than 0.8 were considered as being in the high risk-class.

In order to classify patients, an ensemble model was constructed from multiple random forest classification models, which were all trained using different combinations of training and test data. The final classification model achieved a value of 76.21% prediction accuracy. Machine learning models that showed good prediction capabilities were incorporated into the final classification ensemble, and they achieved mean prediction accuracy values of 74.1%, 77.3%, 78.1% and 83.6%, which were tested with 5%, 10%, 15% and 20% test samples, respectively.

In conclusion, we have succeeded in creating a machine learning ensemble that is capable of classifying patients based on their risk of death via a fractional flow reserve, which greatly improves prediction capabilities over a single machine learning model, even when using a small amount of available training data. Additionally, feature importance was calculated based on the training weights of the created model, which provides a possible starting point for future research and classification accuracy improvements.

Author Contributions: Conceptualization, M.S.P. and O.P.; methodology, O.P. and I.S.; software, O.P.; validation, M.S.P., F.F., T.G. and T.E.; formal analysis, I.S. and F.F.; investigation, M.S.P.; resources, M.S.P.; data curation, M.S.P.; writing—original draft preparation, O.P., I.S. and M.S.P.; writing—review and editing, O.P. and T.G.; supervision, N.F.; project administration, N.F.; funding acquisition, N.F. All authors have read and agreed to the published version of the manuscript.

Funding: This research was funded by the Ministry of Science, Technological Development and Innovation of the Republic of Serbia (contract number 451-03-47/2023-01/200107) (Faculty of Engineering, University of Kragujevac). This research was also supported by the project that has received funding from the European Union's Horizon 2020 research and innovation programmes under grant agreement no. 952603 (SGABU project). This article reflects only the authors' views. The Commission is not responsible for any use that may be made of the information it contains.

Institutional Review Board Statement: The study was conducted in accordance with the Declaration of Helsinki, and approved by the Ethics Committee of the Clinical Center of Kragujevac (approval code: 01/19/2941, approval date: 12 July 2019).

Informed Consent Statement: Informed consent was obtained from all subjects involved in the study.

Data Availability Statement: The data presented in this study are available on request from the corresponding author. The data are not publicly available due to patient privacy protection and ethical guidelines.

Conflicts of Interest: The authors declare that they do not have any competing interest.

References

1. Reyes-Retana, J.A.; Duque-Ossa, L.C. Acute Myocardial Infarction Biosensor: A Review From Bottom Up. *Curr. Probl. Cardiol.* **2021**, *46*, 100739. [CrossRef]
2. GBD 2017 Causes of Death Collaborators. Global, regional, and national age-sex-specific mortality for 282 causes of death in 195 countries and territories, 1980–2017: A systematic analysis for the Global Burden of Disease Study 2017. *Lancet* **2018**, *392*, 1736–1788. [CrossRef]
3. GBD 2019 Diseases and Injuries Collaborators. Global burden of 369 diseases and injuries in 204 countries and territories, 1990–2019: A systematic analysis for the Global Burden of Disease Study 2019. *Lancet* **2020**, *396*, 1204–1222. [CrossRef]

4. Mechanic, O.J.; Gavin, M.; Grossman, S.A. Acute Myocardial Infarction. August 2022. Available online: https://www.ncbi.nlm.nih.gov/books/NBK459269 (accessed on 26 February 2023).
5. Chan, D.; Leong, L. Biomarkers in acute myocardial infarction. *BMC Med.* **2010**, *8*, 34. [CrossRef]
6. Andreou, I.; Antoniadis, A.P.; Shishido, K.; Papafaklis, M.I.; Koskinas, K.C.; Chatzizisis, Y.S.; Coskun, A.U.; Edelman, E.R.; Feldman, C.L.; Stone, P.H.; et al. How do we prevent the vulnerable atherosclerotic plaque from rupturing? Insights from in vivo assessments of plaque, vascular remodeling, and local endothelial shear stress. *J. Cardiovasc. Farmacol. Ther.* **2015**, *20*, 261–275. [CrossRef]
7. Insull, W., Jr. The pathology of atherosclerosis: Plaque development and plaque responses to medical treatment. *Am. J. Med.* **2009**, *122*, 3–14. [CrossRef]
8. Libby, P.; Pasterkamp, G.; Crea, F.; Jang, I.K. Reassessing the Mechanisms of Acute Coronary Syndromes The "Vulnerable Plaque" and Superficial Erosion. *Circ. Res.* **2019**, *124*, 150–160. [CrossRef]
9. Kristensen, M.S.; Green, A.; Nybo, M.; Hede, S.M.; Mikkelsen, K.H.; Gislason, G.; Larsen, M.L.; Ersbøll, A.K. Lipid-lowering therapy and low-density lipoprotein cholesterol goal attainment after acute coronary syndrome: A Danish population-based cohort study. *BMC Cardiovasc. Disord.* **2020**, *20*, 336. [CrossRef]
10. Solnica, B.; Sygitowicz, G.; Sitkiewicz, D.; Cybulska, B.; Jóźwiak, J.; Odrowąż-Sypniewska, G.; Banach, M. 2020 Guidelines of the Polish Society of Laboratory Diagnostics (PSLD) and the Polish Lipid Association (PoLA) on laboratory diagnostics of lipid metabolism disorders. *Arch. Med. Sci.* **2020**, *16*, 237–252. [CrossRef]
11. Collins, R.; Reith, C.; Emberson, J.; Armitage, J.; Baigent, C.; Blackwell, L.; Blumenthal, R.; Danesh, J.; Smith, G.D.; DeMets, D.; et al. Interpretation of the evidence for the efficacy and safety of statin therapy. *Lancet* **2016**, *388*, 2532–2561. [CrossRef]
12. Mythili, S.; Malathi, N. Diagnostic markers of acute myocardial infarction. *Biomed. Rep.* **2015**, *3*, 743–748. [CrossRef]
13. Fan, J.; Ma, J.; Xia, N.; Sun, L.; Li, B.; Liu, H. Clinical Value of Combined Detection of CK-MB, MYO, cTnI and Plasma NT-proBNP in Diagnosis of Acute Myocardial Infarction. *Clin. Lab.* **2017**, *63*, 427–433. [CrossRef]
14. Chapman, A.; Adamson, P.; Shah, A.; Anand, A.; Strachan, F.; Lee, K.K.; Ferry, A.; Sandeman, D.; Stables, C.; Newby, D.; et al. High-Sensitivity Cardiac Troponin and the Universal Definition of Myocardial Infarction. *Circulation* **2020**, *141*, 161–171. [CrossRef]
15. Farmakis, D.; Mueller, C.; Apple, F.S. High-sensitivity cardiac troponin assays for cardiovascular risk stratification in the general population. *Eur. Heart J.* **2020**, *41*, 4050–4056. [CrossRef]
16. Thygesen, K.; Alpert, J.S.; Jaffe, A.S.; Chaitman, B.R.; Bax, J.J.; Morrow, D.A.; White, H.D. The Executive Group on behalf of the Joint European Society of Cardiology (ESC)/American College of Cardiology (ACC)/American Heart Association (AHA)/World Heart Federation (WHF) Task Force for the Universal Definition of Myocardial Infarction. Fourth Universal Definition of Myocardial Infarction (2018). *Circulation* **2018**, *138*, 618–651.
17. Bettencourt, P.; Ferreira, A.; Pereira, M.; Pardal-Oliveira, N.; Ós, C.Q.; Újo, V.A.; Cerqueira-Gomes, M.; Maciel, M.J. Clinical significance of brain natriuretic peptide in patients with postmyocardial infarction. *Clin. Cardiol.* **2000**, *23*, 921–927. [CrossRef]
18. Jernberg, T.; Stridsberg, M.; Venge, P.; Lindahl, B. N-terminal pro brain natriuretic peptide on admission for early risk stratification of patients with chest pain and no ST-segment elevation. *J. Am. Coll. Cardiol.* **2002**, *40*, 437–445. [CrossRef]
19. Pijls, N.H.; de Bruyne, B.; Peels, K.; van der Voort, P.H.; Bonnier, H.J.; Bartunek, J.; Koolen, J.J. Measurement of fractional flow reserve to assess the functional severity of coronary-artery stenoses. *N. Engl. J. Med.* **1996**, *334*, 1703–1708. [CrossRef]
20. Lo, E.W.; Menezes, L.J.; Torii, R. On outflow boundary conditions for CT-based computation of FFR: Examination using PET images. *Med. Eng. Phys.* **2020**, *76*, 79–87. [CrossRef]
21. Kurata, A.; Fukuyama, N.; Hirai, K.; Kawaguchi, N.; Tanabe, Y.; Okayama, H.; Shigemi, S.; Watanabe, K.; Uetani, T.; Ikeda, S.; et al. On-Site Computed Tomography-Derived Fractional Flow Reserve Using a Machine-Learning Algorithm—Clinical Effectiveness in a Retrospective Multicenter Cohort. *Circulation* **2019**, *83*, 1563–1571. [CrossRef]
22. Coenen, A.; Kim, Y.-H.; Kruk, M.; Tesche, C.; De Geer, J.; Kurata, A.; Lubbers, M.L.; Daemen, J.; Itu, L.; Rapaka, S.; et al. Diagnostic Accuracy of a Machine-Learning Approach to Coronary Computed Tomographic Angiography–Based Fractional Flow Reserve. *Circulation* **2018**, *11*, e007217. [CrossRef]
23. Brandt, V.; Schoepf, U.J.; Aquino, G.J.; Bekeredjian, R.; Varga-Szemes, A.; Emrich, T.; Bayer, R.R.; Schwarz, F.; Kroencke, T.J.; Tesche, C.; et al. Impact of machine-learning-based coronary computed tomography angiography–derived fractional flow reserve on decision-making in patients with severe aortic stenosis undergoing transcatheter aortic valve replacement. *Eur. Radiol.* **2022**, *32*, 6008–6016. [CrossRef]
24. Vukicevic, A.; Cimen, S.; Jagic, N.; Jovicic, G.; Frangi, A.F.; Filipovic, N. Three-dimensional reconstruction and NURBS-based structured meshing of coronary arteries from the conventional X-ray angiography projection images. *Sci. Rep.* **2018**, *8*, 1711. [CrossRef]
25. Milovanovic, A.; Saveljic, I.; Filipovic, N. Numerical vs analytical comparison with experimental fractional flow reserve values of right coronary artery stenosis. *Technol. Health Care* **2023**, *31*, 977–990. [CrossRef]
26. Sakellarios, A.; Correia, J.; Kyriakidis, S.; Georga, E.; Tachos, N.; Siogkas, P.; Sans, F.; Stofella, P.; Massimiliano, V.; Clemente, A.; et al. A cloud-based platform for the non-invasive management of coronary artery disease. *Enterp. Inf. Syst.* **2020**, *14*, 1102–1123. [CrossRef]

27. Modi, B.N.; Rahman, H.; Kaier, T.; Ryan, M.; Williams, R.; Briceno, N.; Ellis, H.; Pavlidis, A.; Redwood, S.; Clapp, B.; et al. Revisiting the Optimal Fractional Flow Reserve and Instantaneous Wave-Free Ratio Thresholds for Predicting the Physiological Significance of Coronary Artery Disease. *Circ. Cardiovasc. Invent.* **2018**, *11*, e007041. [CrossRef]
28. Kojić, M.; Filipović, N.; Stojanović, B.; Kojić, N. *Computer Modeling in Bioengineering: Theoretical Background, Examples and Software*; John Wiley & Sons: Hoboken, NJ, USA, 2008.
29. Pijls, N.H.; Fearon, W.F.; Tonino, P.A.; Siebert, U.; Ikeno, F.; Bornschein, B.; van't Veer, M.; Klauss, V.; Manoharan, G.; Engstrøm, T.; et al. Fractional flow reserve versus angiography for guiding percutaneous coronary intervention in patients with multivessel coronary artery disease: 2-year follow-up of the FAME (Fractional Flow Reserve Versus Angiography for Multivessel Evaluation) study. *J. Am. Coll. Cardiol.* **2010**, *56*, 177–184. [CrossRef]
30. Polkar, R. Ensemble learning. In *Ensemble Machine Learning*; Springer: Berlin/Heidelberg, Germany, 2012; Volume 1, pp. 1–34.
31. Sagi, O.; Rokach, L. Ensemble learning: A survey. *WIREs Data Min. Knowl. Discov.* **2018**, *8*, e1249. [CrossRef]

Disclaimer/Publisher's Note: The statements, opinions and data contained in all publications are solely those of the individual author(s) and contributor(s) and not of MDPI and/or the editor(s). MDPI and/or the editor(s) disclaim responsibility for any injury to people or property resulting from any ideas, methods, instructions or products referred to in the content.

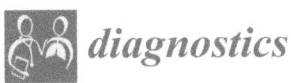

Article

Optimizing Inference Distribution for Efficient Kidney Tumor Segmentation Using a UNet-PWP Deep-Learning Model with XAI on CT Scan Images

P. Kiran Rao [1,2,*], Subarna Chatterjee [2], M. Janardhan [3], K. Nagaraju [4], Surbhi Bhatia Khan [5,6,*], Ahlam Almusharraf [7] and Abdullah I. Alharbe [8]

1 Artificial Intelligence, Department of Computer Science and Engineering, Ravindra College of Engineering for Women, Kurnool 518001, India
2 Department of Computer Science and Engineering, Faculty of Engineering, MS Ramaiah University of Applied Sciences, Bengaluru 560058, India; subarna.cs.et@msruas.ac.in
3 Artificial Intelligence, Department of Computer Science and Engineering, G. Pullaiah College of Engineering and Technology, Kurnool 518008, India; m.janardhan0105@gmail.com
4 Department of Computer Science and Engineering, Indian Institute of Information Technology Design and Manufacturing Kurnool, Kurnool 518008, India; knagaraju@iiitk.ac.in
5 Department of Data Science, School of Science, Engineering and Environment, University of Salford, Salford M5 4WT, UK
6 Department of Electrical and Computer Engineering, Lebanese American University, Byblos 13-5053, Lebanon
7 Department of Business Administration, College of Business and Administration, Princess Nourah bint Abdulrahman University, P.O. Box 84428, Riyadh 11671, Saudi Arabia; aialmusharraf@pnu.edu.sa
8 Department of Computer Science, Faculty of Computing and Information Technology, King Abdulaziz University, Rabigh 21911, Saudi Arabia; aamalharbe@kau.edu.sa
* Correspondence: kiranraocse@gmail.com (P.K.R.); surbhibhatia1988@yahoo.com (S.B.K.)

Abstract: Kidney tumors represent a significant medical challenge, characterized by their often-asymptomatic nature and the need for early detection to facilitate timely and effective intervention. Although neural networks have shown great promise in disease prediction, their computational demands have limited their practicality in clinical settings. This study introduces a novel methodology, the UNet-PWP architecture, tailored explicitly for kidney tumor segmentation, designed to optimize resource utilization and overcome computational complexity constraints. A key novelty in our approach is the application of adaptive partitioning, which deconstructs the intricate UNet architecture into smaller submodels. This partitioning strategy reduces computational requirements and enhances the model's efficiency in processing kidney tumor images. Additionally, we augment the UNet's depth by incorporating pre-trained weights, therefore significantly boosting its capacity to handle intricate and detailed segmentation tasks. Furthermore, we employ weight-pruning techniques to eliminate redundant zero-weighted parameters, further streamlining the UNet-PWP model without compromising its performance. To rigorously assess the effectiveness of our proposed UNet-PWP model, we conducted a comparative evaluation alongside the DeepLab V3+ model, both trained on the "KiTs 19, 21, and 23" kidney tumor dataset. Our results are optimistic, with the UNet-PWP model achieving an exceptional accuracy rate of 97.01% on both the training and test datasets, surpassing the DeepLab V3+ model in performance. Furthermore, to ensure our model's results are easily understandable and explainable. We included a fusion of the attention and Grad-CAM XAI methods. This approach provides valuable insights into the decision-making process of our model and the regions of interest that affect its predictions. In the medical field, this interpretability aspect is crucial for healthcare professionals to trust and comprehend the model's reasoning.

Keywords: adaptive partitioning; explainable AI; kidney tumor segmentation; optimization; weight pruning; UNet-PWP; DeepLabV3+; GCAM-attention

Citation: Rao, P.K.; Chatterjee, S.; Janardhan, M.; Nagaraju, K.; Khan, S.B.; Almusharraf, A.; Alharbe, A.I. Optimizing Inference Distribution for Efficient Kidney Tumor Segmentation Using a UNet-PWP Deep-Learning Model with XAI on CT Scan Images. *Diagnostics* **2023**, *13*, 3244. https://doi.org/10.3390/diagnostics13203244

Academic Editor: Daniele Giansanti

Received: 14 September 2023
Revised: 10 October 2023
Accepted: 10 October 2023
Published: 18 October 2023

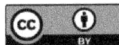

Copyright: © 2023 by the authors. Licensee MDPI, Basel, Switzerland. This article is an open access article distributed under the terms and conditions of the Creative Commons Attribution (CC BY) license (https://creativecommons.org/licenses/by/4.0/).

1. Introduction

The kidneys serve a vital role in the human body by filtering waste products and toxins from the bloodstream [1,2]. Tumors, or cancers, result from the abnormal growth of cells and can manifest differently in individuals, leading to various symptoms. Early detection of kidney tumors (KT) is paramount for mitigating the risk of disease progression and preserving the patient's life [2,3]. Although approximately one third of KT cases are identified after spreading to other areas, many remain asymptomatic and are incidentally discovered during unrelated medical evaluations. Kidney tumors can manifest as masses, cysts, or abdominal discomfort in patients, often unrelated to kidney function [4,5]. Nevertheless, some subtle symptoms or complications may arise due to KT, including low hemoglobin levels, weakness, vomiting, abdominal pain, hematuria (blood in urine), or elevated blood sugar levels. Anemia is also a common occurrence, affecting about 30% of KT patients [6,7]. Unfortunately, tumors and solid masses that develop within the kidneys frequently become cancerous. Detecting the presence of cancer is crucial in selecting the appropriate treatment method, as the prognosis and recovery rate often hinge on early identification. Computed tomography (CT) scans of the abdomen and pelvis are among the essential diagnostic tests used to ascertain the presence of kidney tumors. These scans provide specific characteristics that aid in tumor detection and assessment. Figure 1 illustrates a case of KT, depicting a renal mass lesion in the left kidney measuring approximately 4 cm (with the kidney in red and renal cancer in green). Given the life-threatening nature of tumors, accurate diagnosis is paramount, leading to various procedures aimed at assisting the physician [8,9]. Deep learning (DL) is a remarkably potent machine learning technology capable of autonomously acquiring numerous features and patterns without human intervention [10–12]. DL has empowered the development of predictive models for early tumor disease detection, with scientists relying on established pattern analysis techniques. DL algorithms have demonstrated superiority over traditional machine learning methods, yielding impressive results [13–15]. Furthermore, DL frequently achieves performance levels that match or exceed human capabilities, making it the preferred approach for handling image-related tasks [16,17]. This heightened recognition of DL in image processing, particularly within the medical domain, is attributed to the central role of radiology in extracting valuable insights from images.

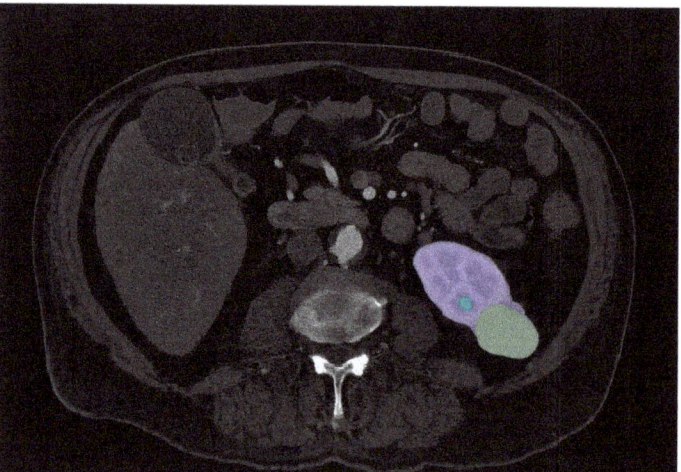

Figure 1. An example of a segmented slice from volume of CT scan Modality. The kidney region is shown in purple, the tumor is shown in green, and the cyst is shown in blue.

Semantic segmentation, a task in computer vision, has witnessed significant advancements with the proliferation of DL techniques. DL has proven highly effective in enhancing image understanding [18,19]. These DL methods for semantic segmentation can be categorized into several approaches, including region-based, fully connected network FCN-based, and semi-supervised methods. Region-based methods follow a pipeline approach, initially extracting free-form regions from input images, followed by region-based classification. Ultimately, these methods assign labels to pixels based on the scored areas [19]. In contrast, FCN-based methods do not require region proposal extraction. Instead, they learn a direct mapping from pixel to pixel, allowing them to handle images of arbitrary sizes [19]. Semi-supervised methods are useful when dealing with datasets requiring extensive time for mask annotation. These methods aim to make the most of the available annotated data while incorporating unsupervised techniques to improve segmentation results [19].

Moreover, in addition to these primary categories, explainable artificial intelligence (XAI) [20] holds promise in shedding new light on disease characteristics, potentially serving as an indicator for assessing responses to exposure or other therapeutic interventions. Nevertheless, it is imperative that XAI offers clarity regarding the comprehensibility of its decisions, explanations, and potential associated errors. Therefore, before XAI can be considered a valuable and reliable tool for testing research hypotheses or aiding clinical decision-making, it must navigate several critical "translational gaps" [20,21]. Furthermore, the recently implemented European Medical Device [22] Regulation (EU MDR) imposes stringent transparency regulations that must be followed before integrating such a tool into clinical practice [23]. XAI thus holds the potential to be a pivotal factor in promoting greater transparency, ethical considerations, unbiased practices, and overall safety and trustworthiness in the deployment of DL algorithms within clinical settings.

Furthermore, in addition to our proposed model architecture, we have also incorporated state-of-the-art networks into our research; notably, the DeepLab V3+ [23] network along with XAI Grad-CAM [20]. Finally, our model's performance has been rigorously assessed and validated using renal CT scans obtained from the KiTS datasets for the years 2019, 2021, and 2023 [24,25].

1.1. Contribution of Our Proposed Work

- Novel Methodology: We propose a novel methodology for medical image segmentation, addressing hardware constraints through adaptive partitioning and weight pruning.
- Progressive Model Construction: Our approach allows us to incrementally deepen UNet submodels while maintaining a consistent number of parameters, maximizing the architecture's potential.
- GCAM-Attention:GCAM-Attention Fusion contributes to a model that excels in segmentation accuracy and computational efficiency and provides transparency and interpretability.
- Enhanced Kidney Tumor Segmentation: Our work focuses on kidney tumor segmentation, significantly improving accuracy and efficiency in this medical task.

1.2. Organization of the Paper

The remainder of this paper is organized as follows: Section 2 encompasses an exploration of related works, offering insights into the existing body of knowledge within the field. It provides a context for the current study by examining prior research endeavors. Section 3 delves into the methodology and materials employed, elucidating the architecture, dataset, and evaluation metrics that underpin our investigation. Section 4 lists the experimental outcomes and their meticulous analysis. The results are presented comprehensively, followed by an insightful exploration of their implications and significance. Concluding our discourse, Section 5 encapsulates the culmination of our study through the presentation of conclusions drawn from the research.

2. Related Works

Despite the numerous traditional CT image segmentation techniques proposed over the past few decades, including manual, threshold-based, atlas-based, graph-based, and hybrid methods, they exhibit limitations in accurately delineating kidneys in CT images. For instance, straightforward approaches like threshold segmentation are highly noise-sensitive and need help handling significant intensity variations in CT scans. Notably, both atlas-based and threshold-based methods require manual intervention and are susceptible to segmentation performance variations due to inter-rater differences.

Ronneberger et al. [26] employed the UNet model for medical image segmentation during the 2015 ISBI competition [26]. However, their approach utilized only a modest dataset of 30 images and data augmentation strategies, achieving a relatively modest error rate and clinching victory in the ISBI competition. Subsequently, various UNet-based algorithms, with adaptations and enhancements, gained prominence across diverse image processing domains consistently yielding commendable results.

In 2021, Heller et al. [27] summarized the top-performing methods in the KiTS19 challenge [23–25]. Notably, the segmentation models of the top contestants were all based on the UNet architecture. Fabian et al. [28] secured the first position with a 3D UNet-based approach, achieving impressive dice scores of 0.974 and 0.851 for kidney and tumor segmentation, resulting in a composite score of 0.912 [29]. Several other researchers [30–34] proposed kidney and tumor segmentation methods, achieving notable results in subsequent studies.

In recent times, researchers have increasingly turned to XAI to perform comprehensive assessments and provide explanations for model outcomes. For instance, Yang et al. [35] employed 3D Convolutional Neural Networks (CNNs) to classify Alzheimer's disease while also offering visual explanations for their model's decisions. Wickstrom et al. [36] utilized Gradient boosting (GB) techniques to improve the explainability of colon polyp classifications. Esmaeili et al. [37] integrated an explainability method based on Grad-CAM into the 2D glioma segmentation task. Saleem et al. [38] extended similar approaches to the realm of 3D image analysis.

Natekar et al. [39] harnessed Grad-CAM to shed light on the process of brain tumor segmentation, providing insights into the model's decision-making process. Adebayo et al. [40] conducted a sanity check and discovered that class activation mapping (CAM)-based methods offer superior performance in classification tasks. Pereira et al. [41] put forward an explainability methodology that combines global and local information to enhance tumor segmentation, employing both GB and CAM techniques in brain tumor detection. Their experiments revealed that GB excels at identifying critical areas rather than categories, whereas CAM performs admirably in both tasks.

Furthermore, Narayanan et al. [42] utilized GoogLeNet and ResNet to detect various medical conditions such as malaria, diabetic retinopathy, brain tumors, and tuberculosis across different imaging modalities. They leveraged class activation mappings to provide visualizations that enhance the comprehension of these deep neural networks' decisions. Moving forward to the KiTS21 challenge [25], Shen et al. [33] employed the COTRNet model for kidney segmentation, achieving a kidney dice score of 0.923. Adam et al. [25] used a 3D U-ResNet method for kidney segmentation and reached the 12th position in KiTS21. Zhao et al. [24] secured the first position in KiTS21 with a nnU-Net-based framework, attaining remarkable dice scores for kidney, mass, and tumor segmentation.

In conclusion, while various approaches have been explored for kidney segmentation, most kidney tumor segmentation studies rely on cascaded architectures as their primary models. However, 3D models demand significant computational resources, while 2D models may need more crucial spatial information. This paper introduces a novel segmentation approach for kidneys and tumors to address the computational complexity associated with 3D CNNs while maintaining high segmentation accuracy. The goal is to enhance the neural network architecture without compromising accuracy, presenting a versatile methodology applicable to kidney tumor segmentation. Beyond just KiTS19, KiTS21, and KiTs23 [24,25], our focus extends to aiding physicians in the rapid diagnosis of patients through improved segmentation results.

3. Materials and Methods

This section presents the methodology employed for kidney tumor segmentation using the KiTs variant dataset [25]. Our approach harnesses the power of deep neural networks, specifically UNet, combined with XAI, adaptive partitioning, and weight-pruning techniques to achieve accurate and validate the segmentation of kidney tumors.

3.1. Data Pre-Processing

The evaluation of kidney tumor segmentation techniques often leverages the KiTs 19, 21, and 23 variant datasets [25], a well-established benchmark for assessing the efficacy of such methodologies. This dataset comprises high-contrast CT images [2] acquired between 2010 and 2020 at the University of Minnesota Medical Center [2]. It encompasses data from 489 patients who underwent partial or radical nephrectomy for one or more kidney tumors. The dataset offers a rich diversity of scans featuring varying in-plane resolutions (ranging from 0.437 to 1.04 mm) and slice thicknesses (ranging from 0.5 to 5.0 mm). Each instance within this dataset is accompanied by ground-truth masks representing malignant tumors and healthy kidney tissue, as depicted in Figure 2. The meticulous creation of these masks involved the collaboration of medical students guided by expert radiologists—notably, the manual annotation process utilized solely the axial projections of the CT images. The dataset adheres to the NIFTI format and is defined by dimensions specifying the number of slices, height, and width. It has garnered widespread recognition as a standard benchmark for evaluating kidney tumor segmentation approaches, including the model proposed in this study.

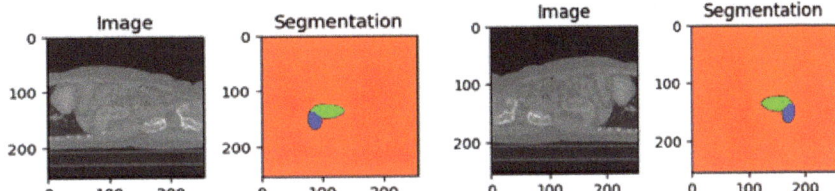

Figure 2. Visualization of kidney and tumor region segmentation using deep learning semantic segmentation.

In addition to the KiTS23 dataset [23,24], variants such as KiTS19 [23] and KiTS21 [24] play a crucial role in refining the evaluation process. Including these variant datasets enriches the evaluation process by capturing a broader spectrum of challenges and scenarios encountered in clinical practice. This comprehensive assessment not only strengthens the validation of the proposed model but also underscores its potential to address the complexities inherent in kidney tumor segmentation tasks.

3.2. Enhancing Kidney Tumor Segmentation: UNet Partitioning, Weight Pruning, and GCAM-Attention Fusion

The proposed model begins by constructing a complex Standard UNet model [28] for kidney tumor segmentation with deeper layers to extract the features. Let X represent the input CT scan [23,26] image, and Y be the corresponding ground-truth segmentation mask. The UNet model takes X as input and produces pixel-wise predictions $\hat{Y}$ for kidney tumor regions. The output of UNet is expressed as in Equation (1)

$$\hat{Y} = UNet(X) \qquad (1)$$

3.2.1. Adaptive Partitioning for Scalable Submodels

The 3D-UNet architecture [26] is a highly intricate model with numerous layers, depth, and ten million parameters. Due to its complexity, it can be challenging to fit into standard GPU configurations. To overcome this limitation, an adaptive partitioning approach is employed to evaluate the intricacy of each UNet layer based on the interplay between the number of learnable parameters and computations performed during inference. This evaluation guides the division of the UNet into submodels, each with its own depth. Within this context, the complexity of each layer is described by the balance between the number of learnable parameters (P_i) and the computations carried out during inference via floating-point operations ($FLOPs_i$).

$$\text{Complexity of layer } L_i = P_i \times FLOPs_i \quad (2)$$

The parameter max_c denotes the upper bound on the allowable complexity for each submodel, and max_p signifies the envisaged number of partitions. Through mathematical analysis, we determine the target complexity $target_c$ as elucidated by the formula:

$$target_c = \frac{\text{Total Complexity}}{max_p} \quad (3)$$

Target complexity ($target_c$) is computed to ensure each submodel balances complexity and resource constraints. This process results in smaller, more manageable portions of the original UNet, each designed to fit within standard GPU memory limitations.

3.2.2. Weight Pruning for Efficient Resource Utilization

To enhance submodel efficiency, we employ a technique known as weight pruning, as referenced in [43–45]. This involves selectively reducing the number of parameters within a submodel by setting specific weight values to zero. By doing so, we can improve computational efficiency while also simplifying the submodel's structure and preserving its ability to capture critical data features.

To provide further insight, let us consider a submodel represented by a set of parameters denoted as W. Weight pruning, as described in [46], identifies less impactful parameters based on their magnitudes. We can prune by assigning a value of zero to W_{ij} for specific neurons, resulting in a sparser weight matrix. This process occurs after the incremental layer addition and fine-tuning phases. To balance model complexity and performance, we iteratively prune less influential parameters and fine-tune the submodel. This results in a more concise, resource-friendly submodel. Our methodology aims to optimize deep neural networks for practical use cases, particularly those with limited computational resources. This approach has significantly contributed to the effectiveness of our progressively trained UNet submodels in tasks such as biomedical image segmentation.

3.2.3. Gradient-Weighted Class Activation Mapping(Grad-CAM)

Grad-CAM is an explainable AI technique designed for convolutional neural networks (CNNs) to visualize the regions in an input image that are important for the network's classification decision [47–49]. Grad-CAM generates heatmaps that highlight the most relevant areas in the image, making it easier to understand the model's focus and reasoning. Assuming a CNN model as f and an input image x, the goal of Grad-CAM [40] is to generate a heatmap that highlights the important regions in the image for the predicted class c. Grad-CAM follows these steps:

1. Identify the target layer: Grad-CAM focuses on the last convolutional layer of the CNN, which contains the high-level features that are most relevant to the classification task. Let A be the activation map of this layer with dimensions $H \times W$, where H and W are the height and width of the map, respectively.

2. Compute the gradients: Calculate the gradients of the score for the predicted class c (denoted as Y_c) with respect to the activation map A. The gradients ($\frac{\partial Y_c}{\partial A}$) represent the importance of each activation for the predicted class.
3. Calculate the weights: Compute the weights α by global average pooling the gradients over the height and width dimensions [6].

$$\alpha_k = \frac{1}{H \cdot W} \sum_{i=1}^{H} \sum_{j=1}^{W} \frac{\partial Y_c}{\partial A_{i,j,k}} \quad (4)$$

where k is the index of the k-th feature map, and $A_{i,j,k}$ is the activation at location (i, j) of the k-th feature map.

4. Compute the weighted activation map: Multiply each feature map in A by its corresponding weight α_k, and sum the weighted feature maps to obtain the weighted activation map L.

$$L = \sum_k \alpha_k A_k \quad (5)$$

5. Generate the heatmap: Apply a ReLU function to the weighted activation map L to eliminate the negative values and obtain the final heatmap H.

$$H = \text{ReLU}(L) \quad (6)$$

The resulting heatmap H highlights the regions in the input image [49] that contributed the most to the predicted class c. Grad-CAM can provide insights into the model's decision-making process, enabling users to identify potential biases, verify the model's focus on relevant features, and ensure that the model does not rely on irrelevant or spurious patterns. Grad-CAM is specifically designed for CNNs and may not be applicable to other types of neural networks or machine learning models [23]. However, it has been widely used for explainability in image classification tasks and can be adapted for other tasks such as object detection or semantic segmentation.

3.3. Generating Attention Heatmap

The attention heatmap visualization technique highlights the regions within an input kidney tumor CT scan that receive the most focus from a neural network during the segmentation process. The generation of an attention heatmap begins with an input image represented as a 2D array with dimensions $H(height)$ and $W(width)$. In this process, a predefined center of attention, indicated by the coordinates ($attention_{center_x}, attention_{center_y}$), plays a pivotal role. Initially, an empty attention heatmap, denoted as A, is created with dimensions matching the input image's dimensions. Subsequently, a Gaussian filter is applied to the attention heatmap A. This filter emphasizes the regions of interest surrounding the designated center of attention [50], and its extent is determined by a specified standard deviation (σ). In the next step, the Gaussian filter operation is applied as $A' = G\sigma * A$, where A' represents the filtered attention heatmap and $G\sigma$ is the Gaussian filter. Following applying the Gaussian filter, the attention heatmap A' is subjected to a normalization process to ensure that pixel values correspond to the intensity of attention. Normalization is achieved by mapping the pixel values from A' to the range [0, 1]. This step enhances the interpretability [51–54] of the heatmap, allowing it to effectively convey the relative importance or relevance of different regions within the input image. The normalization of the filtered attention heatmap A' is performed using the equation $A_{normalized} = (A' - min(A'))/(max(A') - min(A') + \epsilon)$, where $A_{normalized}$ represents the final normalized attention heatmap, $min(A')$ signifies the minimum pixel value in A, $max(A')$ denotes the maximum pixel value in A', and ϵ is a small positive constant introduced to prevent division by zero. The resulting $A_{normalized}$ serves as the attention heatmap, effectively highlighting areas of increased importance or focus as determined by the selected center of attention and the Gaussian filter. This methodology offers a systematic and mathematical approach to generating attention heatmaps, valuable for visualizing the regions of interest within images, particularly in applications such as computer vision and image analysis.

3.4. GCAM-Attention Fusion:

The fusion process seamlessly combines the Grad-CAM with attention heatmaps. It starts by taking an equal-weighted combination of the Grad-CAM heatmap and the attention heatmap. This balanced fusion ensures that both sources contribute equally to the final interpretability heatmap. The resulting fused heatmap represents a harmonious blend of the Grad-CAM's focus on prediction-influential regions and the attention heatmap's emphasis on areas of interest as given in Equation (7).

$$H_{\text{fusion}}(i,j) = (H_{\text{Grad-CAM}}(i,j) + H_{\text{attention}}(i,j))/2 \tag{7}$$

In the context of kidney tumor segmentation and other medical image analysis tasks, this fusion methodology can be instrumental in providing healthcare professionals with transparent, interpretable, and trustworthy insights into the model's decision-making process. It bridges the gap between complex deep-learning models and human interpretability, ultimately enhancing the model's utility and impact in critical applications.

Proposed UNet-PWP with XAI (GCAM-Attention Fusion)

Our proposed approach, "UNet-PWP with GCAM-Attention Fusion", leverages advanced neural network models to segment kidney tumors in medical images precisely. Our primary objective is to attain high precision and efficiency while considering hardware resource constraints. Although the 3D-UNet architecture [31] inherently possesses complexity with multiple layers and millions of parameters, deploying it on standard GPU configurations can be daunting. In response to this challenge, we employ adaptive partitioning techniques that assess the complexity of each UNet layer. This approach balances model complexity and available computational resources, aligning with our primary goal and interpretability.

Our methodology involves incremental depth augmentation, wherein we introduce new layers (L_{new}) to a submodel (M_k). This augmentation enhances the submodel's capacity to capture intricate data features while retaining the benefits of smaller submodel sizes achieved through initial adaptive partitioning. Subsequently, we fine-tune submodel performance (M_k) by precisely adjusting submodel weights using advanced optimization techniques, such as the Adam optimizer. Additionally, we systematically apply weight pruning [34] techniques guided by established principles to reduce the number of parameters, thus enhancing model efficiency without compromising performance.

Our approach follows a structured sequence in which submodels undergo incremental refinement. We create a compact 3D-UNet architecture through adaptive partitioning and gradually increase depth through subsequent applications of adaptive partitioning. The result is a submodel with the original UNet's depth but fewer trainable parameters, making it compatible with standard hardware configurations. We can refer to Figure 3 for a visual representation of our process. By incorporating "GCAM-Attention Fusion" into our approach, we enhance the interpretability and visualization aspects of the UNet-PWP model, allowing for deeper insights into the segmentation process while maintaining computational efficiency.

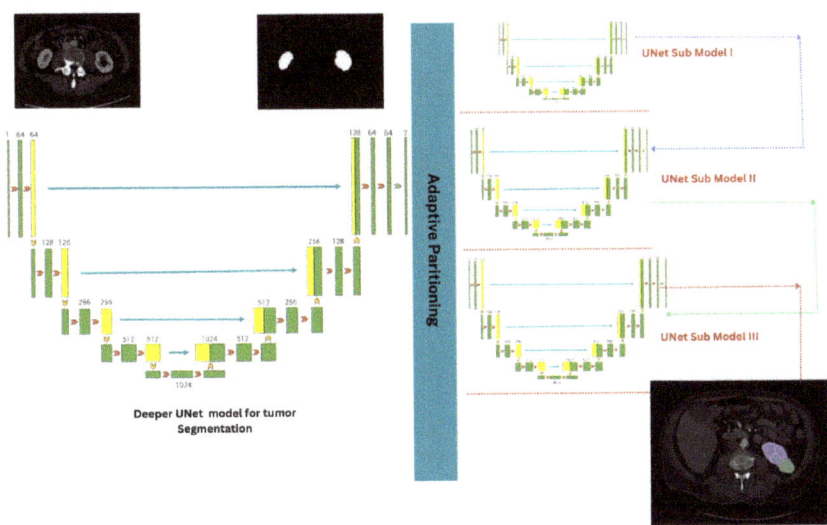

Figure 3. Adaptive Partitioning with Weight Pruning: Visualizing Progressive Submodels in a Complex UNet Architecture (UNet-PWP).

4. Results

In this section, we present the comprehensive results obtained from our proposed methodology, which effectively combines adaptive partitioning and weight pruning [34] techniques applied to the UNet model for kidney tumor segmentation. The evaluation is focused on assessing the effectiveness of the partitioned and weight-pruned submodels in terms of segmentation accuracy and computational efficiency. Our experimentation encompassed the utilization of variant KiTS datasets [23,25], namely KiTS19, KiTS21, and KiTS23.

4.1. Experimental Setup

Our experiment utilized a high-performance workstation equipped with an Intel Core i9-10900K CPU and an NVIDIA GeForce RTX 3050 GPU with 6 GB memory. To train our models, we implemented the UNet architecture [26], along with partitioning and weight-pruning algorithms [34], using Python and TensorFlow. Our dataset consisted of CT scan images of kidney tumors from the KiTs19, KiTs21, and KiTs23 variants [24]. We divided these datasets into training, validation, and test sets, with 342 cases allocated for training, 73 cases for validation, and 73 for testing. We preprocessed the datasets to ensure consistent input dimensions and normalized pixel values [43].

Throughout the training process, we employed the Adam optimizer to minimize the dice loss function. Our models were trained for 100 epochs with a batch size of 12, and we utilized data augmentation techniques such as random rotations and flips to enhance model generalization. To implement our proposed partitioning and weight-pruning methodology, we set the maximum complexity of each submodel to 10 million FLOPs and the maximum number of partitions to 3. Our pruning ratio was determined empirically at 0.2, indicating that 20% of the weights were pruned.

4.2. Ablation Study

In this ablation study, we conduct a comprehensive assessment of various modifications to the UNet architecture, with the overarching goal of facilitating informed design choices within the context of kidney tumor segmentation. Our primary aim is to pinpoint the most effective model configuration, all the while carefully considering the trade-offs between computational efficiency and segmentation accuracy.

We introduce four distinct modifications, each designed to enhance the original UNet architecture:

- UNet: The baseline UNet architecture [26] serves as our starting point, with a total of 100,000,000 trainable parameters.
- UNet (Adaptive Partitioning + Weight Pruning): In this modification, we apply adaptive partitioning and weight-pruning techniques to the initial UNet model [26]. The result is a more streamlined model with a total of 10,000,000 trainable parameters, significantly reducing computational demands.
- UNet (Adaptive Partitioning + Weight Pruning + Depth Increase): Here, we not only apply adaptive partitioning and weight pruning but also augment the UNet model [26] by increasing its depth with previously trained weights. The resulting architecture maintains the same total and trainable parameters of 10,000,000 million, which can fit with the same computational demands, albeit with enhanced capacity for intricate feature extraction.
- UNet (Adaptive Partitioning + Weight Pruning + Depth Increase + GCAM-Attention Fusion): To further enhance the interpretability and visualization aspects of our UNet-PWP model, we introduce the innovative 'GCAM-Attention Fusion' component. This fusion technique is integrated into the UNet architecture, extending the model's region-specific analysis and understanding capabilities.

The performance of these modifications, including 'UNet (Adaptive Partitioning + Weight Pruning + Depth Increase + GCAM-Attention Fusion),' is meticulously documented and compared against the original UNet architecture, DeepLab v3+, and our proposed UNet-PWP model. The comprehensive evaluation results are presented in Tables 1–3, while the visual representation of these findings can be observed in Figures 4 and 5. This holistic assessment provides valuable guidance for optimizing kidney tumor segmentation models and showcases the significance of 'GCAM-Attention Fusion' in achieving superior interpretability and performance.

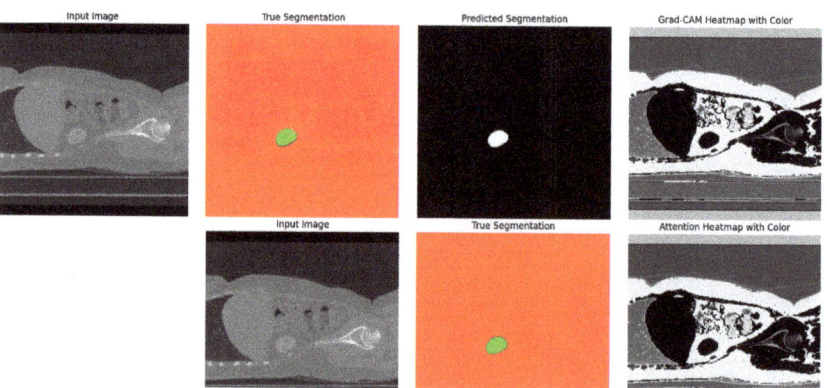

Figure 4. Cognitive Heatmaps for Kidney and Tumor Regions.

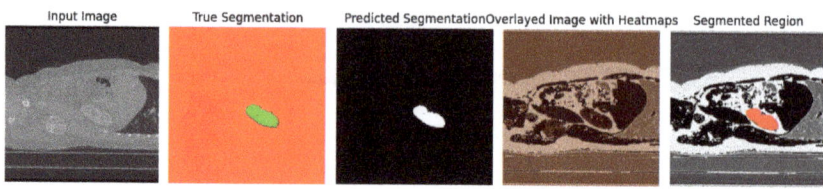

Figure 5. GCAM-Attention Fusion Visualization for Kidneys and Tumor Regions.

4.3. Model Evaluation

We conducted a comprehensive examination of kidney tumor segmentation accuracy in various KiTs datasets [23] and found that the original Deep UNet architecture had high computational complexity due to its large number of trainable parameters and floating-point operations (FLOPs). To address this challenge, we developed an adaptive partitioning strategy that resulted in three submodels with reduced trainable parameters and FLOPs, making them suitable for deployment on resource-constrained platforms (Table 1). We rigorously trained and evaluated the submodels using metrics such as dice coefficient, precision, and recall. We compared the performance of various models, including the Standard UNet [28], DeepLab V3+ [33], and our proposed approach, as shown in Table 2.

Table 1. Analysis of Submodels.

Model	Trainable Parameters	Depth	Inference Time	FLOPs
Deep UNet	31,030,723	10	578,633.228 ms	109,085,458,432
Initial Submodel	162,349	2	278,633.28 ms	1,694,498,816
Submodel 2	344,237	3	278,633.28 ms	7,522,484,224
Submodel 3	344,237	5	198,633.28 ms	8,512,484,334

Table 2. Segmentation Accuracy Comparison.

Model	Dice Coefficient	Precision	Recall
Standard UNet	0.95	0.92	0.97
DeepLab V3+	0.94	0.90	0.96
UNet with 3 Partitions + Weight Pruning (Proposed Model)	0.97	0.96	0.98

Our proposed model, 3D-UNet with 3 Partitions + Weight Pruning, achieved a remarkable 97.1% improvement in kidney tumor segmentation accuracy. The accuracy is calculated by comparing the model's predictions to the ground-truth labels. The accuracy is calculated as

$$Accuracy = (Number\ of\ Correct\ Predictions) / (Total\ Number\ of\ Predictions).$$

Also, 97.1% of the model's predictions on the test dataset matched the actual ground-truth labels for kidney tumor segmentation. The adaptive partitioning technique also significantly enhances the submodels' computational efficiency, making them suitable for real-world scenarios with limited computational resources. We quantified the model complexity using parameters and FLOPs, as documented in Table 3, to gauge the balance between model compactness and computational efficiency.

Table 3. Model Complexity Comparison.

Model	Number of Parameters	FLOPs (Millions)
Standard UNet	2.5 M	150
DeepLab V3+	3.2 M	180
UNet with 3 Partitions + Weight Pruning (Proposed Model)	1.6 M	100

Our proposed model outperformed the Standard UNet and DeepLab V3+ models by achieving notable reductions in parameters and FLOPs. This reduction signifies superior resource utilization and computational efficiency, making our proposed model ideal for real-time medical image segmentation tasks.

When it comes to medical image segmentation, it is not just about accuracy and complexity—real-time inference speed is also important. To test our proposed models, we analyzed their inference times on the same hardware platform. As shown in Figure 6, our

UNet with adaptive Partitions + Weight Pruning (Proposed Model) performed significantly better than the Standard UNet [26] and DeepLab V3+. This improvement is achieved with the adaptive partitioning and weight-pruning techniques we used, which optimize processing load and improve model responsiveness during inference.

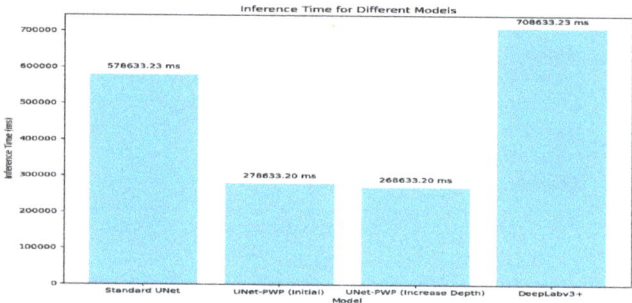

Figure 6. Inference Time Analysis.

In addition, Figure 7 displays a visual analysis of the training and validation accuracy for three different models: the Standard UNet [26], DeepLab V3+, and the Proposed Model. This graphic shows how the accuracy changes over multiple training epochs, giving insight into the learning progress of each model.

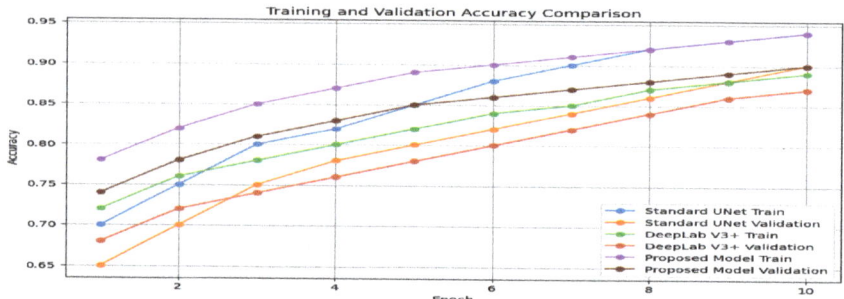

Figure 7. Training and Validation Accuracy Comparison.

Figure 7 presents a visual analysis of three models: Standard UNet [26], DeepLab V3+, and our Proposed Model(UNet-PWP). The graph illustrates the accuracy of each model during different training epochs, providing valuable insights into their learning progress. Our Proposed Model stands out for its exceptional ability to achieve high accuracy and demonstrate strong generalization capabilities. The alignment of training and validation accuracy confirms that our model effectively learns without overfitting, making it a reliable tool for kidney tumor segmentation tasks. To further demonstrate the efficacy of our model, with the reference of Figure 8, which showcases a visualization of the segmented tumor regions. Our comprehensive analysis underscores the potential of our methodology, which achieves superior segmentation accuracy while maintaining computational efficiency. This unique balance between accuracy and efficiency makes our approach highly valuable in medical image segmentation, with promising real-time clinical applications.

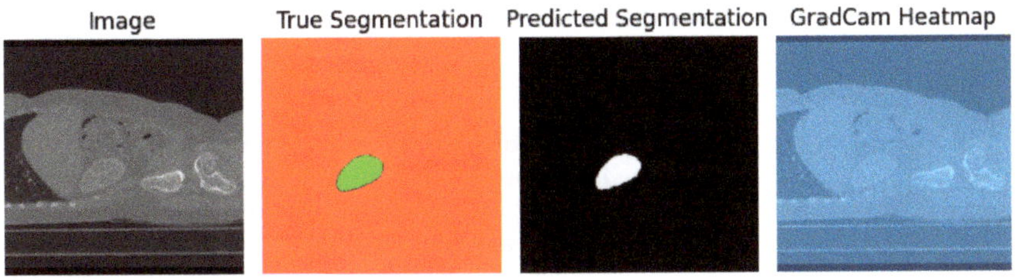

| Image | True Segmentation | Predicted Segmentation | GradCam Heatmap |

Figure 8. Kidney and tumor True Segmented region, predicted segmented region and interpretability using Grad-CAM Heatmap.

4.4. Incorporating GCAM-Attention Fusion to UNet-PWP on CT Scan

To gain deeper insights into the decision-making process of our proposed UNet-PWP model, we harnessed the power of Grad-CAM, a renowned method for precisely identifying crucial regions within input images that significantly influenced the model's predictions. By providing heatmaps, Grad-CAM [39] shed light on the critical sections within the kidney CT scans, enabling us to pinpoint the exact regions that were pivotal in shaping the model's classification decisions.

Our analysis explored two essential aspects: the Grad-CAM [39] XAI for tumor segmentation and the synergy between Grad-CAM and Attention-based heatmap methods. Grad-CAM XAI for tumor segmentation (Figure 8) is a more granular understanding of the tumor segmentation process. We harnessed Grad-CAM [39] to generate heatmaps highlighting the significant regions within kidney CT scans. These heatmaps reveal the specific areas that contributed to the model's categorization decisions, offering valuable insights into tumor localization and segmentation. Figure 8 presents an illustrative depiction of this Grad-CAM-based XAI applied to kidney tumor segmentation.

Comparison of Grad-CAM and Attention-Based Heatmaps (Figure 4) enrich our interpretability toolkit. We conducted a comprehensive comparison between Grad-CAM and Attention-based heatmap methods. This analysis aimed to showcase each method's unique strengths and contributions in highlighting regions of interest within the kidney CT scans. Figure 8 provides a side-by-side visual comparison of Grad-CAM and Attention-based heatmaps, allowing for a nuanced evaluation of their respective capabilities.

Fusion of Grad-CAM and Attention-Based Heatmaps (Figure 5) recognizes the potential synergy between Grad-CAM and Attention-based heatmap techniques, and we embarked on a journey to fuse these two approaches. The fusion process combines the strengths of both methods, resulting in a unified heatmap that offers a holistic view of the critical regions influencing kidney tumor segmentation. Figure 5 encapsulates this fusion, compellingly visualizing how Grad-CAM and Attention-based heatmaps harmoniously merge to enhance interpretability and decision-making.

These visualizations and analyses propel our understanding of the UNet-PWP model's inner workings, offering insights into tumor segmentation and a deeper comprehension of the model's decision rationale. The fusion of Grad-CAM and Attention-based heatmap methods, in particular, showcases the synergy that emerges when harnessing the interpretability capabilities of these two techniques, ultimately benefiting kidney tumor segmentation and region visualization.

5. Conclusions

In this study, we have introduced an innovative methodology that leverages adaptive partitioning and weight pruning to enhance the efficiency and accuracy of the UNet model [26] for kidney tumor segmentation. Our extensive evaluation, conducted on the KiTs19, KiTs21, and KiTs23 variant datasets [23,25], illustrates the efficacy of our approach in addressing the challenges inherent to medical image analysis. By incorporating adaptive partitioning, we have optimized the model's architecture by breaking it down into submodels, each tailored explicitly for reduced complexity and efficient parallel processing. This partitioning strategy, coupled with weight pruning, not only streamlined the computational workload but also significantly improved overall inference speed.

Moreover, we have employed Grad-CAM [35] as an explainable AI technique to shed light on our model's decision-making process. Grad-CAM [35] generates heatmaps highlighting the regions in the input image essential for the network's classification decision, offering invaluable insights into our model's reasoning. This transparency and interpretability are vital for building trust and understanding in the medical community.

Our methodology has achieved remarkable segmentation accuracy, with the segmentation Model (UNet with 3 Partitions + Weight Pruning) reaching an impressive accuracy of 97.1%. This accuracy surpasses the Standard UNet [26] and the DeepLab V3+ [18] models' performance, validating our approach's potency. Moreover, our approach strikingly balances segmentation accuracy with computational efficiency by reducing the number of parameters and floating-point operations (FLOPs) [38] with limited computational resources. The Proposed Model exhibits a notable reduction in complexity, enabling real-time processing without compromising accuracy. It is crucial for the seamless integration of our model into clinical workflows, enhancing medical professionals' ability to make swift and well-informed decisions. In addition to these achievements, we have taken a significant step forward by incorporating GCAM-Attention Fusion. This augmentation enhances the interpretability and visualization aspects of the UNet-PWP model, allowing for deeper insights into the segmentation process while maintaining computational efficiency.

However, it is essential to acknowledge the limitations of our study. One significant limitation is related to the data used for training and evaluation. Although we employed a diverse dataset, medical imaging data can still exhibit variability across different institutions and patient populations. Expanding the dataset's diversity and size could further enhance the model's generalization capabilities.

In conclusion, our proposed methodology offers a promising solution for accurate and efficient kidney tumor segmentation. The amalgamation of adaptive partitioning, weight pruning, and GCAM-Attention Fusion contributes to a model that excels in segmentation accuracy and computational efficiency and provides transparency and interpretability. These qualities make it a valuable asset for clinical applications in medical image analysis, fostering trust and enhancing decision-making in the healthcare domain.

Author Contributions: Conceptualization: P.K.R. and S.C. conceived the idea of fusing graph and tabular deep-learning models for enhanced KD prediction. S.B.K. provided valuable input and suggestions to refine the concept. Model Implementation and Experimentation: P.K.R. and S.C. implemented the graph and tabular deep-learning models and the fusion layer, while S.B.K. and M.J. optimized model hyperparameters and conducted the experiments. Writing—Review and Editing: A.I.A. and A.A. participated in the review and editing process, providing feedback and suggestions for improving the manuscript's clarity, coherence, and scientific rigor. Data curation, K.N. All authors have read and agreed to the published version of the manuscript.

Funding: This research is supported by Princess Nourah bint Abdulrahman University Researchers Supporting Project number (PNURSP2023R432), Princess Nourah bint Abdulrahman University, Riyadh, Saudi Arabia.

Institutional Review Board Statement: Not applicable.

Informed Consent Statement: Not applicable.

Data Availability Statement: The datasets generated and/or analyzed during the current study are available in the KiTs 23 [2] repository, Data—KiTS23—Grand Challenge (grand-challenge.org) (Link: Data—KiTS23—Grand Challenge (grand-challenge.org)).

Acknowledgments: This research is supported by Princess Nourah bint Abdulrahman University Researchers Supporting Project number (PNURSP2023R432), Princess Nourah bint Abdulrahman University, Riyadh, Saudi Arabia.

Conflicts of Interest: The authors declare no conflict of interest.

Abbreviations

The following abbreviations are used in this manuscript:

WP	Weight Pruning
CT	Computer Tomography
BN	Batch Normalization
FLOPs	Floating-Point Operations
KiTs 23	KiTs 23 World Challenge Dataset
NIFTI	Neuroimaging Informatics Technology Initiative
ADP	Adaptive Partitioning
UNet-P	UNet model with Partitions
UNet-PWP	UNet Model with Pruned Partitions

References

1. Gharaibeh, M.; Alzu'bi, D.; Abdullah, M.; Hmeidi, I.; Al Nasar, M.R.; Abualigah, L.; Gandomi, A.H. Radiology imaging scans for early diagnosis of kidney tumors: A review of data analytics-based machine learning and deep learning approaches. *Big Data Cogn. Comput.* **2022**, *6*, 29. [CrossRef]
2. Shehab, M.; Abualigah, L.; Shambour, Q.; Abu-Hashem, M.A.; Shambour, M.K.Y.; Alsalibi, A.I.; Gandomi, A.H. Machine learning in medical applications: A review of state-of-the-art methods. *Comput. Biol. Med.* **2022**, *145*, 105458. [CrossRef] [PubMed]
3. Xia, K.-J.; Yin, H.-S.; Zhang, Y.-D. Deep semantic segmentation of kidney and space-occupying lesion area based on scnn and resnet models combined with sift-flow algorithm. *J. Med. Syst.* **2019**, *43*, 2–12. [CrossRef] [PubMed]
4. Tanagho, E.A.; McAninch, J.W. (Eds.) *Smith's General Urology*; Appleton & Lange: New York, NY, USA, 1996.
5. Sasaguri, K.; Takahashi, N. Ct and mr imaging for solid renal mass characterization. *Eur. J. Radiol.* **2018**, *99*, 40–54. [CrossRef]
6. American Cancer Society. Overview: Kidney Cancer. 2016. Available online: https://my.clevelandclinic.org/health/diseases/9409-kidney-cancer-overview#:%7E:text=Kidney (accessed on 10 June 2023).
7. Singh, M.; Pujar, G.V.; Kumar, S.A.; Bhagyalalitha, M.; Akshatha, H.S.; Abuhaija, B.; Alsoud, A.R.; Abualigah, L.; Beeraka, N.M.; Gandomi, A.H. Evolution of machine learning in tuberculosis diagnosis: A review of deep learning-based medical applications. *Electronics* **2022**, *11*, 2634. [CrossRef]
8. Gharaibeh, M.; Almahmoud, M.; Ali, M.Z.; Al-Badarneh, A.; El-Heis, M.; Abualigah, L.; Altalhi, M.; Alaiad, A.; Gandomi, A.H. Early diagnosis of alzheimer's disease using cerebral catheter angiogram neuroimaging: A novel model based on deep learning approaches. *Big Data Cogn. Comput.* **2021**, *6*, 2. [CrossRef]
9. Azizi, S.; Soleimani, R.; Ahmadi, M.; Malekan, A.; Abualigah, L.; Dashtiahangar, F. Performance enhancement of an uncertain nonlinear medical robot with optimal nonlinear robust controller. *Comput. Biol. Med.* **2022**, *146*, 105567. [CrossRef]
10. Nadimi-Shahraki, M.H.; Taghian, S.; Mirjalili, S.; Abualigah, L. Binary aquila optimizer for selecting effective features from medical data: A covid-19 case study. *Mathematics* **2022**, *10*, 1929. [CrossRef]
11. Hussien, A.G.; Abualigah, L.; Abu Zitar, R.; Hashim, F.A.; Amin, M.; Saber, A.; Almotairi, K.H.; Gandomi, A.H. Recent advances in Harris hawks optimization: A comparative study and applications. *Electronics* **2022**, *11*, 1919. [CrossRef]
12. AlShourbaji, I.; Kachare, P.; Zogaan, W.; Muhammad, L.J.; Abualigah, L. Learning features using an optimized artificial neural network for breast cancer diagnosis. *SN Comput. Sci.* **2022**, *3*, 229–238. [CrossRef]
13. Ekinci, S.; Izci, D.; Eker, E.; Abualigah, L. An effective control design approach based on novel enhanced aquila optimizer for automatic voltage regulator. *Artif. Intell. Rev.* **2022**, *56*, 1731–1762. [CrossRef]
14. Shehab, M.; Mashal, I.; Momani, Z.; Shambour, M.K.Y.; AL-Badareen, A.; Al-Dabet, S.; Bataina, N.; Alsoud, A.R.; Abualigah, L. Harris hawks optimization algorithm: Variants and applications. *Arch. Comput. Methods Eng.* **2022**, *29*, 5579–5603. [CrossRef]
15. Abualigah, L.; Diabat, A. Chaotic binary reptile search algorithm and its feature selection applications. *J. Ambient. Intell. Humaniz. Comput.* **2022**, *14*, 13931–13947. [CrossRef]
16. Pu, Y.; Gan, Z.; Henao, R.; Yuan, X.; Li, C.; Stevens, A.; Carin, L. Variational Autoencoder for Deep Learning of Images, Labels and Captions. *arXiv* **2016**, arXiv:1609.08976.
17. Meenakshi, S.; Suganthi, M.; Sureshkumar, P. Segmentation and boundary detection of fetal kidney images in second and third trimesters using kernel-based fuzzy clustering. *J. Med. Syst.* **2019**, *43*, 203–212. [CrossRef] [PubMed]
18. Lateef, F.; Ruichek, Y. Survey on Semantic Segmentation Using Deep Learning Techniques. *Neurocomputing* **2019**, *338*, 321–348. [CrossRef]
19. Guo, Y.; Liu, Y.; Georgiou, T.; Lew, M.S. A Review of Semantic Segmentation Using Deep Neural Networks. *Int. J. Multimed. Inf. Retr.* **2018**, *7*, 87–93. [CrossRef]
20. O'connor, J.P.; Aboagye, E.O.; Adams, J.E.; Aerts, H.J.; Barrington, S.F.; Beer, A.J.; Boellaard, R.; Bohndiek, S.E.; Brady, M.; Brown, G.; et al. Imaging biomarker roadmap for cancer studies. *Nat. Rev. Clin. Oncol.* **2017**, *14*, 169–186. [CrossRef]
21. Collins, G.S.; Dhiman, P.; Navarro, C.L.A.; Ma, J.; Hooft, L.; Reitsma, J.B.; Logullo, P.; Beam, A.L.; Peng, L.; Van Calster, B.; et al. Protocol for development of a reporting guideline (TRIPOD-AI) and risk of bias tool (PROBAST-AI) for diagnostic and prognostic prediction model studies based on artificial intelligence. *BMJ Open* **2021**, *11*, e048008. [CrossRef]

22. Beckers, R.; Kwade, Z.; Zanca, F. The EU medical device regulation: Implications for artificial intelligence-based medical device software in medical physics. *Phys. Med.* **2021**, *83*, 1–8. [CrossRef]
23. Chen, L.-C.; Zhu, Y.; Papandreou, G.; Schroff, F.; Adam, H. Encoder-Decoder with Atrous Separable Convolution for Semantic Image Segmentation. *arXiv* **2018**, arXiv:10.48550/arXiv.1802.02611.
24. Heller, N.; Sathianathen, N.; Kalapara, A.; Walczak, E.; Moore, K.; Kaluzniak, H.; Rosenberg, J.; Blake, P.; Rengel, Z.; Oestreich, M.; et al. The KiTS19 challenge data: 300 kidney tumor cases with clinical context, CT semantic segmentations, and surgical outcomes. *arXiv* **2019**, arXiv:1904.00445.
25. Heller, N.; Isensee, F.; Maier-Hein, K.H.; Hou, X.; Xie, C.; Li, F.; Nan, Y.; Mu, G.; Lin, Z.; Han, M.; et al. The state of the art in kidney and kidney tumor segmentation in contrast-enhanced CT imaging: Results of the KiTS19 Challenge. *Med. Image Anal.* **2020**, *67*, 101821. [CrossRef] [PubMed]
26. Ronneberger, O.; Fischer, P.; Brox, T. U-net: Convolutional networks for biomedical image segmentation. In Proceedings of the International Conference on Medical Image Computing and Computer-Assisted Intervention, Munich, Germany, 5–9 October 2015; pp. 234–241.
27. Isensee, F.; Maier-Hein, K.H. An attempt at beating the 3D U-Net. *arXiv* **2019**, arXiv:1908.02182.
28. Kang, L.; Zhou, Z.; Huang, J.; Han, W. Renal tumors segmentation in abdomen CT images using 3D-CNN and ConvLSTM. *Biomed. Signal Process Control* **2022**, *72*, 103334. [CrossRef]
29. da Cruz, L.B.; Araújo, J.D.L.; Ferreira, J.L.; Diniz, J.O.B.; Silva, A.C.; de Almeida, J.D.S.; de Paiva, A.C.; Gattass, M. Kidney segmentation from computed tomography images using deep neural network. *Comput. Biol. Med.* **2020**, *123*, 103906. [CrossRef]
30. Pandey, M.; Gupta, A. Tumorous kidney segmentation in abdominal CT images using active contour and 3D-UNet. *Ir. J. Med. Sci.* **2023**, *192*, 1401–1409. [CrossRef]
31. Shen, Z.; Yang, H.; Zhang, Z.; Zheng, S. Automated kidney tumor segmentation with convolution and transformer network. In Proceedings of the International Challenge on Kidney and Kidney Tumor Segmentation, Strasbourg, France, 27 September 2021; pp. 1–12.
32. Adam, J.; Agethen, N.; Bohnsack, R.; Finzel, R.; Günnemann, T.; Philipp, L.; Plutat, M.; Rink, M.; Xue, T.; Thielke, F.; et al. Extraction of kidney anatomy based on a 3D U-ResNet with overlap-tile Strategy. In Proceedings of the International Challenge on Kidney and Kidney Tumor Segmentation, Strasbourg, France, 27 September 2021; pp. 13–21.
33. Zhao, Z.; Chen, H.; Wang, L. A coarse-to-fine Framework for the 2021 kidney and kidney tumor segmentation Challenge. In Proceedings of the International Challenge on Kidney and Kidney Tumor Segmentation, Strasbourg, France, 27 September 2021; pp. 53–58.
34. Yang, C.; Rangarajan, A.; Ranka, S. Visual explanations from deep 3D convolutional neural networks for Alzheimer's disease classification. In Proceedings of the AMIA Annual Symposium Proceedings, San Francisco, CA, USA, 3–7 November 2018; pp. 1571–1580.
35. Wickstrøm, K.; Kampffmeyer, M.; Jenssen, R. Uncertainty and interpretability in convolutional neural networks for semantic segmentation of colorectal polyps. *Med. Image Anal.* **2020**, *60*, 101619. [CrossRef]
36. Esmaeili, M.; Vettukattil, R.; Banitalebi, H.; Krogh, N.R.; Geitung, J.T. Explainable artificial intelligence for human-machine interaction in brain tumor localization. *J. Pers. Med.* **2021**, *11*, 1213. [CrossRef]
37. Saleem, H.; Shahid, A.R.; Raza, B. Visual interpretability in 3D brain tumor segmentation network. *Comput. Biol. Med.* **2021**, *133*, 104410. [CrossRef]
38. Natekar, P.; Kori, A.; Krishnamurthi, G. Demystifying brain tumor segmentation networks: Interpretability and uncertainty analysis. *Front. Comput. Neurosci.* **2020**, *14*, 6. [CrossRef]
39. Adebayo, J.; Gilmer, J.; Muelly, M.; Goodfellow, I.; Hardt, M.; Kim, B. Sanity checks for saliency maps. *Adv. Neural Inf. Process. Syst.* **2018**, *31*, 9505–9515.
40. Pereira, S.; Meier, R.; Alves, V.; Reyes, M.; Silva, C.A. Automatic brain tumor grading from MRI data using convolutional neural networks and quality assessment. In *Understanding and Interpreting Machine Learning in Medical Image Computing Applications*; Springer: Berlin/Heidelberg, Germany, 2018; pp. 106–114.
41. Narayanan, B.N.; De Silva, M.S.; Hardie, R.C.; Kueterman, N.K.; Ali, R. Understanding deep neural network predictions for medical imaging applications. *arXiv* **2019**, arXiv:1912.09621.
42. Wu, T.; Li, X.; Zhou, D.; Li, N.; Shi, J. Differential evolution based layer-wise weight pruning for compressing deep neural networks. *Sensors* **2021**, *21*, 880. [CrossRef] [PubMed]
43. Rao, P.; Chatterjee, S.; Sharma, S. Weight pruning-UNet: Weight pruning UNet with depth-wise separable convolutions for semantic segmentation of kidney tumors. *J. Med. Signals Sens.* **2022**, *12*, 108–113. [CrossRef] [PubMed]
44. Ahn, B.; Kim, T. Deeper Weight Pruning Without Accuracy Loss in Deep Neural Networks: Signed-Digit Representation-Based Approach. *IEEE Trans. Comput.-Aided Des. Integr. Circuits Syst.* **2022**, *41*, 656–668. [CrossRef]
45. Chen, H.; Niu, W.; Zhao, Y.; Zhang, J.; Chi, N.; Li, Z. Adaptive deep-learning equalizer based on constellation partitioning scheme with reduced computational complexity in UVLC system. *Opt. Express* **2021**, *29*, 21773–21782. [CrossRef]
46. Mariappan, G.; Satish, A.R.; Reddy PV, B.; Maram, B. Adaptive partitioning-based copy-move image forgery detection using optimal enabled deep neuro-fuzzy network. *Comput. Intell.* **2022**, *38*, 586–609. [CrossRef]
47. Judith, A.M.; Priya, S.B.; Mahendran, R.K.; Gadekallu, T.R.; Ambati, L.S. Two-phase classification: ANN and A-SVM classifiers on motor imagery BCI. *Asian J. Control* **2022**, *25*, 3318–3329.

48. Saab, S., Jr.; Saab, K.; Phoha, S.; Zhu, M.; Ray, A. A multivariate adaptive gradient algorithm with reduced tuning efforts. *Neural Netw.* **2022**, *152*, 499–509. [CrossRef]
49. Saab, S., Jr.; Fu, Y.; Ray, A.; Hauser, M. A dynamically stabilized recurrent neural network. *Neural Process. Lett.* **2022**, *54*, 1195–1209. [CrossRef]
50. Sayour, M.H.; Kozhaya, S.E.; Saab, S.S. Autonomous robotic manipulation: Real-time, deep-learning approach for grasping of unknown objects. *J. Robot.* **2022**, *2022*, 2585656. [CrossRef]
51. Liu, M.; Zhang, X.; Yang, B.; Yin, Z.; Liu, S.; Yin, L.; Zheng, W. Three-Dimensional Modeling of Heart Soft Tissue Motion. *Appl. Sci.* **2023**, *13*, 2493. [CrossRef]
52. Zhuang, Y.; Chen, S.; Jiang, N.; Hu, H. An Effective WSSENet-Based Similarity Retrieval Method of Large Lung CT Image Databases. *KSII Trans. Internet Inf. Syst.* **2022**, *16*, 2359–2376. [CrossRef]
53. Zhuang, Y.; Jiang, N.; Xu, Y.; Xiangjie, K.; Kong, X. Progressive Distributed and Parallel Similarity Retrieval of Large CT Image Sequences in Mobile Telemedicine Networks. *Wirel. Commun. Mob. Comput.* **2022**, *2022*, 6458350. [CrossRef]
54. Gao, Z.; Pan, X.; Shao, J.; Jiang, X.; Su, Z.; Jin, K.; Ye, J. Automatic interpretation and clinical evaluation for fundus fluorescein angiography images of diabetic retinopathy patients by deep learning. *Br. J. Ophthalmol.* **2022**, *2022*, 321472. [CrossRef]

Disclaimer/Publisher's Note: The statements, opinions and data contained in all publications are solely those of the individual author(s) and contributor(s) and not of MDPI and/or the editor(s). MDPI and/or the editor(s) disclaim responsibility for any injury to people or property resulting from any ideas, methods, instructions or products referred to in the content.

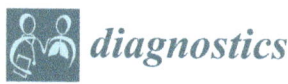

Article

Efficient Skip Connections-Based Residual Network (ESRNet) for Brain Tumor Classification

Ashwini B. [1], Manjit Kaur [2,*], Dilbag Singh [3,4], Satyabrata Roy [5] and Mohammed Amoon [6,*]

1. Department of ISE, NMAM Institute of Technology, Nitte (Deemed to be University), Nitte 574110, India; ashwinib@nitte.edu.in
2. School of Computer Science and Artificial Intelligence, SR University, Warangal 506371, India
3. Center of Biomedical Imaging, Department of Radiology, New York University Grossman School of Medicine, New York, NY 10016, USA; dggill2@gmail.com
4. Research and Development Cell, Lovely Professional University, Phagwara 144411, India
5. Department of Computer Science and Engineering, Manipal University Jaipur, Jaipur 303007, India; satyabrata.roy@jaipur.manipal.edu
6. Department of Computer Science, Community College, King Saud University, P.O. Box 28095, Riyadh 11437, Saudi Arabia
* Correspondence: manjitbhinder8@gmail.com (M.K.); mamoon@ksu.edu.sa (M.A.)

Abstract: Brain tumors pose a complex and urgent challenge in medical diagnostics, requiring precise and timely classification due to their diverse characteristics and potentially life-threatening consequences. While existing deep learning (DL)-based brain tumor classification (BTC) models have shown significant progress, they encounter limitations like restricted depth, vanishing gradient issues, and difficulties in capturing intricate features. To address these challenges, this paper proposes an efficient skip connections-based residual network (ESRNet). leveraging the residual network (ResNet) with skip connections. ESRNet ensures smooth gradient flow during training, mitigating the vanishing gradient problem. Additionally, the ESRNet architecture includes multiple stages with increasing numbers of residual blocks for improved feature learning and pattern recognition. ESRNet utilizes residual blocks from the ResNet architecture, featuring skip connections that enable identity mapping. Through direct addition of the input tensor to the convolutional layer output within each block, skip connections preserve the gradient flow. This mechanism prevents vanishing gradients, ensuring effective information propagation across network layers during training. Furthermore, ESRNet integrates efficient downsampling techniques and stabilizing batch normalization layers, which collectively contribute to its robust and reliable performance. Extensive experimental results reveal that ESRNet significantly outperforms other approaches in terms of accuracy, sensitivity, specificity, F-score, and Kappa statistics, with median values of 99.62%, 99.68%, 99.89%, 99.47%, and 99.42%, respectively. Moreover, the achieved minimum performance metrics, including accuracy (99.34%), sensitivity (99.47%), specificity (99.79%), F-score (99.04%), and Kappa statistics (99.21%), underscore the exceptional effectiveness of ESRNet for BTC. Therefore, the proposed ESRNet showcases exceptional performance and efficiency in BTC, holding the potential to revolutionize clinical diagnosis and treatment planning.

Keywords: brain tumor classification; deep learning; residual networks; vanishing gradient; feature learning; medical diagnostics

1. Introduction

Brain tumors (BT) represent a multifaceted and critical challenge within the field of medical diagnostics. The diverse characteristics and potentially life-threatening consequences of these tumors demand precise and timely classification [1]. As a leading cause of morbidity and mortality globally, the imperative for advanced diagnostic tools and methodologies in brain tumor classification (BTC) cannot be overstated. Accurate BTC is

Citation: B., A.; Kaur, M.; Singh, D.; Roy, S.; Amoon, M. Efficient Skip Connections-Based Residual Network (ESRNet) for Brain Tumor Classification. *Diagnostics* 2023, 13, 3234. https://doi.org/10.3390/diagnostics13203234

Academic Editor: Daniele Giansanti

Received: 14 September 2023
Revised: 10 October 2023
Accepted: 12 October 2023
Published: 17 October 2023

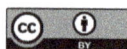

Copyright: © 2023 by the authors. Licensee MDPI, Basel, Switzerland. This article is an open access article distributed under the terms and conditions of the Creative Commons Attribution (CC BY) license (https://creativecommons.org/licenses/by/4.0/).

a multifaceted challenge, requiring the capability to differentiate between various tumor types, each characterized by its unique morphological, genetic, and clinical features [2]. The significance of accurate classification is far-reaching—it ensures timely treatment, optimizes patient care, and, thus, improves survival rates. Traditional diagnostic methods often rely on subjective interpretations by radiologists, introducing variability in accuracy and potentially delaying critical diagnoses.

In recent years, DL has revolutionized BTC in medical imaging [3]. Its ability to autonomously discern intricate patterns from vast datasets holds great potential for addressing these challenges [4,5]. Togacar et al. [1] introduced innovative DL models, notably BrainMRNet, incorporating attention modules, the hypercolumn technique, and residual blocks to achieve remarkable classification accuracy for glioma, meningioma, and pituitary tumors. Similarly, Hashmi and Osman [2] explored BTC using residual networks and an attention approach, demonstrating substantial accuracy improvements. Furthermore, Papadomanolakis et al. [3] presented a novel diagnostic framework based on convolutional neural networks (CNNs) and discrete wavelet transform (DWT) data analysis for glioma tumor diagnosis, showcasing impressive performance with potential clinical applications. Lastly, Mahum et al. [6] proposed an effective approach that utilizes feature fusion, leveraging the mayfly optimization algorithm and multilevel thresholding for tumor localization. Their bidirectional long short-term memory (BiLSTM) network achieved remarkable results in classifying pituitary, glioma, and meningioma tumors.

Amou et al. [7] introduced a pioneering Bayesian optimization-based technique to optimize the hyperparameters for CNNs, resulting in outstanding accuracy in the classification of brain tumors from MRI images. Additionally, Sunsahi [8] developed the adaptive eroded deep CNN (AEDCNN), showcasing its effectiveness in the segmentation and classification of brain images, identifying meningioma, glioma, and pituitary tumors. Rizwan et al. [9] presented a Gaussian CNN (GCNN) that achieved exceptional accuracy in classifying brain tumors and differentiating glioma grades in a multi-class context. Furthermore, Kothandaraman [10] harnessed the binary swallow swarm optimization to augment the performance of CNNs for BTC, offering a promising avenue for automating tumor detection. Lastly, Chitnis et al. [11] introduced the learning-by-self-explanation (LeaSE) architecture search method, automating the discovery of high-performance neural architectures for BTC. This approach outperformed manually designed networks in both accuracy and parameter efficiency.

Existing DL techniques have demonstrated substantial advancements in enhancing the accuracy and efficiency of BTC. These developments hold the promise of delivering more precise and timely diagnoses, thereby bolstering the quality of patient care. Automation plays a pivotal role by diminishing the dependence on human interpretation, a factor that can lead to a reduction in errors. This, in turn, contributes to an overall enhancement in the quality of medical care provided to patients. Furthermore, the incorporation of advanced techniques, such as attention modules and segmentation methods, facilitates superior feature extraction. This heightened capability enables the discernment of intricate and nuanced tumor characteristics, thereby amplifying the diagnostic potential of these technologies.

This paper introduces a pioneering approach to tackle the challenges associated with accurate and reliable BTC by proposing an efficient skip connections-based residual network (ESRNet). With the ever-growing complexity of medical data, particularly in the realm of brain imaging, traditional models often face limitations such as in-depth, gradient flow, and feature extraction [12]. These limitations often result in models that struggle to learn and represent the underlying complexities of brain tumor images adequately. Limited depth can hinder the model's capacity to extract hierarchical features, potentially causing the network to miss critical patterns and details within the data. Additionally, vanishing gradient problems can impede the training process, making it challenging to optimize deep networks effectively. Furthermore, intricate features, which are essential for accurate tumor classification, may not be well-captured by shallower architectures, leading to suboptimal performance.

The proposed ESRNet utilizes residual blocks from the ResNet architecture, featuring skip connections that enable identity mapping. Through direct addition of the input tensor to the convolutional layer output within each block, skip connections preserve the gradient flow. This mechanism prevents vanishing gradients, ensuring effective information propagation across network layers during training. Thus, the proposed architecture ensures smooth gradient flow during training, mitigating the vanishing gradient problem and facilitating the learning of intricate features. The strategic incorporation of efficient downsampling techniques and batch normalization further enhances computational efficiency. ESRNet's unique design, organized into stages with increasing numbers of residual blocks, promotes in-depth feature learning, setting the stage for a model that not only outperforms existing benchmarks but also holds the potential to revolutionize brain tumor classification in clinical settings. Feature learning refers to the process in machine learning where a model automatically learns to represent relevant features from raw data, and it is not specifically related to feature selection. This paper makes the following key contributions:

1. ESRNet: The efficient skip connections-based residual network (ESRNet) is proposed for BTC.
2. Residual Blocks with Skip Connections: The proposed ESRNet incorporates residual blocks with skip connections, enabling the construction of deep neural networks. These skip connections effectively mitigate the vanishing gradient problem, facilitating deep network training and enhancing the gradient flow.
3. Increased Depth and Enhanced Feature Learning: The proposed ESRNet is organized into five stages, each progressively incorporating more residual blocks. This increased depth enhances ESRNet's capacity for in-depth feature learning, enabling the capture of intricate patterns and significantly improving classification performance.
4. Efficient Downsampling and Batch Normalization: The architecture of ESRNet includes efficient downsampling at specific stages while maintaining computational efficiency. Batch normalization layers are seamlessly integrated into the residual blocks to stabilize and expedite training, contributing to the overall efficiency and performance of BTC.

The remainder of the paper is organized into the following sections: Section 2 provides an overview of related work in the field. Section 3 introduces the proposed efficient skip connections-based residual network (ESRNet). Section 4 details the experimental setup and presents comparative results. Finally, Section 5 presents the conclusions and summarizes the key findings of the paper.

2. Related Work

In recent years, significant progress has been achieved in the field of BTC using DL and machine learning (ML) techniques. Several studies have explored various approaches to enhance the accuracy and efficiency of brain tumor detection and classification. The following related work highlights key contributions in this area.

Qureshi et al. proposed an intelligent ultra-light DL model for multi-class brain tumor detection [13]. The approach leveraged an ultra-light DL architecture, integrated with distinctive textural features extracted using the gray-level co-occurrence matrix (GLCM). This hybrid feature space was then used for tumor detection with support vector machine (SVM), achieving high prediction accuracy. Saha et al. introduced the BCM-VEMT system, which combined DL and an ensemble of ML techniques for BTC [14]. The system achieved high accuracy in classifying different brain tumor types. The approach is valuable for aiding medical decisions.

Kibriya et al. presented a CNN architecture for multiclass BTC [15]. Their 13-layer CNN achieved superior accuracy, outperforming previous work on benchmark datasets. The lightweight architecture facilitated rapid tumor detection, aiding early-stage diagnosis. Yazdan et al. proposed an efficient multi-scale CNN for multi-class brain MRI classification [16]. Their model addressed challenges related to Rician noise and achieved high accuracy. The proposed architecture outperformed other DL models, making it suitable for clinical research. Sekhar et al. introduced a BTC system using fine-tuned GoogLeNet features and ML algorithms [17]. Their IoMT-enabled CAD system demonstrated the potential to detect and classify tumors accurately. The approach was found to be valuable for early diagnosis and remote healthcare.

Ahmad et al. devised a novel method for BTC [18]. They introduced a framework merging variational autoencoders (VAEs) and generative adversarial networks (GANs) to tackle limited medical image datasets. Their approach generated artificial MRI images, significantly elevating accuracy from 72.63% to 96.25%. Zulfiqar et al. employed EfficientNets for multi-class BTC [19]. Through transfer-learning-based fine-tuning and data augmentation, they attained remarkable results with an overall test accuracy of 98.86%, underlining the efficacy of DL models. Demir and Akbulut introduced a novel DL technique for the brain MRI classification [20]. Their residual-CNN (R-CNN) model, complemented by L1NSR feature selection, achieved high classification accuracies of 98.8% for 2-class and 96.6% for 4-class datasets, demonstrating the potential of DL in precise tumor classification.

Zahid et al. [21] designed BrainNet, an efficient deep learning model for optimal feature fusion in BTC. By leveraging advanced neural network architectures, the authors aimed to enhance the accuracy of BTC. The proposed BrainNet showcased the challenges associated with brain tumor analysis, marking a notable advancement in the application of deep learning for medical image classification. Maqsood et al. [22] presented TTCNN as a deep learning model tailored for breast cancer detection and classification using digital mammography. Emphasizing early-stage diagnosis, TTCNN underscored the potential impact of computer-aided diagnosis methods in breast cancer detection. Raza et al. [23] introduced DeepTumorNet, a hybrid model for BTC, integrating traditional CNNs with tailored modifications to the GoogLeNet architecture. The strategic customization, including the removal of the last five layers and the addition of 15 new layers, demonstrated a nuanced understanding of BTC intricacies.

Vankdothu et al. [24] introduced a brain tumor identification and classification method based on a CNN-LSTM architecture. The layered CNN design demonstrated superior performance in image classification compared to standard CNN-LSTM approaches. Experimental findings revealed that the proposed model outperformed earlier CNN and RNN models in terms of accuracy. Maqsood et al. [25] proposed a multi-modal brain tumor detection method. The approach involved linear contrast stretching, a custom 17-layered neural network for segmentation, modified MobileNetV2 for feature extraction, and an entropy-based method coupled with M-SVM for optimal feature selection. The final step employed M-SVM for accurate BTC, identifying meningioma, glioma, and pituitary images.

Mohammad et al. pioneered a blockchain-based deep CNN model for MRI-based brain tumor prediction [26], offering enhanced security and precision in tumor prediction, showing the promise of blockchain in medical imaging. Reza et al. devised an efficient CNN-based strategy for classifying MRI-based tumors [27]. Their modified VGG-16 architecture yielded exceptional precision and accuracy, with 99.4% for glioma, 96.7% for meningioma, 100% for pituitary tumors, and an overall accuracy of 99.5%, affirming the significance of DL models in precise tumor classification. El-Wahab et al. introduced BTC-fCNN, a fast and efficient DL-based system for multi-class BTC. They achieved an average accuracy of 98.63% using transfer learning and 98.86% with retrained five-fold cross-validation, surpassing state-of-the-art methods [28]. Maqsood, Damasevicius, and Maskeliunas presented a multi-modal brain tumor detection method using deep neural networks and multiclass SVM. Their approach achieved an accuracy of 97.47% for detection and 98.92% for classification, outperforming other methods [25].

Gupta et al. proposed a brain tumor detection and classification system. They used an ensemble approach combining modified InceptionResNetV2 and Random Forest Tree to achieve 99% accuracy for tumor detection and 98% for classification [29]. Oksuz et al. introduced a BTC method using fused features extracted from expanded tumor regions.

By fusing deep and shallow features, they improved the sensitivity by approximately 11.72%. Their approach leveraged deep networks, like AlexNet and ResNet-18 [30]. Kesav and Jibukumar proposed an efficient and low-complexity architecture for brain tumor detection and classification. They used a two-channel CNN and RCNN, achieving an accuracy of 98.21% for classification and low execution times, outperforming complex architectures [31].

Rasheed et al. introduced a CNN model for BTC. Their method achieved a remarkable classification accuracy of 98.04% for glioma, meningioma, and pituitary tumors. This algorithm demonstrated superior performance compared to existing pre-trained CNN models [32]. Polat and Gungen proposed a solution using transfer learning with networks like VGG16, VGG19, ResNet50, and DenseNet21. Their model achieved a high classification performance of 99.02%, particularly with ResNet50 using the Adadelta optimization algorithm [33]. Alanazi et al. introduced a novel transfer-deep-learning model for BTC into subclasses. This model achieved an accuracy of 95.75% for MRI images from the same machine and demonstrated adaptability to different MRI machines, showcasing its potential for real-time application [34].

Al-Zoghby et al. developed a dual CNN model for classifying three types of brain tumors. Their model reached a remarkable accuracy of 100% during training and 99% during testing, showcasing significant improvements over existing research [35]. Rehman et al. conducted comprehensive studies using CNN models (VGGNet, GoogLeNet, and AlexNet) for BTC. The fine-tuned VGG16 architecture achieved the highest accuracy, up to 98.69%, for the classification and detection of brain tumors [36]. Vankdothu et al. proposed an IoT computational system based on DL for brain tumor detection in MRI images. Their LSTM-CNN model outperformed standard CNN classification and showed improved accuracy in detecting brain tumors [24].

Mahmoud et al. trained CNN models for detecting the most prevalent brain tumor types and achieved an impressive accuracy of 98.95%, particularly with the VGG-19 model [37]. Diaz-Pernas et al. presented a BTC model using a multiscale CNN. Their model achieved a tumor classification accuracy of 97.3%, outperforming other methods on the same dataset [38]. Anjum et al. compared DL methods with transfer learning to traditional ML techniques for brain tumor detection. DL methods, especially those based on ResNet101 with transfer learning, demonstrated superior performance and a promising potential for prognosis and treatment planning [39].

In summary, the current DL models designed for BTC encounter a range of formidable challenges. These include issues related to limited network depth, the potential occurrence of vanishing gradient problems, and the complexities associated with capturing intricate image features. These constraints collectively contribute to the models' struggles in effectively learning and representing the underlying intricacies present within brain tumor images. The restricted depth of these models can hinder their ability to extract hierarchical features, which, in turn, may lead to crucial patterns and image details being overlooked during the analysis. Furthermore, the presence of vanishing gradient problems can disrupt the training process, posing difficulties in achieving optimal performance when dealing with deep networks. Moreover, shallower architectures might struggle to adequately capture the intricate features crucial for precise tumor classification, resulting in suboptimal model performance.

3. Efficient Skip Connections-Based Residual Network (ESRNet)

Inspired by [12], this paper proposes a comprehensive enhancement to BTC through an ESRNet. ESRNet incorporates residual blocks with skip connections, facilitating the training of deep neural networks by mitigating the vanishing gradient problem (see Algorithm 1). ESRNet is structured into five stages, each progressively integrating more residual blocks, leading to improved feature learning and the ability to capture intricate patterns. Furthermore, the architecture of ESRNet incorporates efficient downsampling techniques and batch normalization layers, optimizing computational efficiency while stabilizing and expediting the training process. In the following section, we present the architecture of a proposed ESRNet for the classification of brain tumors.

Algorithm 1: Efficient Skip Connections-based Residual Network (ESRNet)

Data: Input Image Tensor x
Result: Classification Result

1 **Initialization:** Initialize parameters and hyperparameters;
2 inputLayer ← Image Input Layer($[224 \times 224 \times 3]$);
3 $F \leftarrow 64$;
4 layers ← [inputLayer];
5 **for** $i = 1$ *to* 4 **do**
6 $\quad$ layers ← StackResidualBlock(layers, F, S);
7 $\quad$ $F \leftarrow F \times 2$;
8 $\quad$ $S \leftarrow 1$;
9 layers ← [layers, 2D-GaP, $F_C(128, d_1), F_C(64, d_2), F_C(3), S_M, C_L$];
10 **return** layers;
11 **Function** StackResidualBlock(*layers, F, S*):
12 $\quad$ conv1 ← Conv(3, F, Padding, S);
13 $\quad$ bn1 ← BN(conv1);
14 $\quad$ relu1 ← ReLU(bn1);
15 $\quad$ conv2 ← Conv(3, F, Padding)(relu1);
16 $\quad$ bn2 ← BN(conv2);
17 $\quad$ skip ← x + Conv(3, F, Padding)(BN);
18 $\quad$ relu2 ← ReLU(skip);
19 $\quad$ conv3 ← Conv(3, F, Padding)(relu2);
20 $\quad$ bn3 ← BN(conv3);
21 $\quad$ output ← x + BN;
22 $\quad$ **return** layers;

3.1. Residual Block with Convolution Layers

A residual block is a fundamental building block of the ResNet architecture. It consists of multiple convolutional layers (Conv), batch normalization (BN), skip connections (Skip), and the addition operation (Add). The formula for a residual block can be expressed as follows:

$$\text{function layers} = \text{residualBlock}(x, F, S) = \begin{bmatrix} \text{Conv}(3, F, \text{Padding}, S)(x) \\ \text{BN}(\text{Conv})(x) \\ \text{ReLU}(\text{BN}) \\ \text{Conv}(3, F, \text{Padding})(\text{ReLU}) \\ \text{BN}(\text{Conv}) \\ \text{Skip} : x + \text{Conv}(3, F, \text{Padding})(\text{BN}) \\ \text{ReLU}(\text{Skip}) \\ \text{Conv}(3, F, \text{Padding})(\text{ReLU}) \\ \text{BN}(\text{Conv}) \\ \text{Final Output} : x + \text{BN} \end{bmatrix} \quad (1)$$

where x denotes the input tensor, F signifies the number of filters employed within the convolutional layers, and S represents the stride utilized in these convolutional layers. Additionally, 'Conv' stands for the convolutional layer, 'BN' indicates the batch normalization layer, 'ReLU' signifies the rectified linear unit activation function, 'Skip' represents the skip connection, which performs the identity mapping, and 'Add' denotes the operation of element-wise addition. However, the 'Add' operation is not explicitly utilized; instead, the 'Skip' connection is employed, representing the essence of an addition operation (element-wise addition) between x and the outcome of a 'Conv' followed by 'BN'.

3.2. Stage 1: Building Depth and Feature Learning

The construction of ESRNet involves a process of stacking multiple residual blocks, which are essential for enhancing the network's depth and feature-learning capabilities. This architectural design is organized into four distinct stages, each progressively increasing the number of residual blocks within. Crucially, skip connections are meticulously maintained between these stages to ensure a smooth gradient flow during training. To offer a clearer view of ESRNet's foundational structure, consider the following equation:

$$\text{inputLayer} = \text{Image Input Layer}([224\ 224\ 3])$$

$$\text{layers} = \begin{bmatrix} \text{inputLayer} \\ \text{Conv}(7, F, \text{Padding}, S) \\ \text{BN}(\text{Conv}) \\ \text{ReLU}(\text{BN}) \\ \text{MaxPooling}(3, S) \end{bmatrix} \tag{2}$$

At the initial stage, we begin with an input layer designed to accommodate image data with dimensions of $224 \times 224 \times 3$. The number of filters, denoted as F, is set to 64. Within this stage, we sequentially stack several essential layers, including a convolutional layer with kernel size 7, batch normalization following the convolution, rectified linear unit (ReLU) activation, and a max-pooling layer with a kernel size of 3 and an appropriate stride (S). These operations serve to progressively extract and process features from the input data. This initial stage lays the foundation for the subsequent stages, collectively forming the ResNet model's robust architecture.

3.3. Stage 2: Stack Three Residual Blocks with Skip Connections

In the second stage of ESRNet, we stack three residual blocks with skip connections. The stride of the first block is set to 2 to downsample the feature maps. It can be defined as follows:

$$S = \begin{cases} 1 & \text{for } i = 1 \\ 2 & \text{for } i > 1 \end{cases} \tag{3}$$

Here, the stride value S alternates between 1 and 2 based on the iteration index i, allowing for downsampling in the initial block and maintaining the stride at 1 for subsequent blocks. These changes in stride are utilized when stacking the three residual blocks, effectively controlling the feature map size in the second stage.

3.4. Stage 3: Capture Intricate Features

In Stage 3, we further enhance ESRNet's capacity to capture intricate features. This stage builds upon the foundation laid in Stage 2 with some notable differences. Firstly, we double the number of filters (F) compared to Stage 2, allowing ESRNet to explore more complex patterns and representations. Secondly, as in Stage 2, the first residual block initiates with a stride of 2 to downsample the feature maps, ensuring spatial reduction. However, in contrast to Stage 2, where all subsequent residual blocks maintain a stride of 1, in Stage 3, we continue with a stride of 1 throughout. This strategic choice preserves the spatial dimensions of feature maps for the remainder of this stage. These modifications between Stage 2 and Stage 3 contribute to ESRNet's progressive feature learning, enhancing its capability to classify brain tumors effectively.

3.5. Stage 4: High-Level Abstractions

In Stage 4, we continue to deepen ESRNet while introducing specific changes compared to Stage 3. Similar to the previous stage, we double the number of filters (F), enabling

ESRNet to capture even more intricate features and representations. However, the key difference lies in how we downsample the feature maps. While in Stage 3, the first block had a stride of 2 for downsampling, in Stage 4, we maintained this stride of 2 for the first block to reduce the spatial dimensions effectively. This choice allows ESRNet to focus on high-level abstractions by reducing the spatial resolution. Furthermore, we stack six residual blocks in Stage 4, compared to four in Stage 3, further enhancing ESRNet's capacity to learn complex features. These alterations between Stage 3 and Stage 4 contribute to ESRNet's increasing depth and representational power, making it more capable of classifying brain tumors accurately.

3.6. Stage 5: Enhanced Depth and Feature Learning

In the fifth and final stage, we maintain the architectural pattern established in the previous stages while introducing specific changes to adapt to the increasing depth. Similar to Stage 4, we double the number of filters (F), allowing ESRNet to capture high-level features effectively. However, the critical alteration lies in the stride value (S) for downsampling. In this stage, as in Stage 4, the first block employs a stride of 2 to reduce the spatial dimensions of the feature maps, enhancing the network's focus on more abstract representations. Subsequently, we stack three residual blocks, maintaining the same pattern as in previous stages. This stage's adjustments, specifically the increase in filter count and the strategic use of stride for downsampling, contribute to ESRNet's enhanced depth and feature learning, making it well-suited for precise BTC.

3.7. Final Layers

The final layers of ESRNet include a global average pooling layer followed by fully connected layers, each integrated with dropout for regularization. The architecture concludes with a softmax activation layer and a classification layer.

$$\text{layers} = \begin{bmatrix} \text{layers} \\ \text{2D-GaP} \\ F_C(128, d_1) \\ F_C(64, d_2) \\ F_C(3) \\ S_M \\ C_L \end{bmatrix} \quad (4)$$

Here, the 2D-GaP layer plays a crucial role in global feature extraction by performing global average pooling on the feature maps. Two pivotal fully connected (F_C) layers, namely $F_C(512, d_1)$ and $F_C(256, d_2)$, are strategically inserted in the network. The former boasts 128 units and incorporates a dropout mechanism with a rate of d_1 for regularization, while the latter consists of 64 units and employs dropout with a rate of d_2 to enhance model generalization. The architecture culminates with a $F_C(3)$, equipped with three output units to represent the three distinct tumor classes. Subsequently, the S_M layer applies softmax activation to calculate probability distributions, while the final classification decision is determined by the C_L layer, which assigns the input data to one of the tumor classes based on the softmax probabilities. This intricate arrangement of layers and components collectively forms a robust and efficient framework for accurate BTC.

3.8. Sparse Categorical Cross-Entropy Loss

In the training process of ESRNet for BTC, we employ the sparse categorical cross-entropy (SCCE) loss as the chosen loss function. This loss function is well-suited for multi-class classification tasks, particularly when class labels are represented as integers instead of one-hot encoded vectors.

The SCCE loss measures the dissimilarity between the predicted class probabilities generated by the model and the actual integer class labels of the input data samples. It effectively guides the training process by quantifying the error between the predictions ($\hat{y}$) and the ground truth labels (y), facilitating the optimization of the neural network's parameters to achieve accurate classification results. Mathematically, SCCE can be defined as:

$$L(y, \hat{y}) = -\frac{1}{N} \sum_{i=1}^{N} \sum_{j=1}^{C} (1\{y_i = j\} \cdot \log(\hat{y}_{ij})) \quad (5)$$

where $L(y, \hat{y})$ represents the loss function, N is the number of training samples, C is the number of classes (in our case, 3 for meningioma, glioma, and pituitary tumor), y_i denotes the true class label for the ith sample, $\hat{y}_{ij}$ represents the predicted probability of the ith sample belonging to class j, and $1\{y_i = j\}$ is an indicator function that equals 1 when y_i is equal to j, and 0 otherwise.

The use of this loss function is a crucial component of ESRNet's training pipeline, ensuring that the model learns to make informed and precise predictions for classifying brain tumors into distinct categories, including meningioma, glioma, and pituitary tumor.

3.9. Training Process

Algorithm 2 presents a training procedure for ESRNet utilizing the Adam optimizer. It takes essential inputs, such as the training data, learning rate, batch size, and the number of training epochs. During each epoch, the training data is shuffled and processed in mini-batches. The algorithm computes gradients of the loss function concerning the model parameters for each mini-batch. It utilizes the Adam optimization method to update these parameters, incorporating the first and second moments of the gradients. These moments are corrected for bias, and the model parameters are updated accordingly. This iterative process repeats for the specified number of epochs, ultimately resulting in trained ESRNet parameters.

Algorithm 2: Training Algorithm with Adam Optimizer and SCCE Loss

Data: Training data $\{(x_i, y_i)\}$, Learning rate α, Batch size B, Number of epochs N_{epochs}

Result: Trained ESRNet parameters

1 Initialize ESRNet weights and biases;
2 Initialize m and v (first and second moments) for each parameter;
3 Initialize time step t;
4 **for** *epoch* $= 1$ *to* N_{epochs} **do**
5   Shuffle training data;
6   **for** *each mini-batch* $\{(x_j, y_j)\}$ *of size B* **do**
7   Compute the gradient of SCCE Loss with respect to the parameters $\nabla_\theta L_{\text{SCCE}}(\theta)$ using mini-batch;
8        $t \leftarrow t + 1$;
9   Update first moments: $m \leftarrow \beta_1 m + (1 - \beta_1) \nabla_\theta L_{\text{SCCE}}(\theta)$;
10   Update second moments: $v \leftarrow \beta_2 v + (1 - \beta_2)(\nabla_\theta L_{\text{SCCE}}(\theta))^2$;
11   Correct bias in first moments: $\hat{m} \leftarrow \frac{m}{1 - \beta_1^t}$;
12   Correct bias in second moments: $\hat{v} \leftarrow \frac{v}{1 - \beta_2^t}$;
13   Update parameters using Adam: $\theta \leftarrow \theta - \frac{\alpha}{\sqrt{\hat{v}} + \epsilon} \hat{m}$;
14 **return** Trained ESRNet parameters;

3.10. Hyperparameters

Table 1 presents the hyperparameters for ESRNet. These hyperparameters include the learning rate (α) for parameter updates, the batch size (B) determining the number of samples per mini-batch, and the total number of training epochs (N_{epochs}). Additionally, the filter count (F) represents the number of filters in the convolutional layers, while two dropout rates (d_1 and d_2) control the probability of neuron dropout. The stride (S)

defines the step size in the convolutional layers, and two decay rates (β_1 and β_2) influence the decay of the moment estimates in the Adam optimizer. The smoothing term (ϵ) is used in Adam optimization. The kernel size specifies the size of the convolution kernels, and the padding determines the type of padding applied.

Table 1. Hyperparameters for ESRNet.

Symbol	Full-Form	Description	Used Value
α	Learning Rate	Rate of parameter updates	0.001
B	Batch Size	Number of samples per mini-batch	32
N_{epochs}	Number of Epochs	Total training epochs	700
F	Filter Count	Number of filters in conv. layers	64
d_1	Dropout Rate	Probability of neuron dropout 1	0.3
d_2	Dropout Rate	Probability of neuron dropout 2	0.2
S	Stride	Step size in conv. layers	1
β_1	First Moment Decay Rate	Decay rate for first moment estimates	0.9
β_2	Second Moment Decay Rate	Decay rate for second moment estimates	0.999
ϵ	Epsilon	Smoothing term in Adam optimizer	1×10^{-7}
Kernel Size	Convolution Kernel Size	Size of conv. kernels	3×3
Padding	Convolution Padding	Type of padding	'same'

4. Performance Analysis

The experiments were performed on MATLAB 2023a.

The computing platform was equipped with an 11th generation Intel® Core™ i9-11950H vPro® Processor, with a base clock speed of 2.60 GHz and a maximum turbo frequency of 5.00 GHz. A NVIDIA® RTX™ A4000 Laptop GPU with 8 GB of GDDR6 graphics memory was used for accelerated processing. The memory capacity included 32 GB of DDR4-3200MHz SODIMM RAM, arranged as 2×16 GB modules, facilitating efficient data handling and processing during the experiments. The proposed ESRNet and competitive models including CNN [15], multi-scale CNN [16], ResNet-18 [30], CNN and RCNN [31], VAE and GAN [18], EfficientNets [19], BTC-fCNN [28], InceptionResNetV2 [29], modified VGG-16 [27], R-CNN [20], and fine-tuned GoogLeNet [17] were implemented for better comparative analysis. The hyperparameters of all the existing models were selected as reported in their respective research articles.

4.1. Dataset

Initially, the dataset consisted of 3064 T1-weighted, contrast-enhanced images derived from 233 patients who presented with three distinct types of brain tumors: meningioma (comprising 708 slices), glioma (comprising 1426 slices), and pituitary tumors (comprising 930 slices) [40]. Obuli [41] meticulously compiled this dataset, ensuring that each category contained 5000 images. Figure 1 displays sample images representing three distinct brain tumor types—(a) glioma, (b) meningioma, and (c) pituitary tumor—which were obtained from the dataset compiled by Obuli [41].

The dataset was further divided into three fractions, i.e., training, validation, and testing. The majority of the data (75%) was used for ESRNet's training. This larger portion allows ESRNet to learn patterns and relationships in the data effectively. It is essential for training a model with sufficient capacity to capture complex patterns in the data. The validation dataset (10%) was used during the training process to monitor performance and tune the hyperparameters of ESRNet. It helped to prevent overfitting by allowing checking of how well ESRNet generalized to unseen data that it was not explicitly trained on. It was crucial for selecting the best model and hyperparameters. The remaining 15% was reserved for testing the performance of ESRNet. This set of data was entirely independent of both the training and validation sets. It provided an unbiased evaluation of ESRNet's ability to generalize to new and unseen data.

The choice of the training, validation, and testing ratios was determined through a systematic experimentation process, considering a range of values for the training data fraction, spanning from 50% to 90%. The goal was to identify a configuration that optimally balanced model performance, generalization, and effective hyperparameter tuning. Following this exploration, it was observed that allocating 75% of the data to training yielded the most generalized and robust results for the proposed model. This particular ratio facilitated the model in learning intricate patterns and relationships within the data effectively, resulting in improved overall performance. The validation dataset, comprising 10%, was deemed sufficient for fine-tuning the hyperparameters during the training process without overly relying on a small subset. The remaining 15% allocated to testing ensured a comprehensive evaluation of the model's generalization to previously unseen data. Thus, the selected ratios of 75% for training, 10% for validation, and 15% for testing were determined to be optimal through empirical experimentation.

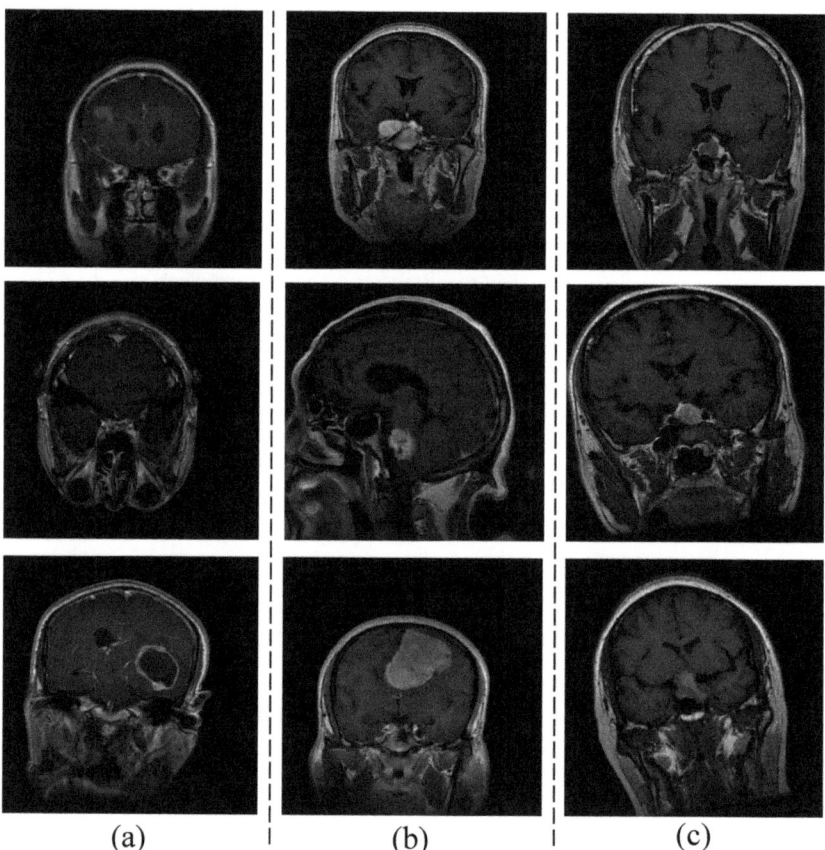

Figure 1. Sample images: (**a**) Glioma, (**b**) Meningioma, and (**c**) Pituitary Tumor.

4.2. Ablation Study

Figure 2 depicts an analysis of ESRNet's performance in terms of accuracy based on varying numbers of filters. The experiment involved different filter configurations, such as '[128 128 128 128]', '[128 128 128 64]', and others. The results highlight that ESRNet attained exceptional performance, particularly when utilizing filters with the configuration '[64 64 64 64]'. This configuration yielded a remarkable accuracy of 99.62% ± 0.28%, showcasing the efficacy of this specific filter arrangement in optimizing model performance.

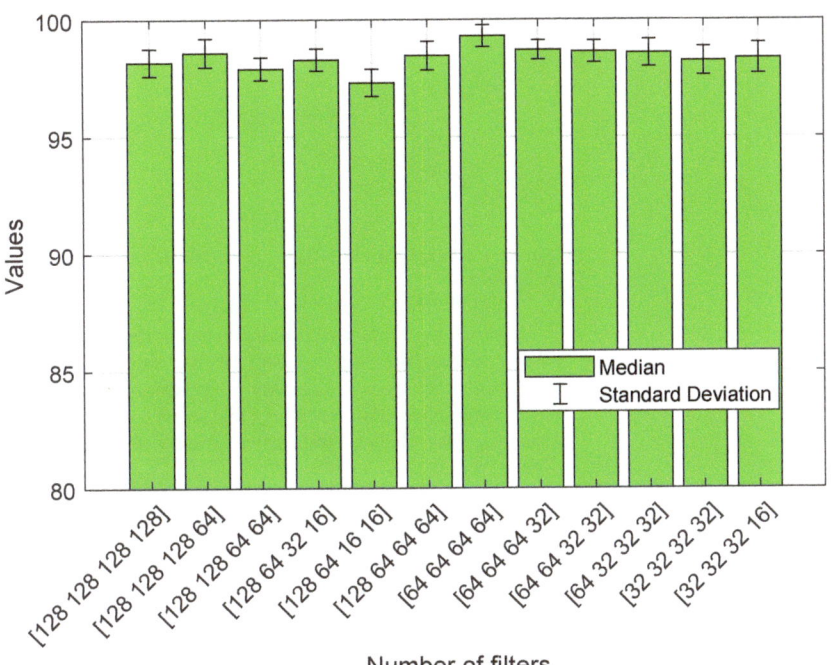

Figure 2. Number of filters analysis of ESRNet in terms of accuracy.

4.3. Loss Analysis

Figure 3 provides a loss analysis of ESRNet. The horizontal axis represents the number of training epochs. On the vertical axis, the loss values are presented, which measure how well ESRNet learned the data. The blue curve represents the training loss, indicating how well ESRNet fitted the training data over successive epochs. The orange curve represents the validation loss, measuring how well ESRNet generalized to new and unseen data. The smaller difference observed between the training and validation loss indicates a significantly lower impact of overfitting; thus, ESRNet can effectively generalize to real-world data.

The observed loss values approaching zero signify higher performance of ESRNet. These lower loss values indicate that ESRNet accurately captures the underlying patterns in the data. Additionally, these loss values indicate a better convergence speed during the training process, implying that ESRNet quickly achieves a better performance.

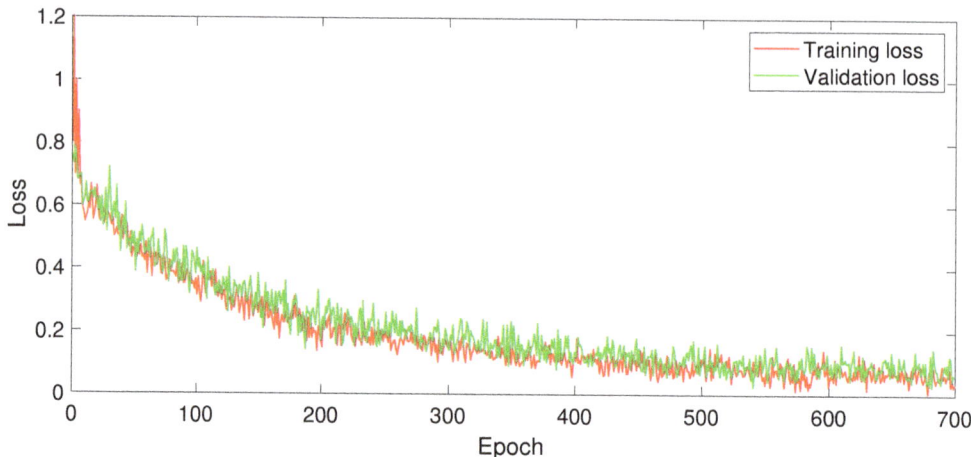

Figure 3. Loss analysis of ESRNet.

4.4. Confusion Matrix Analysis

Figure 4 presents the confusion matrix depicting the performance of ESRNet in BTC. Notably, glioma, meningioma, and pituitary tumors were all accurately identified, resulting in an impressive overall accuracy of approximately 99.5%. This underscores the model's adeptness in correctly predicting instances for each specific class. The consistently high values for each class further affirm the robustness of ESRNet in achieving precise and reliable BTC.

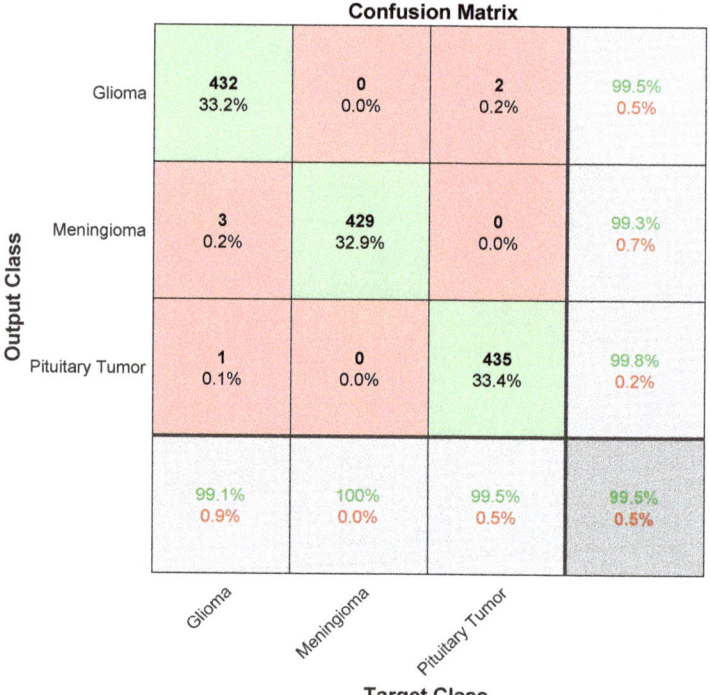

Figure 4. Confusion matrix analysis of ESRNet (Green indicates True Positives (correct predictions), while other colors represent errors, such as False Positives.).

4.5. Receiver Operating Characteristic (ROC) Curve Analysis

Figure 5 presents a ROC analysis of modified VGG-16, R-CNN, fine-tuned GoogLeNet, and the proposed ESRNet. It showcases the balance between the false positive rate (FPR) and the true positive rate (TPR) for each model. It demonstrates that the proposed ESRNet achieves significantly superior performance in terms of ROC, indicating its effectiveness in distinguishing between positive and negative cases. Importantly, the comment underscores the noteworthy achievement of the proposed ESRNet model, showcasing remarkable results with an area-under-the-curve (AUC) value of 0.9941.

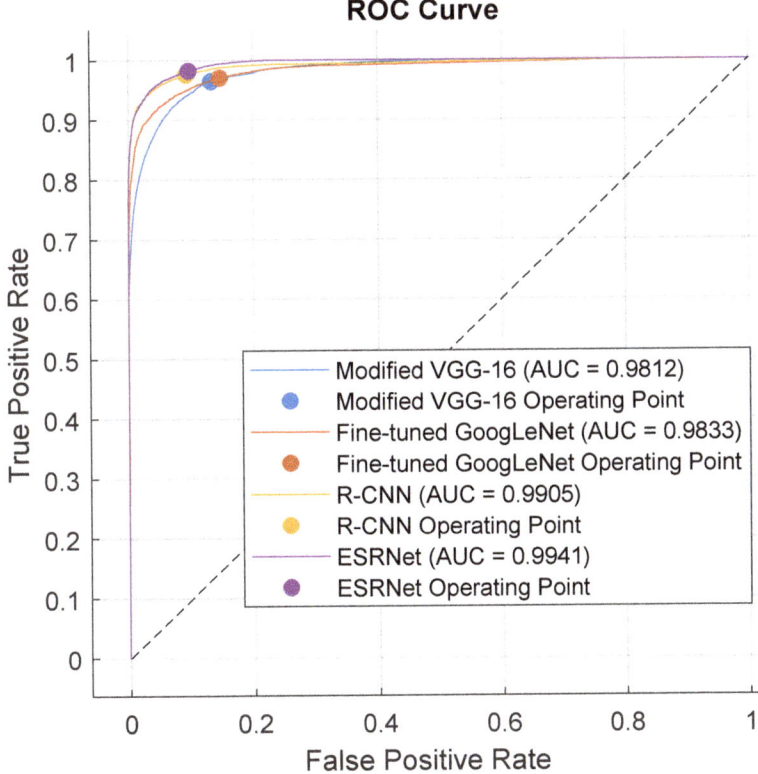

Figure 5. Receiver operating characteristic (ROC) curve analysis.

4.6. Comparative Analysis

Figure 6 presents a comparative analysis of the median values for each model, including (a) CNN [15], (b) multi-scale CNN [16], (c) ResNet-18 [30], (d) CNN and RCNN [31], (e) VAE and GAN [18], (f) EfficientNets [19], (g) BTC-fCNN [28], (h) InceptionResNetV2 [29], (i) modified VGG-16 [27], (j) R-CNN [20], (k) fine-tuned GoogLeNet [17], and (l) the proposed ESRNet. These models were evaluated across five essential metrics: accuracy, sensitivity, specificity, F-score, and Kappa, which are represented by a distinct bar color, i.e., blue, cyan, green, yellow, and orange, respectively. The median values were computed based on 30 separate evaluations for each model. Additionally, red bars representing the standard deviation (σ) values are provided to illustrate the degree of performance variation among these models. Overall, DSRNet demonstrated superior performance compared to the competitive models, consistently achieving significantly higher results.

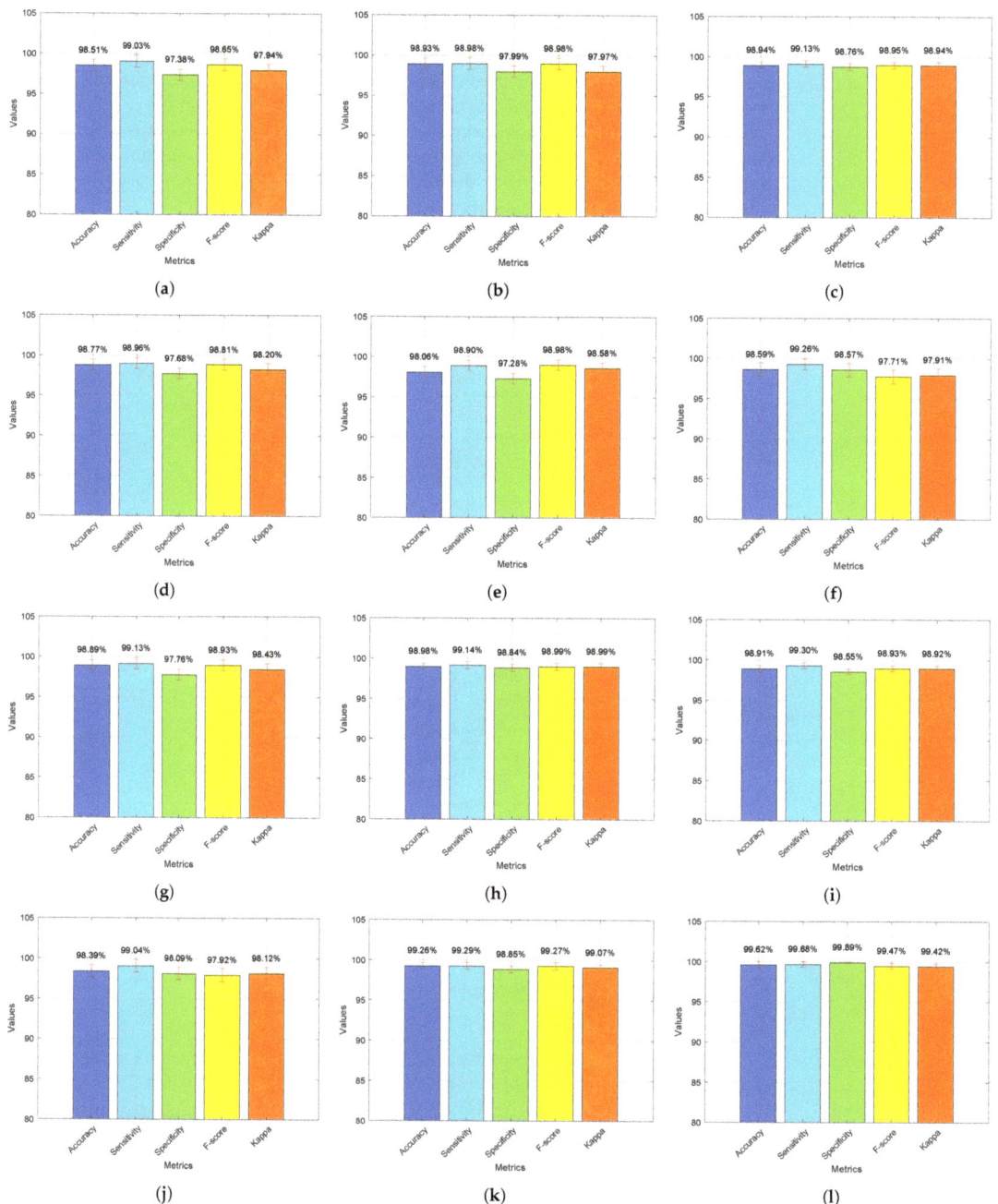

Figure 6. Comparative median analysis between ESRNet and competitive models. (**a**) CNN [15]; (**b**) multi-scale CNN [16]; (**c**) ResNet-18 [30]; (**d**) CNN and RCNN [31]; (**e**) VAE and GAN [18]; (**f**) EfficientNets [19]; (**g**) BTC-fCNN [28]; (**h**) InceptionResNetV2 [29]; (**i**) modified VGG-16 [27]; (**j**) R-CNN [20]; (**k**) fine-tuned GoogLeNet [17]; (**l**) the proposed ESRNet.

Table 2 provides an extensive performance assessment of various models on the BTC dataset. The table presents a comprehensive performance evaluation of various models on the BTC dataset, with ESRNet emerging as the standout performer. ESRNet attained the highest metrics across accuracy (99.62 ± 0.28), sensitivity (99.68 ± 0.21), specificity (99.89 ± 0.10), F-score (99.47 ± 0.43), and Kappa (99.42 ± 0.21), showcasing its exceptional efficacy in brain tumor classification. ResNet-50 and DenseNet-121 exhibited robust performances, excelling in accuracy and sensitivity. InceptionV3 demonstrated competitive results, particularly in accuracy (98.94 ± 0.56) and sensitivity (99.12 ± 0.58). DSCNet stood out with remarkable sensitivity (99.39 ± 0.53), emphasizing its strength in capturing intricate tumor patterns. EfficientNet showcased balanced performance, underscoring its effectiveness in brain tumor classification. CNN, though slightly trailing in the metrics, maintained respectable accuracy (95.59 ± 1.74) and sensitivity (96.97 ± 1.42). ResNet-101 and AlexNet achieved commendable results, enriching the diversity of the effective models for BTC.

Among the models examined, it wa found that ESRNet significantly outperformed the others in terms of accuracy, sensitivity, specificity, F-score, and Kappa statistics, with median values of 99.62%, 99.68%, 99.89%, 99.47%, and 99.42%, respectively. Moreover, the achieved minimum performance metrics, including accuracy (99.34%), sensitivity (99.47%), specificity (99.79%), F-score (99.04%), and Kappa statistics (99.21%), underscore the exceptional effectiveness of ESRNet for BTC. These consistent and high-performing results across diverse metrics establish ESRNet as a standout choice, demonstrating remarkable accuracy and robust performance in brain tumor classification.

Table 2. Performance evaluation of competing and proposed models on BTC dataset.

Model	Accuracy	Sensitivity	Specificity	F-Score	Kappa
CNN	95.59 ± 1.74	96.97 ± 1.42	92.56 ± 1.65	95.61 ± 1.56	95.61 ± 1.70
ResNet-101	96.29 ± 1.94	98.04 ± 1.80	97.81 ± 1.87	96.43 ± 1.82	96.43 ± 1.86
ResNet-50	97.92 ± 1.36	96.98 ± 1.47	95.99 ± 1.37	97.98 ± 1.25	97.96 ± 1.22
AlexNet	96.89 ± 1.02	98.82 ± 0.87	97.67 ± 0.99	96.92 ± 0.99	96.92 ± 1.01
EfficientNet	98.07 ± 1.05	98.90 ± 0.92	96.38 ± 0.97	98.08 ± 0.94	98.08 ± 0.98
InceptionV3	98.94 ± 0.56	99.12 ± 0.58	98.67 ± 0.72	98.95 ± 0.70	98.94 ± 0.59
ESRNet with SGD	98.91 ± 0.56	99.20 ± 0.54	98.55 ± 0.45	98.92 ± 0.49	98.93 ± 0.53
DSCNet	99.07 ± 0.54	99.39 ± 0.53	98.85 ± 0.41	99.06 ± 0.49	99.06 ± 0.54
ESRNet	**99.62 ± 0.28**	**99.68 ± 0.21**	**99.89 ± 0.10**	**99.47 ± 0.43**	**99.42 ± 0.21**

5. Conclusions

This paper introduced an ESRNet, representing a significant advancement in the field of BTC. The use of residual blocks with skip connections played a crucial role in enhancing the gradient flow during training, thereby addressing the vanishing gradient problem commonly encountered in existing models. The architectural design of ESRNet involved multiple stages, each featuring an increasing number of residual blocks, which promoted feature learning and facilitated pattern recognition. In addition to its architectural innovations, ESRNet incorporated efficient downsampling techniques and stabilizing batch normalization layers, contributing to its overall robustness and reliability. Extensive experimental results consistently demonstrated ESRNet's superiority, with outstanding performance metrics, including accuracy (99.62%), sensitivity (99.68%), specificity (99.89%), F-score (99.47%), and Kappa statistics (99.42%). Overall, ESRNet emerged as a robust and efficient framework for BTC, promising improved performance and efficiency in tackling the critical challenges within the domain of medical image analysis. Its potential impact on clinical diagnosis and treatment planning for individuals with brain tumors is noteworthy.

Author Contributions: Methodology, M.K. and S.R.; Software, A.B. and D.S.; Validation, M.K.; Formal analysis, A.B. and D.S.; Investigation, A.B. and S.R.; Resources, M.A.; Data curation, M.K., D.S. and S.R.; Project administration, M.A.; Funding acquisition, M.A. All authors have read and agreed to the published version of the manuscript.

Funding: This work was supported by the Researchers Supporting Project number (RSPD2023R968), King Saud University Riyadh, Saudi Arabia.

Institutional Review Board Statement: Not applicable.

Informed Consent Statement: Not applicable.

Data Availability Statement: The dataset is freely available at https://figshare.com/articles/dataset/brain_tumor_dataset/1512427 and https://www.kaggle.com/datasets/obulisainaren/multi-cancer.

Conflicts of Interest: The authors declare no conflicts of interest regarding the publication of this paper.

References

1. Togacar, M.; Ergen, B.; Comert, Z. Tumor type detection in brain MR images of the deep model developed using hypercolumn technique, attention modules, and residual blocks. *Med. Biol. Eng. Comput.* **2021**, *59*, 57–70. [CrossRef] [PubMed]
2. Hashmi, A.; Osman, A.H. Brain Tumor Classification Using Conditional Segmentation with Residual Network and Attention Approach by Extreme Gradient Boost. *Appl. Sci.* **2022**, *12*, 10791. [CrossRef]
3. Papadomanolakis, T.N.; Sergaki, E.S.; Polydorou, A.A.; Krasoudakis, A.G.; Makris-Tsalikis, G.N.; Polydorou, A.A.; Afentakis, N.M.; Athanasiou, S.A.; Vardiambasis, I.O.; Zervakis, M.E. Tumor Diagnosis against Other Brain Diseases Using T2 MRI Brain Images and CNN Binary Classifier and DWT. *Brain Sci.* **2023**, *13*, 348. [CrossRef] [PubMed]
4. Alnowami, M.; Taha, E.; Alsebaeai, S.; Anwar, S.M.; Alhawsawi, A. MR image normalization dilemma and the accuracy of brain tumor classification model. *J. Radiat. Res. Appl. Sci.* **2022**, *15*, 33–39. [CrossRef]
5. Deepak, S.; Ameer, P.M. Automated Categorization of Brain Tumor from MRI Using CNN features and SVM. *J. Ambient Intell. Humaniz. Comput.* **2021**, *12*, 8357–8369. [CrossRef]
6. Mahum, R.; Sharaf, M.; Hassan, H.; Liang, L.; Huang, B. A Robust Brain Tumor Detector Using BiLSTM and Mayfly Optimization and Multi-Level Thresholding. *Biomedicines* **2023**, *11*, 1715. [CrossRef]
7. Amou, M.A.; Xia, K.; Kamhi, S.; Mouhafid, M. A Novel MRI Diagnosis Method for Brain Tumor Classification Based on CNN and Bayesian Optimization. *Healthcare* **2022**, *10*, 494. [CrossRef]
8. Sunsuhi, G.S. An Adaptive Eroded Deep Convolutional neural network for brain image segmentation and classification using Inception ResnetV2. *Biomed. Signal Process. Control* **2022**, *78*, 103863. [CrossRef]
9. Rizwan, M.; Shabbir, A.; Javed, A.R.; Shabbir, M.; Baker, T.; Obe, D.A.J. Brain Tumor and Glioma Grade Classification Using Gaussian Convolutional Neural Network. *IEEE Access* **2022**, *10*, 29731–29740. [CrossRef]
10. Kothandaraman, V. Binary swallow swarm optimization with convolutional neural network brain tumor classifier for magnetic resonance imaging images. *Concurr. Comput.-Pract. Exp.* **2023**, *35*, e7661. [CrossRef]
11. Chitnis, S.; Hosseini, R.; Xie, P. Brain tumor classification based on neural architecture search. *Sci. Rep.* **2022**, *12*, 19206. [CrossRef] [PubMed]
12. Kaur, M.; AlZubi, A.A.; Jain, A.; Singh, D.; Yadav, V.; Alkhayyat, A. DSCNet: Deep Skip Connections-Based Dense Network for ALL Diagnosis Using Peripheral Blood Smear Images. *Diagnostics* **2023**, *13*, 2752. [CrossRef] [PubMed]
13. Qureshi, S.A.; Raza, S.E.A.; Hussain, L.; Malibari, A.A.; Nour, M.K.; Ul Rehman, A.; Al-Wesabi, F.N.; Hilal, A.M. Intelligent Ultra-Light Deep Learning Model for Multi-Class Brain Tumor Detection. *Appl. Sci.* **2022**, *12*, 3715. [CrossRef]
14. Saha, P.; Das, R.; Das, S.K. BCM-VEMT: Classification of brain cancer from MRI images using deep learning and ensemble of machine learning techniques. *Multimed. Tools Appl.* **2023**. [CrossRef]
15. Kibriya, H.; Masood, M.; Nawaz, M.; Nazir, T. Multiclass classification of brain tumors using a novel CNN architecture. *Multimed. Tools Appl.* **2022**, *81*, 29847–29863. [CrossRef]
16. Yazdan, S.A.; Ahmad, R.; Iqbal, N.; Rizwan, A.; Khan, A.N.; Kim, D.H. An Efficient Multi-Scale Convolutional Neural Network Based Multi-Class Brain MRI Classification for SaMD. *Tomography* **2022**, *8*, 1905–1927. [CrossRef]
17. Sekhar, A.; Biswas, S.; Hazra, R.; Sunaniya, A.K.; Mukherjee, A.; Yang, L. Brain Tumor Classification Using Fine-Tuned GoogLeNet Features and Machine Learning Algorithms: IoMT Enabled CAD System. *IEEE J. Biomed. Health Inform.* **2022**, *26*, 983–991. [CrossRef]
18. Ahmad, B.; Sun, J.; You, Q.; Palade, V.; Mao, Z. Brain Tumor Classification Using a Combination of Variational Autoencoders and Generative Adversarial Networks. *Biomedicines* **2022**, *10*, 223. [CrossRef]
19. Zulfiqar, F.; Bajwa, U.I.; Mehmood, Y. Multi-class classification of brain tumor types from MR images using EfficientNets. *Biomed. Signal Process. Control* **2023**, *84*, 104777. [CrossRef]
20. Demir, F.; Akbulut, Y. A new deep technique using R-CNN model and L1NSR feature selection for brain MRI classification. *Biomed. Signal Process. Control* **2022**, *75*, 103625. [CrossRef]
21. Zahid, U.; Ashraf, I.; Khan, M.A.; Alhaisoni, M.; Yahya, K.M.; Hussein, H.S.; Alshazly, H. BrainNet: Optimal deep learning feature fusion for brain tumor classification. *Comput. Intell. Neurosci.* **2022**, *2022*, 1465173. [CrossRef] [PubMed]
22. Maqsood, S.; Damaševičius, R.; Maskeliūnas, R. TTCNN: A breast cancer detection and classification towards computer-aided diagnosis using digital mammography in early stages. *Appl. Sci.* **2022**, *12*, 3273. [CrossRef]
23. Raza, A.; Ayub, H.; Khan, J.A.; Ahmad, I.; Salama, A.S.; Daradkeh, Y.I.; Javeed, D.; Ur Rehman, A.; Hamam, H. A hybrid deep learning-based approach for brain tumor classification. *Electronics* **2022**, *11*, 1146. [CrossRef]

24. Vankdothu, R.; Hameed, M.A.; Fatima, H. A brain tumor identification and classification using deep learning based on CNN-LSTM method. *Comput. Electr. Eng.* **2022**, *101*, 107960. [CrossRef]
25. Maqsood, S.; Damaševičius, R.; Maskeliūnas, R. Multi-modal brain tumor detection using deep neural network and multiclass SVM. *Medicina* **2022**, *58*, 1090. [CrossRef] [PubMed]
26. Mohammad, F.; Al Ahmadi, S.; Al Muhtadi, J. Blockchain-Based Deep CNN for Brain Tumor Prediction Using MRI Scans. *Diagnostics* **2023**, *13*, 1229. [CrossRef]
27. Reza, A.W.; Hossain, M.S.; Wardiful, M.A.; Farzana, M.; Ahmad, S.; Alam, F.; Nandi, R.N.; Siddique, N. A CNN-Based Strategy to Classify MRI-Based Brain Tumors Using Deep Convolutional Network. *Appl. Sci.* **2023**, *13*, 312. [CrossRef]
28. Abd El-Wahab, B.S.S.; Nasr, M.E.E.; Khamis, S.; Ashour, A.S.S. BTC-fCNN: Fast Convolution Neural Network for Multi-class Brain Tumor Classification. *Health Inf. Sci. Syst.* **2023**, *11*, 3. [CrossRef]
29. Gupta, R.K.; Bharti, S.; Kunhare, N.; Sahu, Y.; Pathik, N. Brain Tumor Detection and Classification Using Cycle Generative Adversarial Networks. *Interdiscip. Sci.-Comput. Life Sci.* **2022**, *14*, 485–502. [CrossRef]
30. Oksuz, C.; Urhan, O.; Gullu, M.K. Brain tumor classification using the fused features extracted from expanded tumor region. *Biomed. Signal Process. Control* **2022**, *72*, 103356. [CrossRef]
31. Kesav, N.; Jibukumar, M.G. Efficient and low complex architecture for detection and classification of Brain Tumor using RCNN with Two Channel CNN. *J. King Saud Univ.-Comput. Inf. Sci.* **2022**, *34*, 6229–6242. [CrossRef]
32. Rasheed, Z.; Ma, Y.K.; Ullah, I.; Al Shloul, T.; Tufail, A.B.; Ghadi, Y.Y.; Khan, M.Z.; Mohamed, H.G. Automated Classification of Brain Tumors from Magnetic Resonance Imaging Using Deep Learning. *Brain Sci.* **2023**, *13*, 602. [CrossRef] [PubMed]
33. Polat, O.; Gungen, C. Classification of brain tumors from MR images using deep transfer learning. *J. Supercomput.* **2021**, *77*, 7236–7252. [CrossRef]
34. Alanazi, M.F.; Ali, M.U.; Hussain, S.J.; Zafar, A.; Mohatram, M.; Irfan, M.; AlRuwaili, R.; Alruwaili, M.; Ali, N.H.; Albarrak, A.M. Brain Tumor/Mass Classification Framework Using Magnetic-Resonance-Imaging-Based Isolated and Developed Transfer Deep-Learning Model. *Sensors* **2022**, *22*, 372. [CrossRef] [PubMed]
35. Al-Zoghby, A.M.; Al-Awadly, E.M.K.; Moawad, A.; Yehia, N.; Ebada, A.I. Dual Deep CNN for Tumor Brain Classification. *Diagnostics* **2023**, *13*, 2050. [CrossRef]
36. Rehman, A.; Naz, S.; Razzak, M.I.; Akram, F.; Imran, M. A Deep Learning-Based Framework for Automatic Brain Tumors Classification Using Transfer Learning. *Circuits Syst. Signal Process.* **2020**, *39*, 757–775. [CrossRef]
37. Mahmoud, A.; Awad, N.A.; Alsubaie, N.; Ansarullah, S.I.; Alqahtani, M.S.; Abbas, M.; Usman, M.; Soufiene, B.O.; Saber, A. Advanced Deep Learning Approaches for Accurate Brain Tumor Classification in Medical Imaging. *Symmetry* **2023**, *15*, 571. [CrossRef]
38. Diaz-Pernas, F.J.; Martinez-Zarzuela, M.; Anton-Rodriguez, M.; Gonzalez-Ortega, D. A Deep Learning Approach for Brain Tumor Classification and Segmentation Using a Multiscale Convolutional Neural Network. *Healthcare* **2021**, *9*, 153. [CrossRef]
39. Anjum, S.; Hussain, L.; Ali, M.; Alkinani, M.H.; Aziz, W.; Gheller, S.; Abbasi, A.A.; Marchal, A.R.; Suresh, H.; Duong, T.Q. Detecting brain tumors using deep learning convolutional neural network with transfer learning approach. *Int. J. Imaging Syst. Technol.* **2022**, *32*, 307–323. [CrossRef]
40. Cheng, J. Brain Tumor Dataset. 2023. Available online: https://figshare.com/articles/dataset/brain_tumor_dataset/1512427 (accessed on 2 June 2023).
41. Naren, O.S. Acute Lymphoblastic Leukemia (ALL) Image Dataset. 2021. Available online: https://www.kaggle.com/datasets/obulisainaren/multi-cancer (accessed on 10 February 2023).

Disclaimer/Publisher's Note: The statements, opinions and data contained in all publications are solely those of the individual author(s) and contributor(s) and not of MDPI and/or the editor(s). MDPI and/or the editor(s) disclaim responsibility for any injury to people or property resulting from any ideas, methods, instructions or products referred to in the content.

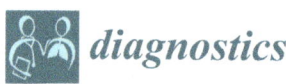

Article

Bone Metastases Lesion Segmentation on Breast Cancer Bone Scan Images with Negative Sample Training

Yi-You Chen [1], Po-Nien Yu [1], Yung-Chi Lai [2], Te-Chun Hsieh [1,3,*] and Da-Chuan Cheng [1,*]

[1] Department of Biomedical Imaging and Radiological Science, China Medical University, Taichung 404, Taiwan; u111202701@cmu.edu.tw (Y.-Y.C.); u111202703@cmu.edu.tw (P.-N.Y.)
[2] Department of Nuclear Medicine, Feng Yuan Hospital, Ministry of Health and Welfare, Taichung 420, Taiwan; daniellai999@hotmail.com
[3] Department of Nuclear Medicine and PET Center, China Medical University Hospital, Taichung 404, Taiwan
* Correspondence: d10119@mail.cmuh.org.tw (T.-C.H.); dccheng@mail.cmu.edu.tw (D.-C.C.); Tel.: +886-4-2205-3366 (D.-C.C.)

Abstract: The use of deep learning methods for the automatic detection and quantification of bone metastases in bone scan images holds significant clinical value. A fast and accurate automated system for segmenting bone metastatic lesions can assist clinical physicians in diagnosis. In this study, a small internal dataset comprising 100 breast cancer patients (90 cases of bone metastasis and 10 cases of non-metastasis) and 100 prostate cancer patients (50 cases of bone metastasis and 50 cases of non-metastasis) was used for model training. Initially, all image labels were binary. We used the Otsu thresholding method or negative mining to generate a non-metastasis mask, thereby transforming the image labels into three classes. We adopted the Double U-Net as the baseline model and made modifications to its output activation function. We changed the activation function to SoftMax to accommodate multi-class segmentation. Several methods were used to enhance model performance, including background pre-processing to remove background information, adding negative samples to improve model precision, and using transfer learning to leverage shared features between two datasets, which enhances the model's performance. The performance was investigated via 10-fold cross-validation and computed on a pixel-level scale. The best model we achieved had a precision of 69.96%, a sensitivity of 63.55%, and an F1-score of 66.60%. Compared to the baseline model, this represents an 8.40% improvement in precision, a 0.56% improvement in sensitivity, and a 4.33% improvement in the F1-score. The developed system has the potential to provide pre-diagnostic reports for physicians in final decisions and the calculation of the bone scan index (BSI) with the combination with bone skeleton segmentation.

Keywords: bone metastasis segmentation; Double U-Net; pre-train; negative mining; transfer learning; deep learning

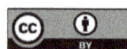

1. Introduction

According to the gender statistics database published by the Gender Equality Committee of the Executive Yuan in Taiwan in 2023, breast cancer was ranked first among the top 10 cancer incidence rates in 2020 [1]. Breast cancer, prostate cancer, lung cancer, and other prevalent cancers account for more than 80% of cases of metastatic bone disease. For patients with breast cancer, late-stage bone metastasis is prone to occur, significantly reducing the prognosis of the patients. A study by Coleman and Rubens reported bone metastasis in 69% of breast cancer patients who died between 1979 and 1984, out of a total of 587 patients [2]. Bone metastasis in breast cancer most commonly occurs in the spine, followed by the ribs and sternum [3]. Radiologically, bone metastases in breast cancer are predominantly osteolytic, leading to severe complications such as bone pain, pathological fractures, spinal cord compression, hypercalcemia, and bone marrow suppression.

Therefore, the early detection and treatment of bone metastasis in breast cancer patients are crucially important.

Current methods for detecting breast cancer metastasis include the clinical observation of distant organ involvement, organ biopsies, diagnostic imaging, and serum tumor markers. One of the primary imaging techniques used in clinics for bone metastasis diagnosis is the whole-body bone scan (WBBS) with vein injection using the Tc-99m MDP tracer [4,5]. WBBS offers the advantages of whole-body examination, cost-effectiveness, and high sensitivity, making it a preferred modality for bone metastasis screening [6]. Unlike X-radiography (XR) and computed tomography (CT) images, which can only detect changes in bone when there is approximately 40–50% mineralization [7], bone scans exhibit higher sensitivity in detecting bone changes, capable of detecting alterations as low as 5% in osteoblast activity. The reported sensitivity and specificity of skeletal scintigraphy for bone metastasis detection are 78% and 48%, respectively [8].

The bone scan index (BSI) is an image biomarker utilized in WBBS to evaluate the severity of bone metastasis in cancer patients. It enables a quantification on the degree of tumor involvement in the skeleton [9,10]. BSI is used for observing disease progression or treatment response. The commercial software EXINI bone (version 1 and version 2, including subversions), developed by EXINI Diagnostics AB, incorporates aBSI (automated bone scan index) technology for the comprehensive automated quantitative assessment of bone scan images [11]. In [11], there exists a strong correlation between manual and automated BSI assessment values ($\rho = 0.80$), which further strengthens ($\rho = 0.93$) when cases with BSI scores exceeding 10 (1.8%) are excluded. This indicates that automated BSI calculations can deliver clinical value comparable to manual calculations. Shimizu et al. has proposed an image interpretation system based on deep learning [12], using BtrflyNets for the hotspot detection of bone metastasis and bone segmentation, followed by automatic BSI calculation. The aBSI technology has now become a clinically valuable tool. Nevertheless, there are still challenges regarding recognition performance (sensitivity and precision) in this technique.

Cheng et al. applied a deep convolutional neural network (D-CNN) for the object detection of bone metastasis from prostate cancer in bone scan images [13]. Their investigation specifically focused on the chest and pelvic regions, and the sensitivity and precision for detecting and classifying chest bone metastasis were determined using bounding boxes to be 0.82 ± 0.08 and 0.70 ± 0.11, respectively. Regarding pelvic bone metastasis classification, the reported sensitivity and specificity were 0.87 ± 0.12 and 0.81 ± 0.11, respectively. Cheng et al. conducted a more detailed study on chest bone metastasis in prostate cancer patients [14]. The average sensitivity and precision for detecting and classifying chest bone metastasis based on lesion locations are reported as 0.72 ± 0.04 and 0.90 ± 0.04, respectively. For classifying chest bone metastasis based on patient-level outcomes, the average sensitivity and specificity are found to be 0.94 ± 0.09 and 0.92 ± 0.09, respectively. Patents filed by Cheng et al. are referenced as [15], which leverage deep learning for the identification of bone metastasis in prostate cancer bone scan images. Since they use bounding boxes, they are unable to calculate BSI.

In a related study [16], a neural network (NN) model based on U-Net++ is proposed for the automated segmentation of metastatic lesions in bone scan images. The anterior–posterior and posterior–anterior views are superimposed, and image segmentation is exclusively performed on the chest region of whole-body bone scan images. The achieved average F1-score is 65.56%.

In this study, we modified the Double U-Net [17] as the fundamental architecture to perform bone metastases segmentation on WBBS. We explored various methods to enhance network performance, including background pre-processing, adding negative samples, and transfer learning. We used Otsu thresholding [18] and negative mining [14] methods for background pre-processing and generating negative samples. Background pre-processing helped eliminate unnecessary background information, while adding negative samples reduced the model's false positive rate. Both of these methods did not require manual labeling or modification, saving time and manpower. Previous studies in the same field [16,19–23] focused only on segmenting bone metastases in specific regions (chest or pelvis) and could only predict either the anterior or posterior view. The datasets we used only excluded the non-metastatic-prone areas below the knees and could simultaneously segment images in both the anterior and posterior views. In comparison, our model was able to provide a more comprehensive assessment of bone metastasis images.

The following points summarize the contributions of this paper:

- We discuss the challenges of lesion segmentation in breast cancer bone scan images.
- We compare and discuss the state-of-the-art methods in the same research field.
- Our experiments have shown that background pre-processing significantly improves a model's performance and adding negative samples enhances model precision. Both methods do not require manual labeling or label modification, saving time and manpower.
- Our segmentation model offers greater comprehensiveness. It can perform lesion segmentation on WBBS images, predicting both anterior and posterior views simultaneously.

2. Related Work

Deep learning has found numerous applications in cancer detection tasks. The authors of Ref. [24] proposed an improved SIFT descriptor with Harris corner to form Bag-Of-Words features in image representation. This study made a significant contribution to medical image classification tasks. For skin lesions, the authors of Ref. [25] conducted a comprehensive comparative study of U-Net and attention-based methods for dermatological image segmentation, aiding in the diagnosis of skin lesions. The authors of Ref. [26] introduced an enhanced deep learning model, SBXception, based on the Xception network to improve skin cancer classification. In the realm of MRI, the authors of Ref. [27] presented a weighted ensemble deep learning model for brain tumor classification. The authors of Ref. [28] explored five machine learning techniques to deepen the understanding of brain tumor classification and enhance its scope and significance.

Some early work has been carried out on automatic segmentation of metastatic lesions using bone scan images [29–33]. The trend of using deep learning for bone scintigraphy image analysis is becoming increasingly evident. In classification tasks, the authors of Ref. [34] introduced an improved ResNet model that combines convolutional block attention module and contextual transformer attention mechanisms to achieve the accurate classification of SPECT images [35] based their work on widely used deep networks, including VGG, ResNet, and DenseNet, by fine-tuning their parameters and structures or by customizing new network architectures. The proposed classifiers performed well in identifying bone metastases through SPECT imaging. The authors of Ref. [36] presented an automated bone metastasis diagnostic model based on multi-view images. The authors of Ref. [37] introduced a new framework in this work, which included data preparation and image classification, for automatically classifying scintigraphy images collected from patients clinically diagnosed with lung cancer.

In object detection tasks, the authors of Ref. [38] employed scaled-YOLOv4 and Detectron2 object detection networks for bone metastasis localization in breast cancer patient nuclear imaging data and for detecting degenerative and pathological findings in whole-body scintigraphy scans. The authors of Ref. [39] proposed an automatic lesion detection model based on single shot multibox object detector for the automatic detection of lung cancer bone metastases in low-resolution SPECT bone scintigraphy images. The authors of Ref. [14] applied D-CNN for object detection of prostate cancer bone metastases in the chest and pelvic regions. As object detection uses bounding boxes, it cannot calculate the BSI as a subsequent quantitative measure.

Compared to classification and object detection tasks, segmentation tasks are more challenging. The authors of Ref. [19] introduced a model called MaligNet, which semantically segments abnormal hotspots in a semi-supervised manner and classifies bone cancer metastases in the chest region. The authors of Ref. [20] built a segmentation model based on U-Net and Mask R-CNN networks by fine-tuning their architectures for identifying and segmenting metastatic hotspots in bone SEPCT images. The authors of Ref. [21] added a methods attention mechanism on top of the original U-Net network's skip connections to enhance feature selection, allowing for the automatic identification and segmentation of bone metastases. The authors of Ref. [16] proposed a neural network model based on U-Net++ for the automatic segmentation of metastatic lesions in bone scan images. The authors of Ref. [22] introduced an improved UNet3+ network that combines attention mechanisms for the automatic segmentation of bone metastatic lesions. The authors of Ref. [23] presented a bone imaging focus segmentation algorithm based on the Swin Transformer, which uses the swin transformer as the backbone network for extracting feature information from bone images. In current research in the same field, segmentation tasks are limited to predicting specific local regions, such as the chest or pelvis, and they cannot simultaneously predict both anterior and posterior views.

3. Materials and Methods

3.1. Materials

In this study, we collected 200 bone scan images from the Department of Nuclear Medicine of China Medical University Hospital. The details of the bone scan images are provided in Table 1. Specifically, D1 is defined as 90 images from breast cancer patients with bone metastasis. D2 is defined as 10 images from breast cancer patients without bone metastasis. D3 is defined as 50 images from prostate cancer patients with bone metastasis. D4 is defined as 50 images from prostate cancer patients without bone metastasis. Figure 1 shows bone scan images of breast cancer patients. This study has been approved by the Institutional Review Board (IRB) of China Medical University and Hospital Research Ethics Committee (CMUH106-REC2-130), approved on 27 September 2017.

Table 1. The details of the bone scan images.

	Breast Cancer	Prostate Cancer
w/metastasis	D1:90	D3:50
w/o metastasis	D2:10	D4:50
Total	100	100

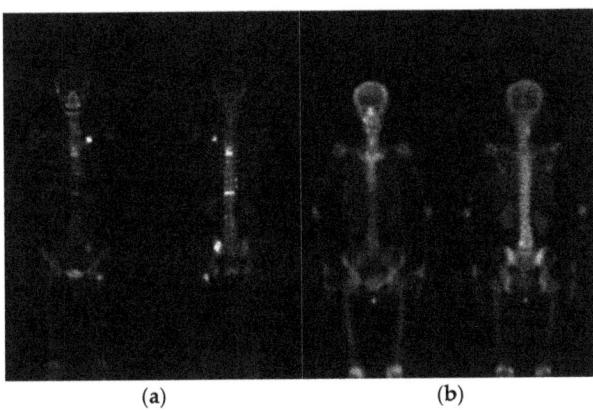

Figure 1. Bone scan images of breast cancer patients. (a) With metastasis; (b) without metastasis.

The WBBS process can be described as follows. Patients undergo WBBS with a gamma camera (Millennium MG, Infinia Hawkeye 4, or Discovery NM/CT 670 system; GE Healthcare, Waukesha, WI, USA). Bone scans are acquired 2–4 h after the intravenous injection of 740–925 MBq (20–25 mCi) of technetium-99m methylene diphosphonate (Tc-99m MDP) with an acquisition time of 10–15 cm/min. The collected WBBS images are saved in DICOM format. The raw images include anterior–posterior (AP) and posterior–anterior (PA) views, with a matrix size of 1024 × 256 pixels.

3.2. Image Labeling

To facilitate labeling the bone scan images, the Labelme (version 4.5.9) software is used as the annotation tool. The manual annotation of bone metastasis images is carried out under the guidance and supervision of nuclear medicine physicians. This process is very time-consuming. The outputs generated by the Labelme software are saved in JSON format, and then converted to the PNG format. Figure 2 represents a schematic of the manually annotated results.

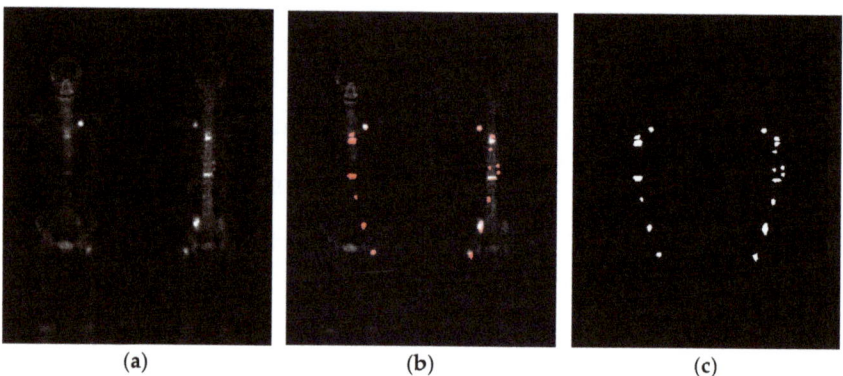

Figure 2. The schematic of the manually annotated results. (**a**) Bone scan image; (**b**) overlay of bone scan image with ground truth; (**c**) ground truth.

3.3. Image Pre-Processing

The raw images possess a large memory size and the DICOM format is not directly suitable for neural network training. Moreover, the raw images exhibit variations in brightness and contrast levels. Thus, the pre-processing of the raw images becomes imperative. The detection of the body range was accomplished using the projection profile, followed by the extraction of two views with dimensions of 950 × 256 pixels through cutting and centering. No scaling or other transformations were applied during this process. We utilized the brightness normalization method proposed in [14] for brightness pre-processing. This method uses a linear transformation to adjust the dynamic range of an image, with the objective of controlling the average intensity of each image within the range of (7, 14). The algorithm for the linear transformation is illustrated in Figure 3. The region below the knees, which is uncommon for bone metastasis, was excluded from the calculation of BSI. To obtain the region above the knees, pixels beyond row 640 were eliminated, resulting in two views with a spatial resolution of 640 × 256 pixels each. Finally, the pre-processed AP (anterior–posterior) and PA (posterior–anterior) view images were horizontally merged, generating images with a spatial resolution of 640 × 512 pixels.

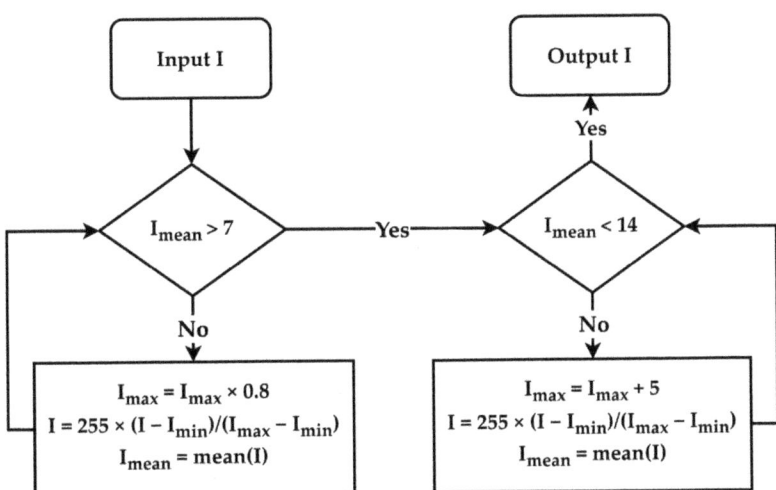

Figure 3. Flowchart of brightness normalization.

3.4. Positive and Negative Samples

According to previous research [14], adding negative samples to the training dataset helps reduce false positives and improve model precision. In this study, we also used negative samples to enhance the model's performance. Positive samples are defined as images with bone metastases (D1 and D3), while negative samples are defined as images without bone metastases (D2 and D4).

For the bone metastasis segmentation task in WBBS images, the background significantly interferes with network training. In this scenario, the background not only includes air but also the non-metastatic (NM) human body regions. Intuitively, NM regions of the human body contain information but do not contain air. Therefore, an alternative approach is to filter out the air to extract NM human body regions to generate NM masks. The generation of NM masks involves two methods, which we briefly explain below.

The Otsu thresholding method is used to generate NM masks for both positive and negative samples. It is important to note that the metastatic (M) regions must be manually excluded from positive samples beforehand. Otsu thresholding can automatically determine the threshold that separates air from the human body.

The negative mining method for generating NM masks involves two steps. First, the baseline network is trained using only positive samples. After training, this model is used to predict negative samples. Since negative samples do not have bone metastatic lesions, all segmentation results produced are false positives. These false positive segmentation results are then treated as NM regions to generate NM masks. The same model is also used to predict positive samples. It is worth noting that the metastatic (M) regions in the positive samples must be manually excluded beforehand.

The initial classes include background and metastasis. After generating NM masks using the two methods mentioned above, the number of classes increases from the original two to three, now including air-background (BG), non-metastatic (NM), and metastatic (M) classes.

3.5. Transfer Learning

Transfer learning is a widely used technique in neural networks to increase their performance. Before applying transfer learning, two crucial factors need to be considered: (1) the size of the target dataset and (2) the similarity between the target dataset and the pre-training dataset.

In this study, the Double U-Net network model was pre-trained using the D3 and D4 datasets. We chose a pre-training dataset that contains highly similar bone scan images of prostate cancer. Subsequently, the model was fine-tuned using the target dataset consisting of breast cancer bone scan images. By leveraging transfer learning and selecting a pre-training dataset closely related to the target dataset, our goal was to utilize shared features between the two datasets to enhance the model's performance on the current specific task.

3.6. Neural Network Model

We adopted the Double U-Net architecture as our network framework. The original Double U-Net architecture was developed for binary segmentation tasks, which we refer to as the baseline network. To adapt the Double U-Net architecture for multi-class segmentation, we modified its network structure following the method described in our previous research [40]. Figure 4 illustrates the modified network architecture. We changed the output layer of network 1 to obtain a SoftMax activation function, enabling it to perform multi-class segmentation. With this modification, the Double U-Net architecture can handle three-class segmentation tasks involving the BG, NM, and M regions.

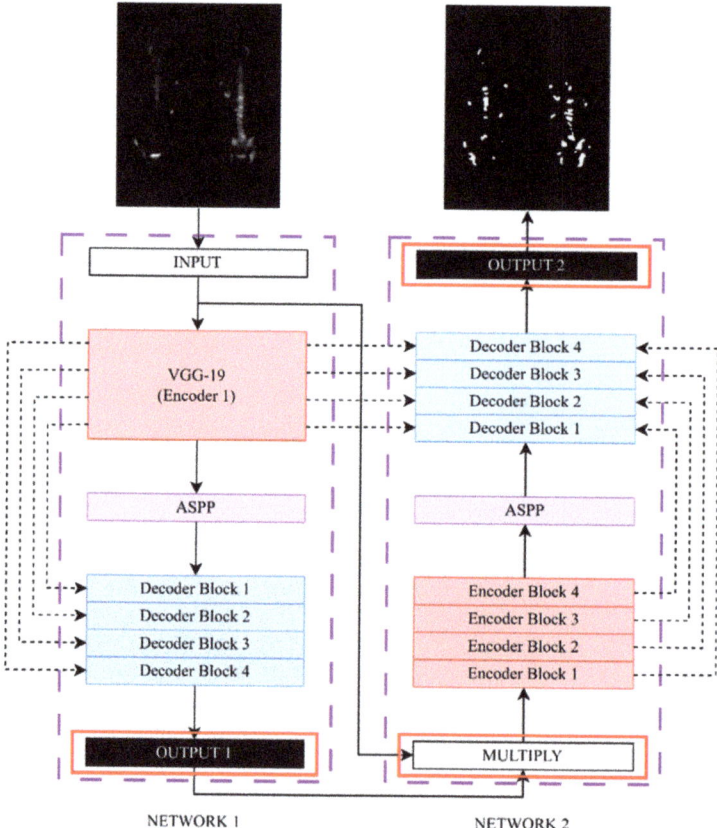

Figure 4. The modified architecture diagram of Double U-Net, the baseline network.

3.7. Loss Function

The selection of an appropriate loss function is a critical aspect in the design of deep learning architectures for image segmentation tasks, as it greatly impacts the learning dynamics of the algorithm. In our study, we consider two loss functions: the Dice loss

(Equation (1)), as originally proposed in [17], and the Focal Tversky loss (Equation (2)). By comparing these loss functions, we aim to explore their respective influences on the model's performance in the context of our specific task.

The dice coefficient is a widely adopted metric in computer vision for assessing the similarity between two images. In our study, we utilize a modified version of the dice coefficient known as the dice loss, which served as a loss function for our model.

$$DL(y, p) = 1 - \frac{2yp}{y + p} \tag{1}$$

where y is true value and p is the predicted outcome.

The focal Tversky loss is particularly well-suited for solving highly imbalanced class scenarios. It incorporates a γ coefficient that allows for the down-weighting of easy samples. Additionally, by adjusting the α and β coefficients, different weights can be assigned to false positives (FP) and false negatives (FN).

$$FTL(y, p) = \left(1 - \frac{yp}{yp + \alpha(1-y)p + \beta y(1-p)}\right)^{\gamma} \tag{2}$$

where $\gamma = 0.75$, $\alpha = 0.3$, and $\beta = 0.7$.

When performing the three-class segmentation task for the BG, NM, and M regions, calculating loss and back-propagating for the BG class is unnecessary and would make model training difficult. Therefore, during the execution of the three-class segmentation task, we do not calculate loss or perform backpropagation for the BG class.

3.8. Experimental Configuration and Evaluation Metrics

All experiments were conducted on four Intel Xeon Gold 6154 CPUs and a 32 GB Nvidia Tesla V100 GPU. The memory capacity configured was 90 GB. Our segmentation system was implemented in Python using Keras with TensorFlow 2.4.1.

The evaluation metrics employed in this study include precision (Equation (3)), sensitivity (Equation (4)), and the overall model assessment based on the F1-score (Equation (5)). The terms true positive (TP), false positive (FP), true negative (TN), and false negative (FN) were defined at the pixel level.

$$\text{Precision} = \frac{TP}{TP + FP} \tag{3}$$

$$\text{Sensitivity} = \frac{TP}{TP + FN} \tag{4}$$

$$\text{F1-score} = 2 \times \frac{\text{Precision} \times \text{Sensitivity}}{\text{Precision} + \text{Sensitivity}} \tag{5}$$

4. Results

All experimental results in tables are obtained through 10-fold cross-validation, with a ratio of 8:1:1 for the training, validation, and testing sets, respectively. The learning rate used for training was 0.0001, batch size was set to 4, and the number of iterations was 500.

4.1. Negative Samples

The qualitative results of two negative samples are illustrated in Figure 5. The Otsu thresholding can extract NM masks easily and produce three classes: BG, NM, and M. Its results are shown in Figure 5a. Nevertheless, negative mining requires two steps, as described in the method. Its results are shown in Figure 5b.

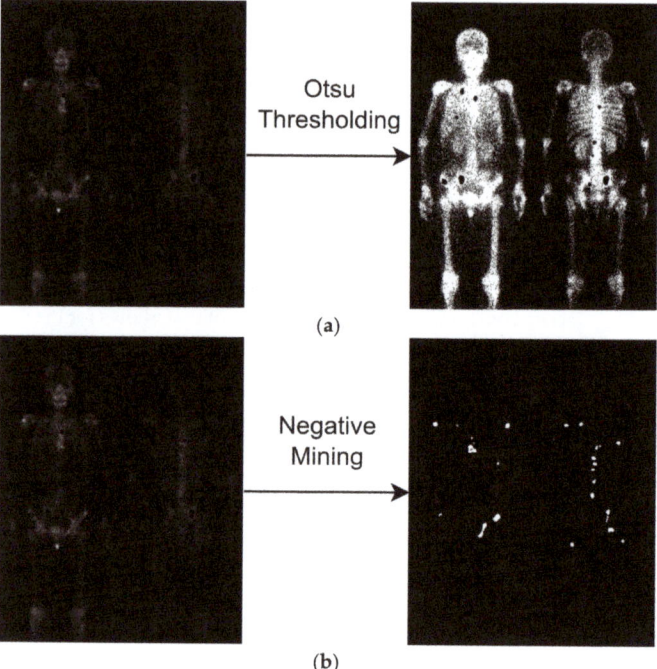

Figure 5. Illustration of negative sample productions. Notably, the metastasis hotspots are eliminated (the black holes), if the image has metastasis. (**a**) Otsu thresholding; (**b**) negative mining.

4.2. Results of the Baseline Network

The original Double U-Net network was trained using the D1 dataset and utilized the dice loss function. The objective of this experiment was to establish the baseline performance of the baseline network.

For comparison, it is essential to evaluate the performance of deep learning models in each task using quantitative metrics. Here, the precision, sensitivity, and F1-score are utilized for performance evaluation. Figure 6 shows the qualitative results, and the quantitative results are shown in Table 2.

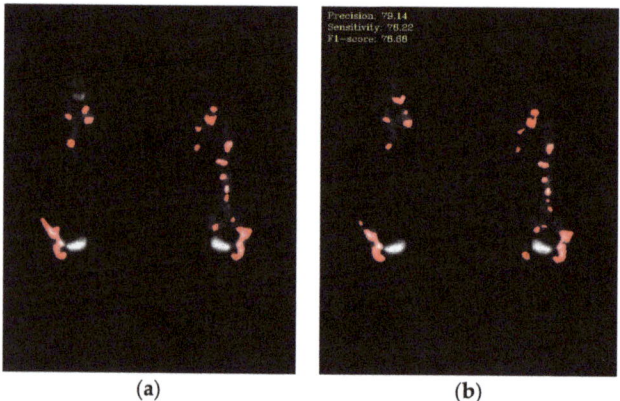

Figure 6. The qualitative result of the baseline network. (**a**) Ground truth; (**b**) segmentation results (precision: 79.14; sensitivity: 78.22; F1-score: 78.68).

Table 2. The quantitative results of the baseline network (dice loss).

Fold Number	Precision	Sensitivity	F1-Score
1	49.21	79.19	60.70
2	58.74	64.98	61.70
3	70.56	60.01	64.86
4	81.69	52.20	63.70
5	60.57	54.06	57.13
6	72.55	45.92	56.24
7	43.63	83.32	57.27
8	49.03	68.21	57.05
9	61.73	60.84	61.28
10	67.89	61.13	64.34
Mean	61.56	62.99	62.27

4.3. The Baseline Network Using Otsu Thresholding

The modified Double U-Net network was trained using the D1 dataset. Before training, we used the Otsu thresholding method on the D1 dataset for background pre-processing, generating the NM mask. Figure 7 illustrates a training sample from the D1 dataset, which includes three classes.

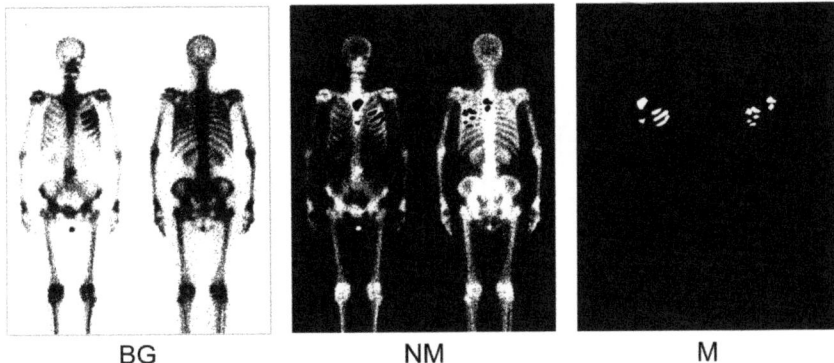

Figure 7. Illustration of applying Otsu thresholding to positive samples to generate NM masks. Three classes are included: BG, NM, and M.

The model's performance is shown in Table 3. In Table 3, we included the focal Tversky loss for comparison. Compared to Table 2, we observe that using the Otsu thresholding method for background pre-processing on the D1 dataset significantly improves the model's performance. In both the dice loss and focal Tversky loss models, the F1-score improved by 3.12% and 4.16%, respectively.

Table 3. The quantitative results for this experiment. Using the Otsu thresholding method for background pre-processing on the D1 dataset.

Fold Number	Dice Loss			Focal Tversky Loss		
	Precision	Sensitivity	F1-Score	Precision	Sensitivity	F1-Score
1	68.74	67.72	68.23	66.95	68.81	67.86
2	71.29	56.75	63.20	69.91	60.70	64.98
3	70.11	64.57	67.23	69.69	68.49	69.09
4	83.92	58.39	68.86	85.19	56.34	67.82
5	64.06	58.32	61.06	65.52	60.17	62.73

Table 3. *Cont.*

Fold Number	Precision	Dice Loss Sensitivity	F1-Score	Precision	Focal Tversky Loss Sensitivity	F1-Score
6	77.01	53.10	62.86	79.24	51.88	62.70
7	60.52	73.99	66.58	60.64	76.05	67.47
8	51.30	65.19	57.41	52.36	68.90	59.50
9	63.24	64.24	63.73	62.55	66.40	64.42
10	66.14	70.58	68.29	66.66	72.67	69.54
Mean	67.63	63.29	65.39	67.87	65.04	66.43

We wanted to investigate the impact of adding negative samples to the training dataset on the model. In this experiment, we first used the Otsu thresholding method for background pre-processing on the D2 dataset, generating the NM mask. Then, we added the D2 dataset to the D1 training dataset in each fold. Figure 8 shows an example training sample from the D2 dataset, which contains three classes.

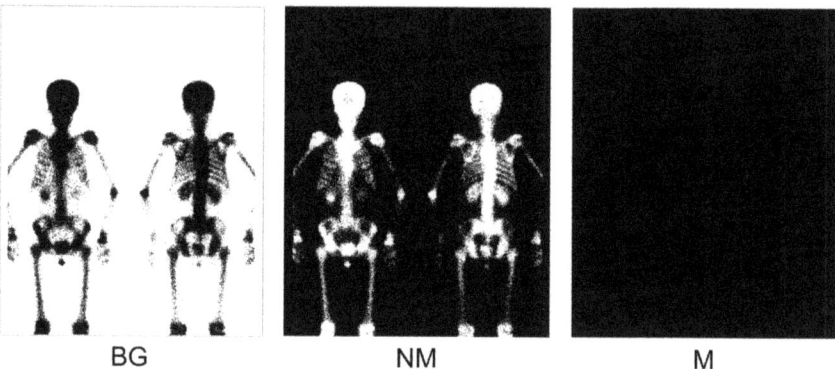

Figure 8. Illustration of applying Otsu thresholding to negative samples to generate NM masks. Three classes are included: BG, NM, and M.

Table 4 presents the model performance when adding the D2 dataset using the Otsu thresholding method. In both the dice loss and focal Tversky loss models, precision improved by 2.61% and 2.09%, respectively. From the results, we did not observe any significant improvement in the F1 score. However, adding negative samples did indeed increase precision, which aligns with our expectations.

Table 4. The quantitative results for this experiment. Using the Otsu thresholding method for background pre-processing on the D2 dataset and adding it to the training set.

Fold Number	Precision	Dice Loss Sensitivity	F1-Score	Precision	Focal Tversky Loss Sensitivity	F1-Score
1	70.41	65.42	67.82	69.66	67.94	68.79
2	70.85	60.72	65.39	70.09	63.16	66.44
3	73.88	64.55	68.90	72.29	67.43	69.78
4	85.21	54.91	66.78	85.29	56.55	68.01
5	71.95	55.89	62.91	72.86	53.82	61.91
6	82.09	49.93	62.10	82.54	51.38	63.34
7	62.14	67.76	64.83	62.22	72.58	67.00
8	54.31	65.79	59.50	54.42	64.25	58.93
9	65.37	63.09	64.21	63.23	64.94	64.07
10	66.14	69.90	67.97	66.98	73.49	70.08
Mean	70.24	61.80	65.75	69.96	63.55	66.60

4.4. The Baseline Network Using Negative Mining

The modified Double U-Net network was trained using the D1 dataset. Prior to training, we applied the negative mining method to pre-process the D1 dataset and generate the NM mask. Figure 9 illustrates a training sample from the D1 dataset, including three classes.

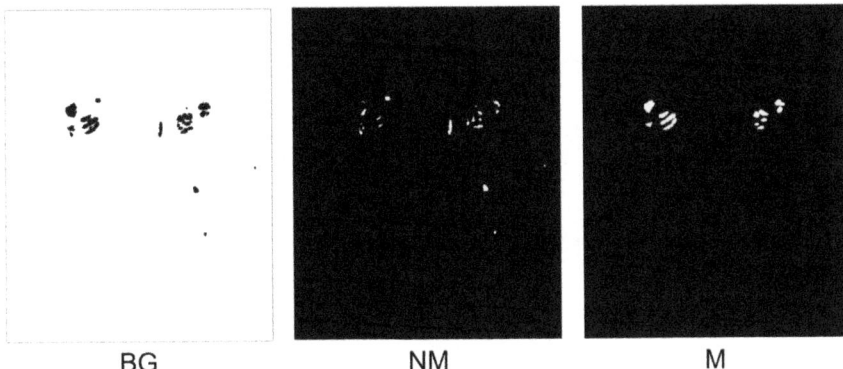

Figure 9. Illustration of applying negative mining to positive samples to generate NM masks. Three classes are included: BG, NM, and M.

The model performance is shown in Table 5. Compared to the baseline (Table 2), negative mining indeed shows significant improvement. In the dice loss and focal Tversky loss models, F1-score improved by 2.14% and 2.27%, respectively.

Table 5. The quantitative results for this experiment. Using the negative mining method for background pre-processing on the D1 dataset.

Fold Number	Dice Loss			Focal Tversky Loss		
	Precision	Sensitivity	F1-Score	Precision	Sensitivity	F1-Score
1	65.94	72.63	69.13	65.01	70.95	67.85
2	71.47	59.26	64.80	65.70	62.18	63.89
3	70.63	61.13	65.54	67.49	68.33	67.91
4	82.85	48.77	61.40	80.04	60.92	69.19
5	57.72	57.81	57.76	40.43	78.88	53.46
6	78.32	45.99	57.95	64.76	60.65	62.64
7	49.50	82.30	61.82	51.50	80.99	62.97
8	50.25	73.06	59.55	48.97	70.11	57.66
9	59.42	68.06	63.45	52.04	74.00	61.11
10	70.00	63.57	66.63	57.81	79.95	67.10
Mean	65.61	63.26	64.41	59.38	70.70	64.54

Next, in this experiment, we first used the negative mining method to pre-process the D2 dataset and generate the NM mask. Then, we added the D2 dataset to the training data of D1 in each fold. Figure 10 shows a training sample from the D2 dataset (containing three classes).

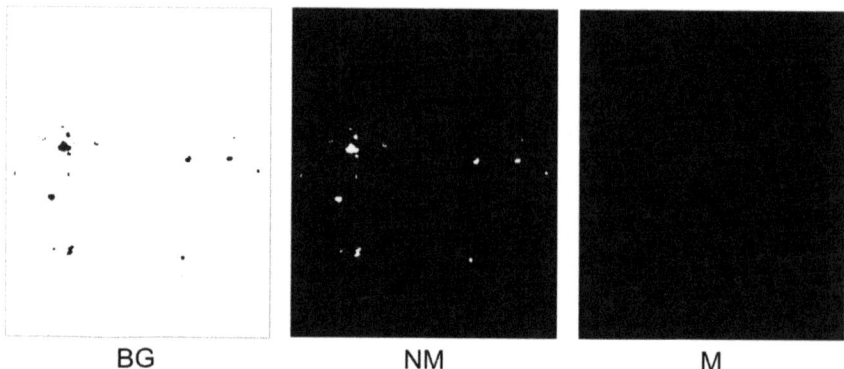

Figure 10. Illustration of applying negative mining to negative samples to generate NM masks. Three classes are included: BG, NM, and M.

The quantitative results of this experiment are shown in Table 6. In both the dice loss and focal Tversky loss models, precision improved by 1.85% and 1.64%, respectively. Similar to Table 4, adding negative samples to the training set led to a slight improvement in precision but a slight decrease in sensitivity. The F1-score remained unchanged, as expected.

Table 6. The quantitative results for this experiment. Using the negative mining method for background pre-processing on the D2 dataset and adding it to the training set.

Fold Number	Dice Loss			Focal Tversky Loss		
	Precision	Sensitivity	F1-Score	Precision	Sensitivity	F1-Score
1	64.79	69.79	67.19	59.59	76.92	67.16
2	70.67	59.40	64.55	59.27	71.75	64.92
3	77.27	48.05	59.26	67.96	62.61	65.18
4	85.56	53.52	65.85	83.36	54.10	65.62
5	57.46	63.47	60.32	46.52	69.61	55.77
6	80.69	46.10	58.68	74.92	59.45	66.29
7	57.06	73.52	64.25	48.79	81.93	61.16
8	54.72	62.98	58.56	50.79	71.00	59.22
9	65.60	62.07	63.79	60.26	65.43	62.74
10	60.75	74.89	67.08	58.71	73.35	65.22
Mean	67.46	61.38	64.28	61.02	68.62	64.59

4.5. Model Performance after Transfer Learning

Based on the previous experiments, we found that using the Otsu threshold method to generate the NM mask leads to better performance improvement. To understand the impact of transfer learning, we pre-trained the modified Double U-Net network using the D3 and D4 datasets. Before pretraining, we used the Otsu threshold method to pre-process the D3 and D4 datasets and generate the NM masks. Then, we added the D4 dataset to the training data of D3 in each fold.

The pre-trained model was fine-tuned by learning from breast cancer patient images. Before fine-tuning, we used the Otsu threshold method to pre-process the D1 and D2 datasets and generate the NM masks. Then, we added the D2 dataset to the training data of D1 in each fold.

The qualitative results of segmentation are shown in Figure 11. Specifically, we compare two loss functions: dice and focal Tversky.

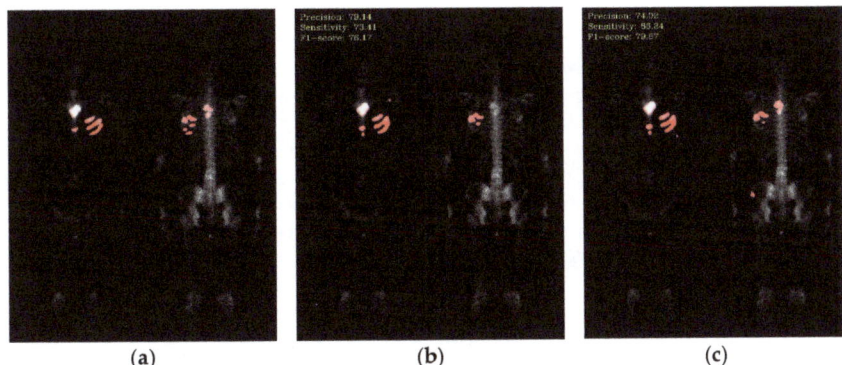

Figure 11. The qualitative results after transfer learning. (**a**) Ground truth; (**b**) segmentation results with dice loss (precision: 79.14, sensitivity: 73.41, F1-score: 76.17); (**c**) segmentation results with focal Tversky loss (precision: 74.02, sensitivity: 86.24, F1-score: 79.67).

The quantitative results are shown in Table 7. Compared to the results without transfer learning (Table 4), a slight improvement can be seen in the F1-score.

Table 7. The model performance with transfer learning.

Fold Number	Dice Loss			Focal Tversky Loss		
	Precision	Sensitivity	F1-Score	Precision	Sensitivity	F1-Score
1	67.81	70.28	69.02	66.51	72.04	69.17
2	71.44	63.75	67.38	70.80	60.64	65.33
3	76.75	60.73	67.80	69.87	69.25	69.56
4	86.56	51.54	64.61	81.80	60.28	69.41
5	68.88	62.84	65.72	51.28	66.78	58.01
6	84.14	43.46	57.31	80.00	52.20	63.18
7	62.07	66.34	64.14	50.69	86.04	63.80
8	51.90	72.17	60.38	43.82	85.62	57.97
9	62.30	64.44	63.35	52.07	77.78	62.38
10	64.98	74.47	69.40	63.92	77.56	70.09
Mean	69.68	63.00	66.17	63.08	70.82	66.72

5. Discussion

In this study, the raw Double U-Net architecture served as the baseline model for performance comparison. Subsequently, two schemes on negative sample extraction are explored to see the impact on the model performance.

Otsu thresholding can easily separate air and body, thus removing the air background. The air background contains no information and wastes computation time. Although we define three classes in training, the BG class does not count into the loss. Another profit is to extract negative samples. In our previous study [14] we found that training with only metastasis (positive) class is not a good idea. It is better to train models with positive and negative samples simultaneously. Our results shown in Tables 3 and 4 have confirmed this again; they are better than the baseline shown in Table 2.

Tables 5 and 6 show the results obtained using negative mining. The model performances seem slightly worse than Otsu thresholding. This might be due to the fact that negative sample areas are significantly smaller than those negative samples produced using the thresholding technique. Thus, they contained less information for training. Moreover, negative mining requires a pre-trained model, and the thresholding technique does not. Our study indicates that while adding negative samples is necessary, there is not only one way to do so. There could be many other ways to create negative samples for training.

We compared our research with other relevant studies in terms of network architecture and results, as shown in Table 8. This table summarizes studies that used deep learning methods for the segmentation of bone metastases in bone scan images. The authors of [20] proposed an improved ResU-Net model for the segmentation of metastatic hotspots in thorax SPECT images, achieving precision, sensitivity, and IoU scores of 77.21%, 67.88%, and 61.03%, respectively. The authors of [21] added a methods attention mechanism to the original U-Net network's skip connections to enhance model performance, resulting in an F1-score of 57.10% and an IoU of 63.30%. The authors of [16] introduced a neural network model based on U-Net++, achieving segmentation performance with a precision of 68.85%, a sensitivity of 62.57%, and an F1-score of 65.56%. The authors of [22] combined the UNet3+ network with an attention mechanism, proposing an improved UNet3+ network that achieved segmentation performance with a precision of 61.20%, a sensitivity of 68.33%, and an F1-score of 64.33%. The authors of [23] utilized a swin transformer as the backbone network and proposed a bone imaging focus segmentation algorithm, achieving an F1-score of 77.81% and an IoU of 35.59%.

Table 8. Comparison with network architecture and analysis results from related studies.

Method	Region	Precision	Sensitivity	F1-Score	IoU
ResU-Net [20]	Thorax	77.21	67.88	-	61.03
U-Net [21]	Thorax	-	-	57.10	63.30
U-Net++ [16]	Thorax	68.85	62.57	65.56	-
UNet3+ [22]	Thorax	61.20	68.33	64.33	-
Swin Transformer [23]	Thorax + Pelvis	-	-	77.81	35.59
Ours	Whole body excluded below knees	69.96	63.55	66.60	-

In Table 8, the improved ResU-Net model used in [20] achieved the best model performance in the segmentation of metastatic lesions in the thorax region. The model based on the swin transformer in [23] achieved the highest F1-score. Our segmented region is the widest in Table 8, and our model's F1-score of 66.60 is second only to [23].

The selection of loss function might play a crucial role in model performance. For complex tasks like segmentation, there is no universally applicable loss function. It largely depends on the properties of the training dataset, such as distribution, skewness, boundaries, etc. For segmentation tasks with extreme class imbalance, focal-related loss functions are more appropriate [41]. Additionally, since the vanilla Double U-Net model has a higher precision than sensitivity, we are keen to use Tversky-related loss functions to balance the false positives (FP) and false negatives (FN) rates. Therefore, we adopt focal Tversky loss as the compared loss function. In the future, further exploration and research should be conducted on the selection of optimizers.

Not all hotspots in bone scan images represent bone metastases; normal bone absorption, renal metabolism, inflammation, and injuries can also cause hotspots in images, leading to false positives in segmentation. In addition to the inherent imaging principles of bone scan images that make training the model challenging, the presence of artifacts in the images is also a crucial factor leading to misclassification. Examples of such artifacts include high-activity areas like the kidneys and bladder, the injection site of the radioactive isotope, and motion artifacts, as shown in Figure 12. Apart from artifacts in breast cancer images, prostate cancer bone scan images also exhibit high-activity artifacts from catheters, urine bags, and diapers, as shown in Figure 13. In the future, appropriate pre-processing can be applied to minimize the impact from artifacts, or additional classes such as benign lesions and artifacts can be introduced to train the model more accurately.

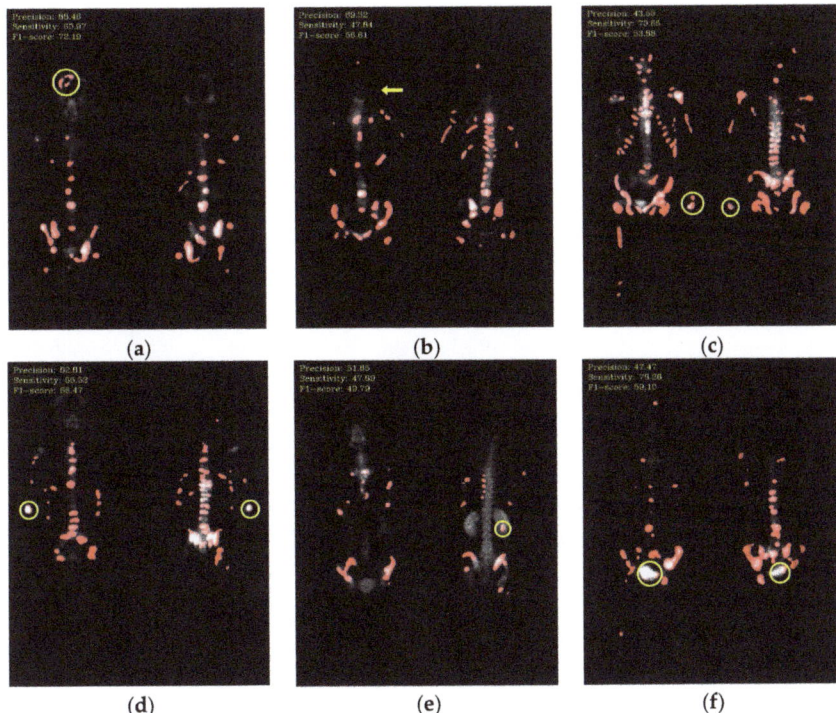

Figure 12. Mis-segmentation of non-metastatic lesions. (**a**) Bone fracture (head region) (precision: 88.46; sensitivity: 60.97; F1-score: 72.19); (**b**) motion artifact (head region) (precision: 69.32; sensitivity: 47.84; F1-score: 56.61); (**c**) injection site (wrist) (precision: 43.55; sensitivity: 70.65; F1-score: 53.88); (**d**) injection site (elbow) (precision: 82.81; sensitivity: 55.52; F1-score: 66.47); (**e**) kidney (precision: 51.85; sensitivity: 47.89; F1-score: 49.79); (**f**) bladder (precision: 47.47; sensitivity: 78.28; F1-score: 59.10).

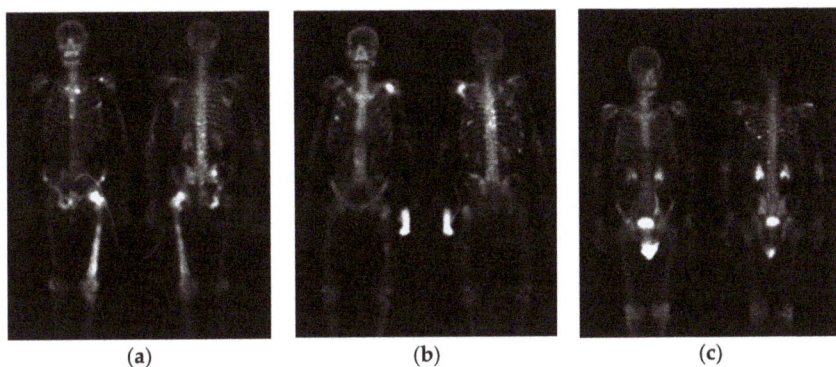

Figure 13. Artifacts in bone scan images of prostate cancer. (**a**) Catheter; (**b**) urinary bag; (**c**) diaper.

The image pre-processing is usually important before using neural networks. Our previous study proposed a pre-processing method where the original images were combined into a 3D image to alleviate the issue of spatial connectivity loss [14]. View aggregation, an operation applied to bone scan images, has been used to enhance areas of high absorption [16]. This method enhances lesions that appear in both anterior and posterior view images and maps lesions that only appear in either anterior or posterior view images. However, that method cannot be applied in this study, since we calculate every pixel here and all errors (sensitivity, precision) are calculated in pixel-wise scale.

6. Conclusions

In this study, we confirm the validity of using negative samples in the task of bone metastatic lesions detection in breast cancer whole body bone scan images. The model is trained using positive and negative samples. We used background pre-processing to remove excess air background information. Adding negative samples improved the model's precision. The images we used only excluded the less common regions below the knees for bone metastatic lesions and could simultaneously perform image segmentation for both anterior and posterior views. Our model is able to provide a more comprehensive evaluation of bone metastasis images. The precision, sensitivity, and F1-score for the segmentation of bone metastatic lesions are calculated on a pixel-level scale and the best results reach 70.24%, 61.80%, and 65.75% for dice loss and 69.96%, 63.55%, and 66.60% for focal Tversky loss, respectively.

The limitation of this study is the use of a small, single-center dataset, comprising only 100 breast cancer patients. This may result in limited model performance and generalizability. In the dataset, only 10 negative samples were collected from breast cancer patients, and the class imbalance between positive and negative samples could also pose a challenge to model performance.

There is still significant room for improvement in the model's performance in this study. In the future, we plan to collect more WBBS images from different centers to further validate the proposed model's performance. We will focus on fine-tuning the hyperparameters of the neural network and optimizing the choice of optimizers to enhance segmentation performance and reduce computational costs. Noise and artifacts in WBBS images are inevitable issues, and we plan to explore more image pre-processing methods to remove false artifacts and image noise to improve image quality, thus enhancing segmentation capabilities. Finally, we will use the interpretations of nuclear medicine physicians as the gold standard to compare the final model with the decisions made by nuclear medicine physicians, aiming to assess any discrepancies in decisions and evaluate the clinical utility of the model.

Author Contributions: Conceptualization, D.-C.C.; methodology, D.-C.C.; software, P.-N.Y. and Y.-Y.C.; validation, P.-N.Y. and Y.-Y.C.; formal analysis D.-C.C.; investigation, Y.-C.L. and T.-C.H.; resources, T.-C.H. and D.-C.C.; data curation, P.-N.Y. and Y.-Y.C.; writing—original draft preparation, Y.-Y.C.; writing—review and editing, D.-C.C.; visualization, D.-C.C.; supervision, D.-C.C.; project administration, D.-C.C.; funding acquisition, D.-C.C. All authors have read and agreed to the published version of the manuscript.

Funding: This research was funded by National Science and Technology Council (NSTC), Taiwan, grant number MOST 111-2314-B-039-040.

Institutional Review Board Statement: The study was approved by the Institutional Review Board (IRB) and the Hospital Research Ethics Committee (CMUH106-REC2-130) of China Medical University.

Informed Consent Statement: Patient consent was waived by IRB due to this being a retrospective study and images were only used without patients' identification.

Data Availability Statement: Not applicable.

Acknowledgments: We thank the National Center for High-performance Computing (NCHC) for providing computational and storage resources.

Conflicts of Interest: The authors declare no conflict of interest.

References

1. Gender Equality Committee of the Executive Yuan. Available online: https://www.gender.ey.gov.tw/gecdb/Stat_Statistics_DetailData.aspx?sn=nLF9GdMD%2B%2Bv41SsobdVgKw%3D%3D (accessed on 24 February 2023).

2. Coleman, R.E.; Rubens, R.D. The clinical course of bone metastases from breast cancer. *Br. J. Cancer* **1987**, *55*, 61–66. [CrossRef] [PubMed]
3. Kakhki, V.R.D.; Anvari, K.; Sadeghi, R.; Mahmoudian, A.S.; Torabian-Kakhki, M. Pattern and distribution of bone metastases in common malignant tumors. *Nucl. Med. Rev.* **2013**, *16*, 66–69. [CrossRef] [PubMed]
4. Hamaoka, T.; Madewell, J.E.; Podoloff, D.A.; Hortobagyi, G.N.; Ueno, N.T. Bone imaging in metastatic breast cancer. *J. Clin. Oncol.* **2004**, *22*, 2942–2953. [CrossRef]
5. Even-Sapir, E.; Metser, U.; Mishani, E.; Lievshitz, G.; Lerman, H.; Leibovitch, I. The detection of bone metastases in patients with high-risk prostate cancer: 99mTc-MDP Planar bone scintigraphy, single- and multifield-of-viewSPECT, 18F-fluoride PET, and 18F-fluoride PET/CT. *J. Nucl. Med.* **2006**, *47*, 287–297.
6. Costelloe, C.M.; Rohren, E.M.; Madewell, J.E.; Hamaoka, T.; Theriault, R.L.; Yu, T.K.; Ueno, N.T. Imaging bone metastases in breast cancer: Techniques and recommendations for diagnosis. *Lancet Oncol.* **2009**, *10*, 606–614. [CrossRef] [PubMed]
7. Vijayanathan, S.; Butt, S.; Gnanasegaran, G.; Groves, A.M. Advantages and limitations of imaging the musculoskeletal system by conventional radiological, radionuclide, and hybrid modalities. *Semin. Nucl. Med.* **2009**, *39*, 357–368. [CrossRef]
8. O'Sullivan, G.J.; Carty, F.L.; Cronin, C.G. Imaging of bone metastasis: An update. *World J. Radiol.* **2015**, *7*, 202. [CrossRef]
9. Imbriaco, M.; Larson, S.M.; Yeung, H.W.; Mawlawi, O.R.; Erdi, Y.; Venkatraman, E.S.; Scher, H.I. A new parameter for measuring metastatic bone involvement by prostate cancer: The Bone Scan Index. *Clin. Cancer Res.* **1998**, *4*, 1765–1772.
10. Erdi, Y.E.; Humm, J.L.; Imbriaco, M.; Yeung, H.; Larson, S.M. Quantitative bone metastases analysis based on image segmentation. *J. Nucl. Med.* **1997**, *38*, 1401–1406.
11. Ulmert, D.; Kaboteh, R.; Fox, J.J.; Savage, C.; Evans, M.J.; Lilja, H.; Larson, S.M. A novel automated platform for quantifying the extent of skeletal tumour involvement in prostate cancer patients using the Bone Scan Index. *Eur. Urol.* **2012**, *62*, 78–84. [CrossRef]
12. Shimizu, A.; Wakabayashi, H.; Kanamori, T.; Saito, A.; Nishikawa, K.; Daisaki, H.; Kawabe, J. Automated measurement of bone scan index from a whole-body bone scintigram. *Int. J. Comput. Assist. Radiol. Surg.* **2020**, *15*, 389–400. [CrossRef] [PubMed]
13. Cheng, D.C.; Liu, C.C.; Hsieh, T.C.; Yen, K.Y.; Kao, C.H. Bone metastasis detection in the chest and pelvis from a whole-body bone scan using deep learning and a small dataset. *Electronics* **2021**, *10*, 1201. [CrossRef]
14. Cheng, D.C.; Hsieh, T.C.; Yen, K.Y.; Kao, C.H. Lesion-based bone metastasis detection in chest bone scintigraphy images of prostate cancer patients using pre-train, negative mining, and deep learning. *Diagnostics* **2021**, *11*, 518. [CrossRef]
15. Cheng, D.C.; Liu, C.C.; Kao, C.H.; Hsieh, T.C. System of Deep Learning Neural Network in Prostate Cancer Bone Metastasis Identification Based on Whole Body Bone Scan Images. U.S. Patent US11488303B2, 1 November 2022.
16. Cao, Y.; Liu, L.; Chen, X.; Man, Z.; Lin, Q.; Zeng, X.; Huang, X. Segmentation of lung cancer-caused metastatic lesions in bone scan images using self-defined model with deep supervision. *Biomed. Signal Process. Control* **2023**, *79*, 104068. [CrossRef]
17. Jha, D.; Riegler, M.A.; Johansen, D.; Halvorsen, P.; Johansen, H.D. Doubleu-net: A deep convolutional neural network for medical image segmentation. In Proceedings of the IEEE 33rd International Symposium on Computer-Based Medical Systems (CBMS), Rochester, MN, USA, 28–30 July 2020; pp. 558–564.
18. Otsu, N. A threshold selection method from gray-level histograms. *IEEE Trans. Syst. Man Cybern.* **1979**, *9*, 62–66. [CrossRef]
19. Apiparakoon, T.; Rakratchatakul, N.; Chantadisai, M.; Vutrapongwatana, U.; Kingpetch, K.; Sirisalipoch, S.; Chuangsuwanich, E. MaligNet: Semisupervised learning for bone lesion instance segmentation using bone scintigraphy. *IEEE Access* **2020**, *8*, 27047–27066. [CrossRef]
20. Lin, Q.; Luo, M.; Gao, R.; Li, T.; Man, Z.; Cao, Y.; Wang, H. Deep learning based automatic segmentation of metastasis hotspots in thorax bone SPECT images. *PLoS ONE* **2020**, *15*, e0243253. [CrossRef]
21. Zhang, J.; Huang, M.; Deng, T.; Cao, Y.; Lin, Q. Bone metastasis segmentation based on Improved U-NET algorithm. In Proceedings of the 4th International Conference on Advanced Algorithms and Control Engineering (ICAACE), Sanya, China, 29–31 January 2021.
22. Liu, C.; Cao, Y.; Lin, Q.; Man, Z.; He, Y.; Peng, L. Segmentation of metastatic lesions on bone scan images based on improved UNet3+ network. In Proceedings of the 4th International Conference on Computer Engineering and Application (ICCEA), Hangzhou, China, 7–9 April 2023; pp. 916–920.
23. Wu, T.; Luo, R.; Lin, H.; Yu, H.; Wang, Q.; Liu, H. Research on focal segmentation of bone scan based on Swin Transformer. In Proceedings of the 4th International Conference on Computer Vision, Image and Deep Learning (CVIDL), Zhuhai, China, 12–14 May 2023; pp. 426–430.
24. Khan, S.A.; Gulzar, Y.; Turaev, S.; Peng, Y.S. A modified HSIFT Descriptor for medical image classification of anatomy objects. *Symmetry* **2021**, *13*, 1987. [CrossRef]
25. Gulzar, Y.; Khan, S.A. Skin lesion segmentation based on vision transformers and convolutional neural networks—A comparative study. *Appl. Sci.* **2022**, *12*, 5990. [CrossRef]
26. Mehmood, A.; Gulzar, Y.; Ilyas, Q.M.; Jabbari, A.; Ahmad, M.; Iqbal, S. SBXception: A Shallower and Broader Xception Architecture for Efficient Classification of Skin Lesions. *Cancers* **2023**, *15*, 3604. [CrossRef]
27. Anand, V.; Gupta, S.; Gupta, D.; Gulzar, Y.; Xin, Q.; Juneja, S.; Shaikh, A. Weighted Average Ensemble Deep Learning Model for Stratification of Brain Tumor in MRI Images. *Diagnostics* **2023**, *13*, 1320. [CrossRef] [PubMed]
28. Khan, F.; Ayoub, S.; Gulzar, Y.; Majid, M.; Reegu, F.A.; Mir, M.S.; Elwasila, O. MRI-Based Effective Ensemble Frameworks for Predicting Human Brain Tumor. *J. Imaging* **2023**, *9*, 163. [CrossRef] [PubMed]

29. Sadik, M.; Jakobsson, D.; Olofsson, F.; Ohlsson, M.; Suurkula, M.; Edenbrandt, L. A new computer-based decision-support system for the interpretation of bone scans. *Nucl. Med. Commun.* **2006**, *27*, 417–423. [CrossRef] [PubMed]
30. Sadik, M.; Hamadeh, I.; Nordblom, P.; Suurkula, M.; Höglund, P.; Ohlsson, M.; Edenbrandt, L. Computer-assisted interpretation of planar whole-body bone scans. *J. Nucl. Med.* **2008**, *49*, 1958–1965. [CrossRef]
31. Aslantas, A.; Dandil, E.; Sağlam, S.; Çakiroğlu, M. CADBOSS: A computer-aided diagnosis system for whole-body bone scintigraphy scans. *J. Cancer Res. Ther.* **2016**, *12*, 787–792. [CrossRef]
32. Elfarra, F.G.; Calin, M.A.; Parasca, S.V. Computer-aided detection of bone metastasis in bone scintigraphy images using parallelepiped classification method. *Ann. Nucl. Med.* **2019**, *33*, 866–874. [CrossRef]
33. Calin, M.A.; Elfarra, F.G.; Parasca, S.V. Object-oriented classification approach for bone metastasis mapping from whole-body bone scintigraphy. *Phys. Medica* **2021**, *84*, 141–148. [CrossRef]
34. Feng, Q.; Cao, Y.; Lin, Q.; Man, Z.; He, Y.; Liu, C. SPECT bone scan image classification by fusing multi-attention mechanism with deep residual networks. In Proceedings of the 4th International Conference on Computer Vision, Image and Deep Learning (CVIDL), Zhuhai, China, 12–14 May 2023; pp. 47–51.
35. Lin, Q.; Li, T.; Cao, C.; Cao, Y.; Man, Z.; Wang, H. Deep learning based automated diagnosis of bone metastases with SPECT thoracic bone images. *Sci. Rep.* **2021**, *11*, 4223. [CrossRef]
36. Pi, Y.; Zhao, Z.; Xiang, Y.; Li, Y.; Cai, H.; Yi, Z. Automated diagnosis of bone metastasis based on multi-view bone scans using attention-augmented deep neural networks. *Med. Image Anal.* **2020**, *65*, 101784. [CrossRef]
37. Li, T.; Lin, Q.; Guo, Y.; Zhao, S.; Zeng, X.; Man, Z.; Hu, Y. Automated detection of skeletal metastasis of lung cancer with bone scans using convolutional nuclear network. *Phys. Med. Biol.* **2022**, *67*, 015004. [CrossRef]
38. Moustakidis, S.; Siouras, A.; Papandrianos, N.; Ntakolia, C.; Papageorgiou, E. Deep learning for bone metastasis localisation in nuclear imaging data of breast cancer patients. In Proceedings of the 12th International Conference on Information, Intelligence, Systems & Applications (IISA), Chania Crete, Greece, 12–14 July 2021; pp. 1–8.
39. Lin, Q.; Chen, X.; Liu, L.; Cao, Y.; Man, Z.; Zeng, X.; Huang, X. Detecting multiple lesions of lung cancer-caused metastasis with bone scans using a self-defined object detection model based on SSD framework. *Phys. Med. Biol.* **2022**, *67*, 225009. [CrossRef] [PubMed]
40. Yu, P.N.; Lai, Y.C.; Chen, Y.Y.; Cheng, D.C. Skeleton segmentation on bone scintigraphy for BSI computation. *Diagnostics* **2023**, *13*, 2302. [CrossRef] [PubMed]
41. Jadon, S. A survey of loss functions for semantic segmentation. In Proceedings of the IEEE Conference on Computational Intelligence in Bioinformatics and Computational Biology (CIBCB), Via del Mar, Chile, 27–29 October 2020; pp. 1–7.

Disclaimer/Publisher's Note: The statements, opinions and data contained in all publications are solely those of the individual author(s) and contributor(s) and not of MDPI and/or the editor(s). MDPI and/or the editor(s) disclaim responsibility for any injury to people or property resulting from any ideas, methods, instructions or products referred to in the content.

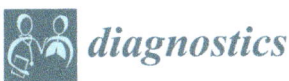

Article

One-Stage Detection without Segmentation for Multi-Type Coronary Lesions in Angiography Images Using Deep Learning

Hui Wu [1,†], Jing Zhao [2], Jiehui Li [3,†], Yan Zeng [4], Weiwei Wu [5], Zhuhuang Zhou [1,*], Shuicai Wu [1,*], Liang Xu [6], Min Song [3], Qibin Yu [3], Ziwei Song [1] and Lin Chen [1]

1. Department of Biomedical Engineering, Faculty of Environment and Life, Beijing University of Technology, Beijing 100124, China
2. Department of Geriatrics, The Third Medical Center of Chinese PLA General Hospital, Beijing 100039, China
3. State Key Laboratory of Cardiovascular Disease, Department of Cardiac Surgery, National Center for Cardiovascular Diseases, Fuwai Hospital, Chinese Academy of Medical Sciences, Peking Union Medical College, Beijing 100037, China
4. Department of Research Center, Shanghai United Imaging Intelligence Co., Ltd., Shanghai 201807, China
5. College of Biomedical Engineering, Capital Medical University, Beijing 100069, China
6. State Key Laboratory of Cardiovascular Disease, Department of Structural Heart Disease, National Center for Cardiovascular Diseases, Fuwai Hospital, Chinese Academy of Medical Sciences, Peking Union Medical College, Beijing 100037, China
* Correspondence: zhouzh@bjut.edu.cn (Z.Z.); wushuicai@bjut.edu.cn (S.W.)
† These authors contributed equally to this work and share first authorship.

Abstract: It is rare to use the one-stage model without segmentation for the automatic detection of coronary lesions. This study sequentially enrolled 200 patients with significant stenoses and occlusions of the right coronary and categorized their angiography images into two angle views: The CRA (cranial) view of 98 patients with 2453 images and the LAO (left anterior oblique) view of 176 patients with 3338 images. Randomization was performed at the patient level to the training set and test set using a 7:3 ratio. YOLOv5 was adopted as the key model for direct detection. Four types of lesions were studied: Local Stenosis (LS), Diffuse Stenosis (DS), Bifurcation Stenosis (BS), and Chronic Total Occlusion (CTO). At the image level, the precision, recall, mAP@0.1, and mAP@0.5 predicted by the model were 0.64, 0.68, 0.66, and 0.49 in the CRA view and 0.68, 0.73, 0.70, and 0.56 in the LAO view, respectively. At the patient level, the precision, recall, and F_1 scores predicted by the model were 0.52, 0.91, and 0.65 in the CRA view and 0.50, 0.94, and 0.64 in the LAO view, respectively. YOLOv5 performed the best for lesions of CTO and LS at both the image level and the patient level. In conclusion, the one-stage model without segmentation as YOLOv5 is feasible to be used in automatic coronary lesion detection, with the most suitable types of lesions as LS and CTO.

Keywords: coronary angiography; deep learning; coronary artery stenosis detection; convolutional neural network; one-stage detection; without segmentation

1. Introduction

Coronary artery disease (CAD) is one of the most common types of cardiovascular disease. It could cause stenoses and occlusions of coronary arteries, which will finally lead to severe endpoints such as myocardial ischemia and infarction. It is also the leading cause of mortality in the world, which is responsible for 16% of the total 55.4 million deaths in recent years [1]. Coronary angiography (CAG), which is recommended as the most important examination for CAD, is considered the gold standard for the diagnosis and treatment of ischemic heart disease [2–4]. CAG images can provide detailed anatomical information of vessels from multiple angle views, which is better than other examinations such as coronary CT angiography (CCTA) and cardiac magnetic resonance imaging (cMRI).

However, compared to CCTA and cMRI, CAG images still have some limitations: (1) Instantaneous contrast agent inhomogeneity makes the images fuzzy, with poor contrast

Citation: Wu, H.; Zhao, J.; Li, J.; Zeng, Y.; Wu, W.; Zhou, Z.; Wu, S.; Xu, L.; Song, M.; Yu, Q.; et al. One-Stage Detection without Segmentation for Multi-Type Coronary Lesions in Angiography Images Using Deep Learning. Diagnostics 2023, 13, 3011. https://doi.org/10.3390/diagnostics13183011

Academic Editor: Daniele Giansanti

Received: 7 August 2023
Revised: 12 September 2023
Accepted: 18 September 2023
Published: 21 September 2023

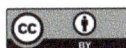

Copyright: © 2023 by the authors. Licensee MDPI, Basel, Switzerland. This article is an open access article distributed under the terms and conditions of the Creative Commons Attribution (CC BY) license (https://creativecommons.org/licenses/by/4.0/).

between vessels and surrounding tissues; (2) irregular angle views cause images to change continuously; (3) complex vessel structures in two-dimensional images cause different coronary arteries to overlap and make them difficult to distinguish. Even so, given its extensive clinical application and significant diagnostic value, many studies still try to perform studies of artificial intelligence (AI)-assisted diagnosis of CAG via the deep learning (DL) method. The method of segmentation before detection has been mostly employed in previous studies. As described in the limitations of CAG images, difficulties in defining and detecting lesions caused by overlapped coronary arteries were the major challenges in the one-stage detection of multi-type coronary lesions. However, right coronary arteries rarely encounter these challenges due to less overlap.

Currently, segmenting the coronary arteries followed by diameter measurements or stenosis evaluations is the most studied method [5–7]. Zhao et al. [8] classified the lesions by performing image segmentation of the vessel centerline, calculating vessel diameters, and measuring the degree of stenoses. Liu et al. [9] performed vessel boundary-aware segmentation, branch node localization, coronary artery tree construction, and vessel diameter fitting, and ultimately accomplished stenosis detection. Algarni et al. [10] employed image noise removal, contrast enhancement, and Otsu thresholding as pre-processing techniques and used attention-based nested U-Net and VGG-16 for vessel segmentation and lesion detection. Their method only generated a binary classification of normal and abnormal images. However, both vessel segmentation and the extraction of coronary artery centerlines require significant work regarding manual annotation. Meanwhile, providing pixel-level specific lesion annotations for each frame reduces the robustness of lesion assessment and limits its clinical use and applications with large datasets.

Furthermore, some studies have stepped further by incorporating the automatic selection of contrast-enhanced images to extract the key frames of diagnosis for AI analysis. Cong et al. [11] employed convolutional neural networks (CNNs) and long short-term memory (LSTM) networks for automatic detection and key frame sampling. Then, they used the modified pre-trained Inception-V3 network [12] and employed the anchor-based feature pyramid network (FPN) for stenosis localization. Similarly, Moon et al. [13] used weakly supervised DL to extract key frames and performed the classification of regions of 50% stenosis. Then, they used the convolutional block attention module (CBAM) [14] to achieve the precise localization of vessel stenosis.

Some other studies have also employed multiple types of network models to improve detection performance. Ling et al. [15] used ResNet, Mask R-CNN, and RetinaNet to construct a system that includes functionalities of classification, segmentation, and detection. Du et al. [16] designed a multi-scale CNN to extract texture features of different scales from CAG images. They used the Faster R-CNN [17] framework for the detection and localization of stenoses. Danilov et al. [18] also trained and tested eight different detectors based on various network architectures and confirmed the feasibility of DL methods for the real-time detection of coronary stenoses by the intercomparisons among them.

On the other hand, studies also used artificially synthesized data because of the significant manual pre-processing steps of CAG images. Antczak et al. [19] trained a patch-based classification model with an artificial dataset and then tuned up the network using real-world patches to improve its accuracy. Ovalle-Magallanes et al. [20] proposed a pre-trained CNN model based on transfer learning for segmentation, along with fine-tuning by artificial and real-world data, to introduce a novel method for automated stenosis detection. The relevant studies are summarized in Table 1.

Table 1. Related studies are summarized in four aspects: Methods, data, classes, and results.

Ref.	Methods	Data	Classes	Results
Zhao et al. (2021) [8]	FP-U-Net++, arterial centerline extraction, diameter calculation, arterial stenosis detection	99 patients, 314 images	1–24%, 25–49%, 50–69%, 70–100%	Precision = 0.6998, recall = 0.6840,
Liu et al. (2023) [9]	AI-QCA	3275 patients, 13,222 images	0–100%	Precision = 0.897, recall = 0.879
Algarni et al. (2022) [10]	ASCARIS model	130 images	normal and abnormal	Accuracy = 97%, recall = 95%, specificity = 93%
Cong et al. (2023) [11]	Inception-v3 and LSTM, redundancy training, and Inception-V3, FPN	230 patients, 14,434 images	<25%, 25–99%, CTO	Accuracy = 0.85, recall = 0.96, AUC = 0.86
Moon et al. (2020) [13]	GoogleNet Inception-v3, CBAM, Grad-CAM	452 clips	Stenosis ≥ 50%	AUC = 0.971, accuracy = 0.934
Ovalle-Magallanes et al. (2020) [20]	pre-trained CNN via Transfer Learning, CAM	10,000 artificial images, 250 real images	Stenosis	Accuracy = 0.95, precision = 0.93, sensitivity = 0.98, specificity = 0.92, F_1 score = 0.95
Antczak et al. (2021) [19]	A patch-based CNN for stenosis detection	10,000 artificial images, 250 real images	Stenosis	Accuracy = 90%
Du et al. (2021) [21]	A DNN for the recognition of lesion morphology	10,073 patients, 20,612 images	Stenotic lesion, total occlusion, calcification, thrombus, and dissection	F_1 score = 0.829, 0.810, 0.802, 0.823, 0.854
Ling et al. (2023) [15]	DLCAG diagnose system	949 patients, 2980 images	Stenosis	mAP = 86.3%
Danilov et al. (2021) [18]	Comparison of state-of-the-art CNN (N = 8)	100 patients, 8325 images	Stenosis ≥ 70%	mAP = 0.94, F_1 score = 0.96, prediction speed = 10 fps
Pang et al. (2021) [22]	Stenosis-DetNet with SFF and SCA	166 sequence, 1494 images	Stenosis	Accuracy = 94.87%, sensitivity 82.22%

However, these studies still have some limitations: (1) Data in these studies are collected from patients with CAD who might undergo medical therapy or percutaneous coronary intervention (PCI) only. Lesions of them may be mild and simple, which could not represent the real world. (2) These studies lack detailed analysis of lesions as stenoses in detailed types. Du et al. [21] segmented the coronary arteries into more than 20 segments and explored various manifestations, such as stenosis, occlusion, calcification, thrombosis, and dissection. However, they did not analyze stenoses more comprehensively, of which lesions are the most common and important in clinical practice. (3) These studies all performed detection based on segmentation. Compared to direct detection, their approaches still involved more learning steps and more complex structures. Too many methods were employed to enhance model efficiency, which leaves space for further modification.

Inspired by this, we intended to develop a strategy to overcome these shortcomings in this study. We classified vascular lesions into four categories: Local stenosis, diffuse stenosis, bifurcation stenosis, and chronic total occlusion. We conducted a multi-view analysis of angiographies from candidates and adopted YOLOv5 as the key model for segmentation-free DL study of lesion detection, localization, and classification. Furthermore, we also employed the technique of gradient-weighted class activation mapping (Grad-CAM) for the visual explanations to evaluate the model performance and the feasibility of one-stage lesion detection without segmentation.

The contributions of this study are as follows:

1. This study enrolled angiography images from patients who were candidates for coronary artery bypass (CAB) surgery for the first time to evaluate the detection performance of DL techniques with complex lesions.
2. A single-stage detection model by the region-free approach was employed for the first time to detect vascular lesions directly, aiming to improve detection efficiency.
3. A more detailed classification of vascular stenoses was performed, providing a comprehensive evaluation of the network model's performance among different types of lesions.

2. Materials and Methods

2.1. Dataset Characteristics

Two hundred and fourteen patients who were potential candidates for CAB surgery were enrolled from a single cardiac center (Fuwai Hospital, Beijing, China). This study was reviewed and approved by the ethics committee of Fuwai Hospital. There were some exclusion criteria when collecting data: (1) Combined with other cardiovascular diseases except atrial septal defect, ventricular septal defect, patent ductus arteriosus, and valvular heart disease; (2) combined with other diseases requiring surgical treatment; (3) emergency coronary artery bypass grafting or clinically unstable coronary artery disease (e.g., myocardial infarction within 30 days, preoperative implantation of the aorta counterpulsation, the need for continuous pumping of nitrates, etc.); (4) preoperative critical condition; (5) history of cardiovascular pulmonary resuscitation (CPR). The dataset was built by patients' angiographies, which were saved as Digital Imaging and Communications in Medicine (DICOM) files and contained several angle views for left and right coronaries. Finally, images of the right coronary were analyzed in this study. Two major angle views were analyzed separately: The LAO (left anterior oblique) view is approximately 45° in the left anterior oblique view, which can display the proximal segment and middle segment well, and the CRA (cranial) view is approximately 20° in the cranial view, which can display the distal segment and posterior descending branch well. Fourteen patients had normal imaging findings with no lesion in the right coronary. Ninety-eight patients had lesions in the CRA view, and 176 patients had lesions in the LAO view. The final dataset had 2453 images in the CRA view and 3338 images in the LAO view. They were randomly divided into training sets and validation sets at the patient level by a ratio of 7:3. The enrollment profile is shown in Figure 1.

Four types of lesions (Figure 2) were analyzed in this study: (1) Local stenosis (LS): A local stenosis defined as any stenosis under 20 mm in length; (2) diffuse stenosis (DS): A diffuse stenosis defined as any stenosis over 20 mm in length, which was also named long lesion [23,24]; (3) bifurcation stenosis (BS): A bifurcation stenosis defined as any stenosis adjacent to, and/or involving, the origin of a significant side branch [25]; (4) chronic total occlusion (CTO): A chronic total occlusion defined as 100% occlusion of a coronary artery for a duration of greater than or equal to 3 months based on angiographic evidence. The details of image distribution are shown in Table 2.

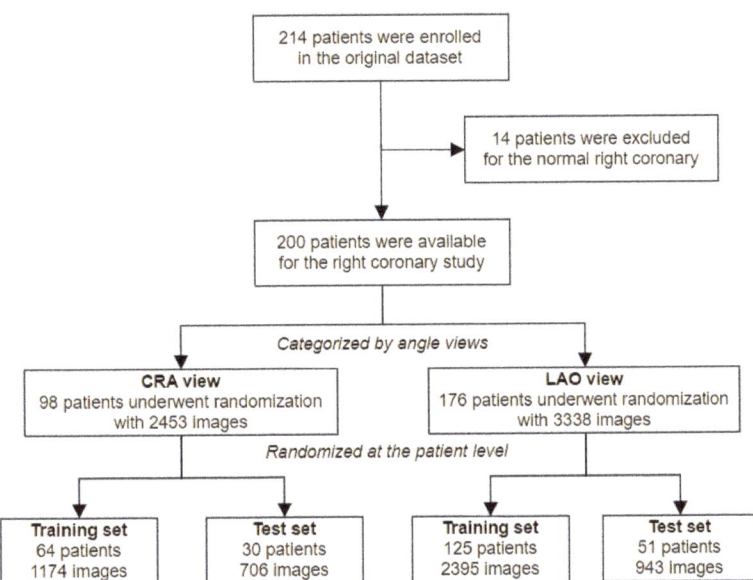

Figure 1. Flow chart of the study enrollment. CRA: cranial; LAO: left anterior oblique.

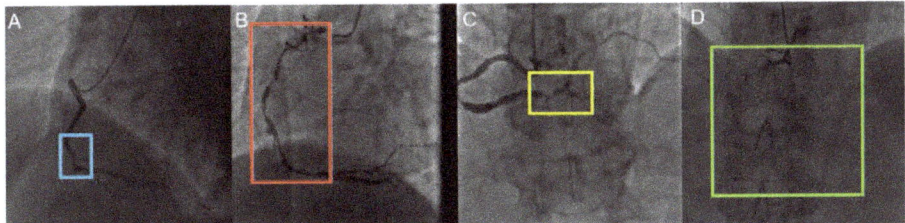

Figure 2. Four types of lesions on the right coronary artery. (**A**) Local stenosis (blue rectangular box); (**B**) diffuse stenosis (red rectangular box); (**C**) bifurcation stenosis (yellow rectangular box); (**D**) chronic total occlusion (green rectangular box).

Table 2. Distributions of images and lesions in the CRA and LAO angle views.

	The CRA View	The LAO View	p Value
Age, years	63 ± 8	64 ± 9	0.54
Gender			
Male (%)	68 (69%)	118 (67%)	0.72
Images	2453	3338	0.66
Training Set (%)	1747	2395	
Test Set (%)	706	943	
Lesions			
Training Set	3259	1529	<0.01
LS	2003	1005	
DS	376	96	
BS	500	375	
CTO	380	53	
Test Set	3874	1262	<0.01
LS	2187	433	
DS	405	273	
BS	411	174	
CTO	871	382	

CRA: cranial; LAO: left anterior oblique; LS: local stenosis; DS: diffuse stenosis; BS: bifurcation stenosis; CTO: chronic total occlusion.

2.2. Reference Standard and Annotation Procedures

We treated manual annotations by cardiologists and radiologists as the reference standard to evaluate the diagnostic performance of the model. Firstly, a researcher converted the DICOM files into JPG image files. Then, the images of the right coronary were selected from these files and handed over to two well-trained cardiologists or radiologists with over 10 years of experience in CAG to choose ideal frames and label the lesions. The lesions were classified into four types: LS, DS, BS, and CTO. In cases of conflicting annotations, the cardiologist and the radiologist collaborated and reached a consensus to determine the final type.

2.3. Experimental Environment and Methodology

Our experiments were conducted on a graphics workstation with Intel(R) Xeon Gold 6132 CPU@2.60 GHz 2.59 GHz, and NVIDIA TITAN RTX 24 G. Python 3.8 and PyTorch 1.13 were chosen as the DL framework. Figure 3 shows the flowchart of the DL procedure. DICOM Files were first exported into serial images. Ideal frames were chosen by our researcher and datasets were subsequently established. The manual annotation procedure was performed in the ways mentioned above, and the labeled images were sent to the network for training and testing. It outputs three vectors containing the predicted box class, confidence, and coordinate location in CAG images. Coronary lesions were directly detected, eliminating the requirement for time-consuming processes like segmentation and blood vessel extraction in previous studies. The types of coronary lesions were simplified to four with discriminative characteristics. To the best of our knowledge, the proposed method is the first to employ the single-stage YOLOv5 model with the region-free method to directly detect coronary lesions in CAG images. Moreover, Grad-CAM was incorporated to visualize the distinguishing area of specific lesion types for network interpretation.

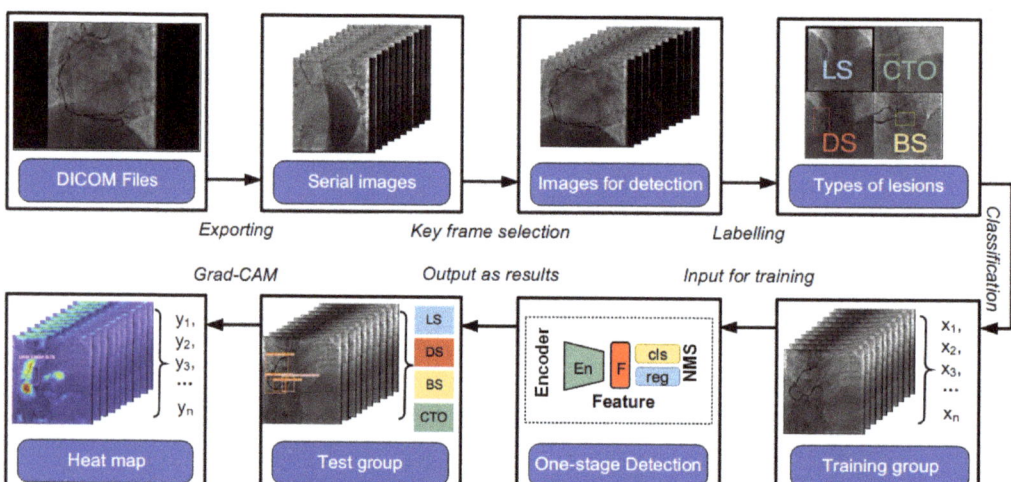

Figure 3. Flowchart of the proposed method. DICOM: digital imaging and communications in medicine; LS: local stenosis; DS: diffuse stenosis; BS: bifurcation stenosis; CTO: chronic total occlusion; NMS: non-max suppression; Grad-CAM: gradient-weighted class activation mapping.

We performed experiments both at the image level and the patient level. Because of the tiny changes in images in the same angle view of one single patient, it might be treated as one lesion for those found in the same position in the serial images. We defined that the prediction was correct at the patient level if one correct prediction of the lesion was found in one of the images in the serial.

2.4. Architecture of Models

2.4.1. The YOLOv5x Model

Figure 4 shows the structure of the YOLOv5x [26]. The input was uniform-size CAG image data, which were sent to the one-stage segmentation-free CNN. The network automatically learned the most class-related discriminant region highlighted to detect lesions directly, skipping the time-consuming classification and location in two steps. Finally, the network directly returned the size, position, and category of the target lesion, achieving end-to-end predictions.

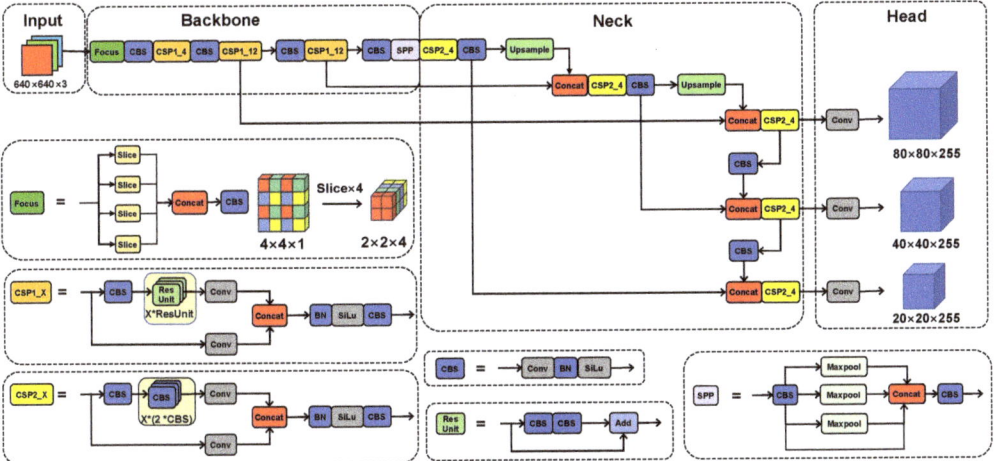

Figure 4. Overview of the YOLOv5x model architecture. The whole architecture contains 4 general modules, namely, an input terminal, a backbone, a neck, and a prediction network, along with 6 basic components: Focus, CSP1_X, CSP2_X, CBS, Res Unit, and SPP.

The YOLOv5x consisted of a backbone feature extraction network, a neck network, and a head target prediction network. The Mosaic data enhancement method was used to augment the data, which makes the network more robust. The backbone network was mainly composed of a focus structure, a cross-stage-partial (CSP) module, and a spatial pyramid pooling (SPP) module. The focus structure sliced the input CAG images and stitched the sliced result, which reduces the loss of lesion information and effectively improves the quality of feature extraction of contrast maps. Two CSP structures were employed to speed up the inference, decrease computation, and improve lesion detection. The feature pyramid network (FPN) [27] and path aggregation network (PAN) [28] were used in the neck to realize multi-scale lesion feature fusion. Three branches of target detection heads were used in the procedure, which could detect lesions on small, medium, and large targets, respectively. The dense anchor frame could significantly increase the network's ability to identify targets, which is obvious for small target detection. The network directly outputs results with predictions of lesion types and confidence to realize the automatic integrated prediction of the lesion type and position.

In this study, the batch size was 16 for the training set and 32 for the test set. A total of 100 epochs of training were conducted. LambdaLR was used as the learning rate updating strategy, and the stochastic gradient descent (SGD) optimizer and an initial learning rate of 10^{-4} were used. Box loss, obj (object) loss, and cls (class) loss were used:

$$Loss = CIoULoss + \sum_{i=0}^{S\times S}\sum_{j=0}^{B} I_{ij}^{obj}[C_i\log(C_i)+(1-C_i)\log(1-C_i)]$$
$$-\sum_{i=0}^{S\times S}\sum_{j=0}^{B} I_{ij}^{noobj}[C_i\log(C_i)+(1-C_i)\log(1-C_i)] \quad (1)$$
$$+\sum_{i=0}^{S\times S}\sum_{j=0}^{B} I_{ij}^{obj}\sum_{c\in classes}[p_i(c)\log(p_i(c))+(1-p_i(c))\log(1-p_i(c))]$$

where S represents the size of the final layer of feature maps and B is the number of detection boxes. I_{ij}^{obj} stands for items in the grid (i, j) and I_{ij}^{noobj} for objects not present in the grid (i, j).

YOLOv5 used *CIoUloss* [29] as the loss function of bounding box coordinate regression, which addresses the issue of slow convergence speed and imprecision regression in *IoU* and *GIoU* [30]. Additionally, while conducting non-maximum suppression, weighted non-maximum suppression (NMS) was employed, which effectively detects some overlapping vessels in coronary angiography images without consuming more processing resources.

2.4.2. The Grad-CAM Technique

We used the Grad-CAM [31] for visual explanations after lesion detection to identify the discriminative regions in each trained model that have varied contribution weights for its classification decision. Grad-CAM can be considered mathematically as a modification of CAM and can be utilized to extend to any CNN-based network.

To understand the significance of each neuron to a specific lesion category c (e.g., the local stenosis), Grad-CAM used the gradient information flowing into the ultimate convolutional layer of the CNN. The neuron importance weights α_k^c were obtained by an averaged pooling of gradients via backpropagation from category c:

$$\alpha_k^c = \frac{1}{Z}\sum_i\sum_j \frac{\partial y^c}{\partial A_{ij}^k} \quad (2)$$

where Z is a normalization operation. The output of Grad-CAM is generated when all feature maps of the same size are weighted and added in accordance with their respective weights. Then, a rectified linear unit (*ReLU*) was applied to the linear combination to reject feature maps with negative activation values (A^k):

$$L_{Grad-CAM}^c = ReLU\left(\sum_k \alpha_k^c \cdot A^k\right) \quad (3)$$

2.5. Performance Evaluation

The detection performance was evaluated by the confusion matrix, precision-recall (P-R) curve, precision, recall, F_1 score, and mean average precision (*mAP*) at the image level and the precision, recall, F_1 score, and *mFP* at the patient level. They were defined as

$$Precision = \frac{TP}{TP+FP} \quad (4)$$

$$Recall = \frac{TP}{TP+FN} \quad (5)$$

$$F_1\ score = 2\times \frac{Precision \times Recall}{Precision + Recall} \quad (6)$$

$$IoU = \frac{|A\cap B|}{|A\cup B|} \quad (7)$$

$$mFP = \frac{FP}{n} \tag{8}$$

where A is the predicted label from YOLOv5x and B is the reference label. A true positive (TP) represents the correct classification of lesions with the intersection over union (IoU) $\geq$ threshold. A false positive (FP) represents the incorrect classification of lesions OR with the intersection over union (IoU) < threshold. The mean false positive (mFP) represents the mean number of FPs for each patient. A false negative (FN) is an undetected reference label. We also employed mAP@0.1 (IoU = 0.1) and mAP@0.5 (IoU = 0.5) in the study.

2.6. Statistics

Descriptive factors were summarized as the mean and standard deviation. Pearson's Chi-square tests and Student's t-tests were conducted for categorical and continuous factors, respectively. A two-sided p-value < 0.05 was considered statistically significant. Statistical Product Service Solutions (SPSS) 25.0 was used for statistical analysis.

3. Results

3.1. The Image Level

Details of the results are presented in Table 3. In the general statistics, the precision, recall, mAP@0.1, and mAP@0.5 predicted by the model were 0.64, 0.68, 0.66, and 0.49 in the CRA view, respectively. Meanwhile, the precision, recall, mAP@0.1, and mAP@0.5 predicted by the model were 0.68, 0.73, 0.70, and 0.56 in general in the LAO view, respectively. The results of CTO showed the best performance with F_1 scores of 0.65 and 0.86 in the four types of lesions in both angle views, compared to the results of LS of 0.67 and 0.50 for the opposite.

Table 3. Results of four lesions with two angle views at the image level.

	Lesions	Number	Precision	Recall	mAP@0.1	mAP@0.5	F_1 Score
CRA	LS	1055	0.685	0.647	0.643	0.405	0.665
	DS	96	0.458	0.844	0.687	0.677	0.594
	BS	374	0.656	0.658	0.675	0.625	0.657
	CTO	53	0.75	0.566	0.647	0.263	0.645
	All	1578	0.637	0.679	0.663	0.493	0.657
LAO	LS	433	0.426	0.617	0.479	0.273	0.504
	DS	273	0.648	0.868	0.773	0.688	0.742
	BS	174	0.699	0.655	0.694	0.521	0.676
	CTO	382	0.927	0.796	0.87	0.749	0.857
	All	1262	0.675	0.734	0.704	0.558	0.703

mAP@0.1: mean average precision (IoU = 0.1); mAP@0.5: mean average precision (IoU = 0.5); CRA: cranial; LAO: left anterior oblique; LS: local stenosis; DS: diffuse stenosis; BS: bifurcation stenosis; CTO: chronic total occlusion.

The confusion matrices for YOLOv5x (Predicted) and manual annotations (True) of four types of lesions are shown in Figure 5 (IoU = 0.1). All the detected regions were taken into account when calculating the confusion matrix's values, similar to other studies on YOLO [32–34]. Two angle views of the right coronary showed the same performance. In the CRA view, the probability of correct localization and classification for DS was 0.81, which was the best, and 0.54, 0.66, and 0.47 for LS, BS, and CTO, respectively. However, it was noted that 51% of the real CTO was predicted as background, while the background was also treated as LS, which represented 66% of the predicted LS. In the LAO view, the probability of correctly locating and classifying DS was 0.79, which was also the best, followed by 0.60, 0.58, and 0.77 for LS, BS, and CTO, respectively. However, like the performance in the CRA view, it could be found that 51% of the background was treated as LS in the LAO results.

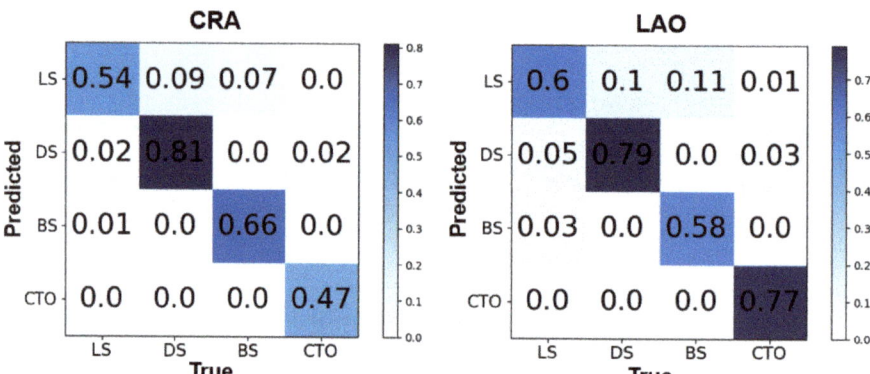

Figure 5. Confusion matrices of the CRA view and the LAO view. The horizontal axis represents the ground truth, and the vertical axis represents the prediction. CRA: cranial; LAO: left anterior oblique; LS: local stenosis; DS: diffuse stenosis; BS: bifurcation stenosis; CTO: chronic total occlusion.

The P-R curves of the two angle views shown in Figure 6 were performed for the situation of $IoU = 0.1$. The area under the curve (AUC) in general was 0.663 (mAP@0.1) in the CRA view and 0.704 (mAP@0.1) in the LAO view. It could be found in Figure 6 that in the LAO view, the result of CTO had an excellent performance, compared to the result of LS on the opposite. Meanwhile, in the CRA view, four types of lesions had the same performance.

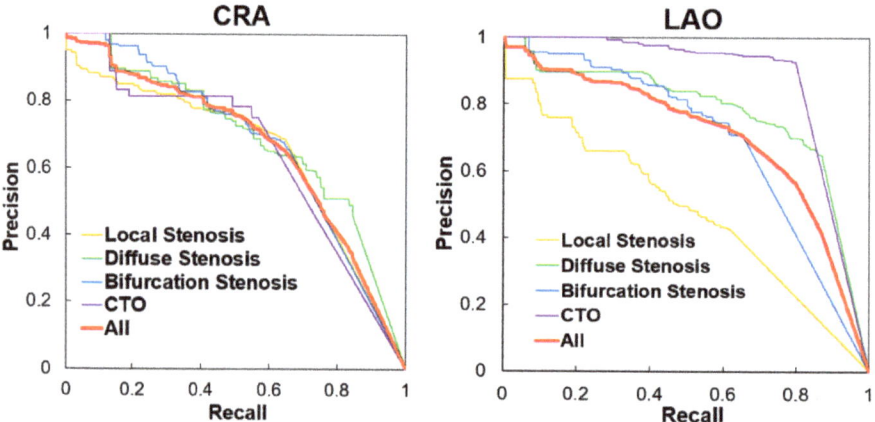

Figure 6. Precision-recall curves of the CRA view and the LAO view. CRA: cranial; LAO: left anterior oblique; CTO: chronic total occlusion.

Figure 7 shows the effect of YOLOv5x-detected lesions in CRA and LAO views. From the test results, it could be found that the model's detection was close to the manual annotations of physicians. With the value of confidence displayed in the following, the model showed good consistency with the reference standard.

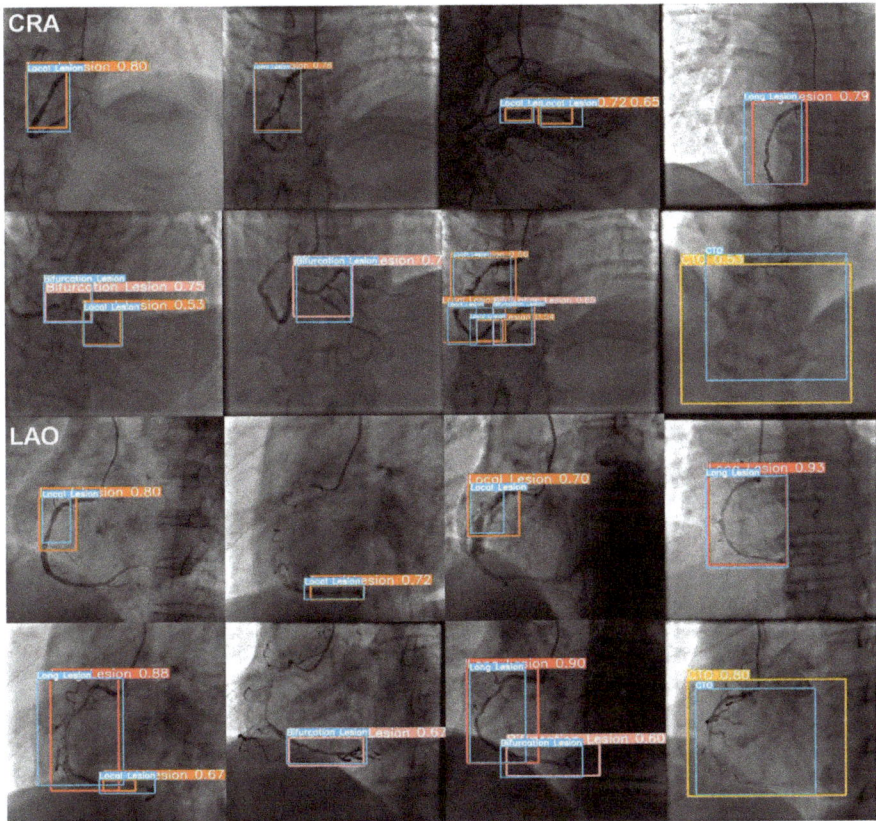

Figure 7. Representative coronary lesion detection results using YOLOv5 in the test set. The bounding boxes contain images of coronary lesions. CRA: cranial; LAO: left anterior oblique; Blue box: the manual annotation; Orange box: predicted local stenosis; Red box: predicted diffuse stenosis (long lesion); Pink box: predicted bifurcation stenosis; Yellow box: predicted CTO; Value: confidence.

3.2. The Patient Level

At the patient level, the model yielded the results of the precision, recall, and F_1 score as 0.52, 0.91, and 0.65 in the CRA view and 0.50, 0.94, and 0.64 in the LAO view, respectively. The results of CTO showed the best performance with an F_1 score of 0.77 and 0.88 in four types of lesions in both angle views, compared to the results of 0.54 for BS and 0.44 for LS on the opposite. We also calculated the mFP in two angle views. The performance of LS made the most mistakes across the four types of lesions. The model performed the best in the CTO with 0.07 and 0.10 of mFP in both views. Moreover, the mFP was 2.47 in the CRA view and 1.86 in the LAO view. Table 4 shows the details of the results ($IoU = 0.1$).

Table 4. Results of four lesions with two angle views at the patient level.

	Lesions	TP + FN	TP	FN	FP	P	R	F_1 Score	mFP
CRA	LS	59	55	4	44	0.556	0.932	0.696	1.467
	DS	6	6	0	8	0.429	1.000	0.600	0.267
	BS	15	13	2	20	0.394	0.867	0.542	0.667
	CTO	6	5	1	2	0.714	0.833	0.769	0.067
	All	86	79	7	74	0.523	0.908	0.652	2.467
LAO	LS	28	24	4	57	0.296	0.857	0.440	1.118
	DS	18	18	0	17	0.514	1.000	0.679	0.333
	BS	11	10	1	16	0.385	0.909	0.541	0.314
	CTO	19	19	0	5	0.792	1.000	0.884	0.098
	All	76	71	5	95	0.497	0.942	0.636	1.863

TP: true positive; FN: false negative; FP: false positive; P: precision; R: recall; mFP: mean predicted positive; CRA: cranial; LAO: left anterior oblique; LS: local stenosis; DS: diffuse stenosis; BS: bifurcation stenosis; CTO: chronic total occlusion.

The Grad-CAM technique always provided valuable information on the model learning procedure. We generated the heat map of Grad-CAM to consequently testify the regions of interest for YOLOv5x in both angle views. As shown in Figures 8 and 9, the activated regions (the highlighted area) corresponded to the regions that the model labeled. The model was confirmed to have a robust performance even with mild lesions. It was found that the model could learn the characteristics of lesions well and locate and classify the lesions precisely.

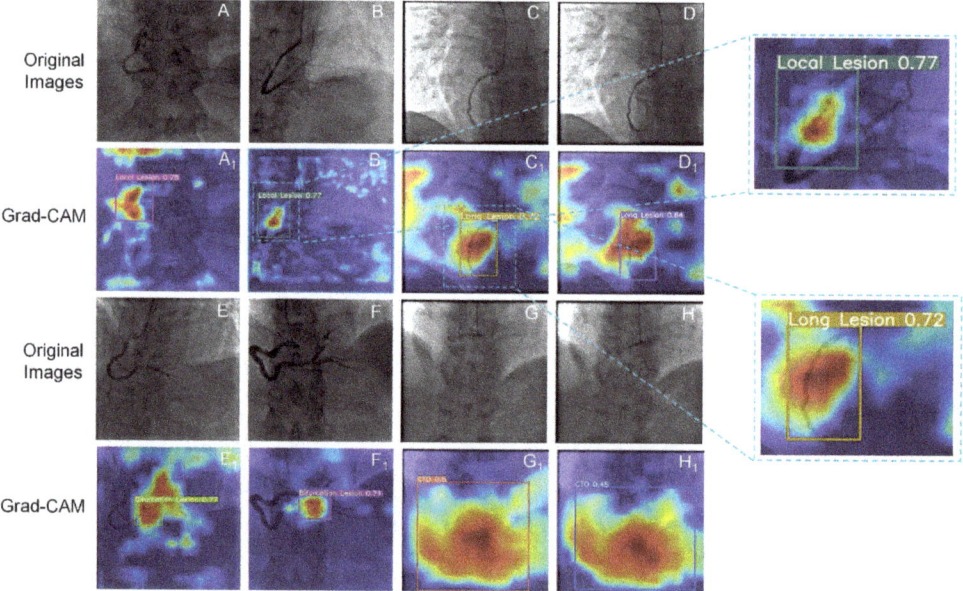

Figure 8. Heatmaps of Grad-CAM generated in the CRA view. The bounding boxes contain images of coronary lesions. (A–H) Original images with local stenosis (local lesion), diffuse stenosis (long lesion), bifurcation stenosis, and CTO; (A_1–H_1) heatmap of Grad-CAM with lesions; Value: confidence.

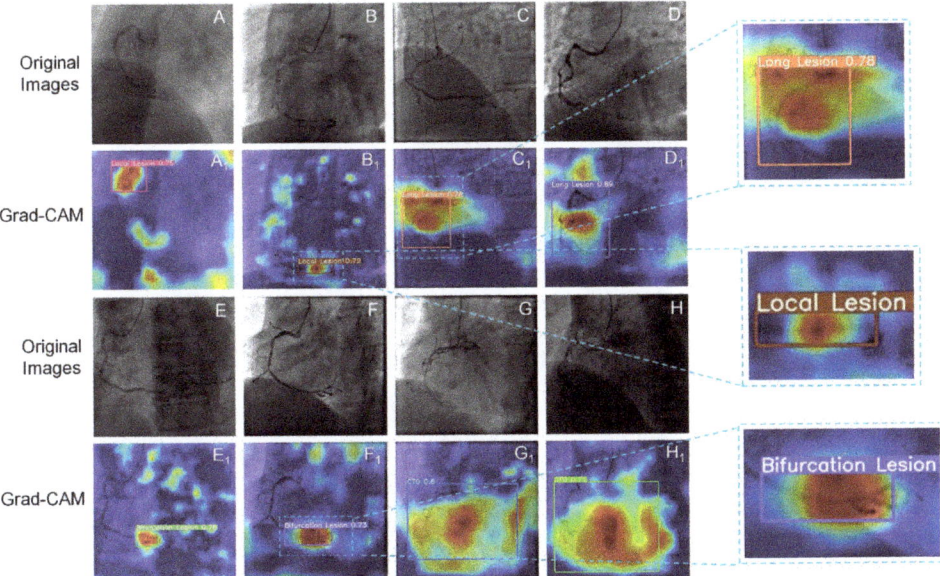

Figure 9. Heatmaps of Grad-CAM generated in the LAO view. The bounding boxes contain images of coronary lesions. (**A–H**): Original images with local stenosis (local lesion), diffuse stenosis (long lesion), bifurcation stenosis, and CTO; (**A$_1$–H$_1$**) heatmap of Grad-CAM with lesions; Value: confidence.

4. Discussion

This study used a single-stage model via the region-free method for the first time to detect coronary lesions directly in CAG images. We also classified common vascular abnormalities into four types: LS, DS, BS, and CTO. Our results showed that direct detection models like YOLOv5x can effectively identify vessel lesions. Meanwhile, because of the segmentation-free feature, YOLOv5x offered a more concise processing procedure, and hence it could maintain a good balance between model performance and detection efficiency in general.

In previous studies, the YOLO series of models have mostly been applied in tumor detection and retinal fundus disease evaluation. However, the fundus vessel lesion evaluation shows similarity compared to the coronary stenoses during the DL processing procedure [35–37]. Santos et al. [36] also used YOLOv5 as the detection model. In their public datasets of diabetic retinopathy images, YOLOv5 generated mAP@0.5 of 0.154 and an F_1 score of 0.252. In our study, the detection of lesions achieved a precision of 0.675, a recall rate of 0.734, an mAP@0.1 of 0.558, and an F_1 score of 0.703 in the LAO view at the image level. Meanwhile, at the patient level, the detection of lesions reached a precision of 0.792, a recall rate of 100%, an F_1 score of 0.884, and a maximum mFP of 0.466.

Generally, it can be found that the YOLO series of models demonstrates promising performance in the automatic detection of coronary artery lesions. The high precision and recall rates at both the image and patient levels indicate the model's reliability in identifying vascular abnormalities in CAG images. The impressive F_1 scores further validate the model's ability to balance precision and recall effectively. The low mFP also suggests that the model minimizes false-positive detections, which is crucial for accurate diagnosis and reducing unnecessary interventions. Overall, these findings highlight the potential of using YOLO-based direct detection models for the efficient and reliable detection of coronary artery abnormalities in medical imaging applications.

In the subgroup analysis of the four lesions, the CTO group and the DS group showed good results. They achieved a precision of 0.927, a recall rate of 0.796, mAP@0.1 of 0.870, and an F_1 score of 0.857 for the CTO group in the LAO view at the image level and a precision of 0.648, a recall rate of 0.868, mAP@0.1 of 0.773, and an F_1 score of 0.742 for the DS group. Du et al. [16] tested the performances of four models (CALD-Net, ZF-Net+Faster R-CNN, VGG+Faster R-CNN, and ResNet50+Faster R-CNN), finding recall rates of 0.88, 0.41, 0.50, and 0.62. Pang et al. [22] tested the performances of five models (Faster R-CNN, Guided Anchoring, Libra R-CNN, Cascade R-CNN, and Stenosis-DetNet), finding F_1 scores of 0.80, 0.79, 0.81, 0.78, and 0.88. Even in the analysis with a large dataset comprising 20,612 CAG images of 10,073 patients, it had a precision of 0.769 for the stenosis and 0.757 for the CTO lesion [21]. Our study showed that the direct detection of lesions like CTO and diffuse stenoses had the same performance compared to these studies. Consequently, it might be concluded that single-stage detection models like YOLOv5 could generate a stable result, which is similar to, or even better than, detection models combining segmentation in suitable situations.

However, in our study, the performance in the LS group showed an unsatisfactory result. In the LAO view of the image level, the LS group had a precision of 0.426, a recall rate of 0.617, a mAP@0.1 of 0.479, and an F_1 score of 0.504. At the patient level, the LS group also had the highest mFP compared to other groups with results of 1.467 in the CRA view and 1.118 in the LAO view, which meant more than one false labeling of LS for each patient. Correspondingly, the mFP in the CTO group was just 0.067 in the CRA view and 0.098 in the LAO view. Moon et al. [13] used the internal dataset and external dataset in their study. They showed a similar performance, with a mean accuracy of diffuse lesions better than focal lesions in each dataset. These results might be related to factors such as low-range stenosis, which is inconspicuous, susceptibility to background noises, and small lesion characteristics resulting in confusion with the visual features of normal arteries. Therefore, it is necessary to perform segmentation before the detection of local stenoses in the DL procedure.

Grad-CAM demonstrated the network-learned lesion characteristics, located the identification details of lesions, and visualized the distinguishing area of specific lesion types in the image based on DL. The low-heat region and high-heat region in the heatmap are determined based on the contribution of the regions in the image to the identification of lesions, with the high-heat region playing a decisive part in the network's inferential decision-making. The network has successfully learned the characteristics of the lesion, allowing the lesion area to receive adequate attention in Grad-CAM, as indicated by the position of the intact area with high heat (darker part) and the detection box being consistent. Figures $8B_1$ and $9B_1$ show that the model effectively learned the tiny characteristics of local stenoses and classified them correctly. Moreover, high-heat areas were only visible in the stenosis area but not in normal blood vessels. As can be observed in the wide array of high-heat areas in Figures $8G_1, H_1$ and $9G_1, H_1$, CTO exhibited a greater range of characteristics than local stenosis, which was also identified by the model. However, Grad-CAM struggles to show only the complicated regions that require attention. Some noise might be produced, which manifests as comparatively low-heat areas like the edge regions in C1 of Figure 8.

This study has several limitations. (1) We only performed the DL analysis in the right coronary. Lesions in the right coronary are always simpler than in the left. The YOLO series of models might face much bigger challenges, and their robustness should be tested in more complex circumstances. (2) The CAG images of candidate patients were collected in primary hospitals in our country, which might make it difficult to control the quality of angiography. It could be an important confounding factor that would impact the final performance of network models. (3) Our dataset should be enriched in future studies. The YOLOv5 model performed better for the local stenosis in the CRA view than for the CRA view, accompanied by a dataset of 1055 lesions compared to 433 lesions. It could be supposed that the performance of YOLOv5 could be better in a huge dataset of CAG images.

5. Conclusions

Our study used the one-stage strategy to detect coronary lesions in a segmentation-free manner and demonstrated that the YOLOv5 model could be feasible in CAG analysis using the DL method, with good robustness. We also found in the subgroup study that lesions of CTO and DS were most suitable for direct detection without segmentation, which could shorten processing time and improve working efficiency.

Author Contributions: Conceptualization: J.L. and S.W.; methodology: H.W., J.Z., Y.Z. and Z.Z.; software: H.W. and J.Z.; validation: Y.Z. and Z.Z.; formal analysis: H.W. and J.Z.; investigation: J.Z., Z.S. and L.C.; resources: L.X., M.S. and Q.Y.; data curation: J.Z., L.X., M.S. and Q.Y.; writing—original draft preparation: H.W., J.Z., J.L. and Y.Z.; writing—review and editing: W.W., Z.Z. and S.W.; project administration: J.L., W.W., Z.Z. and S.W.; funding acquisition, W.W. All authors have read and agreed to the published version of the manuscript.

Funding: This research was funded by the R&D Program of the Beijing Municipal Education Commission (No. KM202310025019).

Institutional Review Board Statement: The study was conducted according to the guidelines of the Declaration of Helsinki and approved by the Ethics Committee of Fuwai Hospital, Beijing, China (protocol code: 2021-1546; date of approval: 29 August 2022).

Informed Consent Statement: Patient consent was waived for this retrospective study.

Data Availability Statement: The raw data supporting the conclusions of this article may be provided upon reasonable requests for scientific research purposes.

Acknowledgments: The authors would like to thank the anonymous reviewers for their valuable comments and suggestions.

Conflicts of Interest: Z.Y. is an employee of Shanghai United Imaging Intelligence Co., Ltd. The authors declare no conflict of interest. The funders had no role in the design of the study; in the collection, analyses, or interpretation of data; in the writing of the manuscript, or in the decision to publish the results.

Abbreviations

The following abbreviations are used in the manuscript:

AI	Artificial Intelligence
BS	Bifurcation Stenosis
CAB	Coronary Artery Bypass
CAD	Coronary Artery Disease
CAG	Coronary AngioGraphy
CNN	Convolutional Neural Network
CPR	Cardiovascular Pulmonary Resuscitation
CRA	CRAnial
CTO	Chronic Total Occlusion
DICOM	Digital Imaging and COmmunications in Medicine
DL	Deep Learning
DS	Diffuse Stenosis
FN	False Negative
FP	False Positive
Grad-CAM	Gradient-weighted Class Activation Mapping
IoU	Intersection over Union
LAO	Left Anterior Oblique
LS	Local Stenosis
mAP	mean Average Precision
mFP	mean False Positive
PCI	Percutaneous Coronary Intervention
PR	Precision-Recall
TN	True Negative
TP	True Positive

References

1. The Top 10 Causes of Death. 2020. Available online: https://www.who.int/news-room/fact-sheets/detail/the-top-10-causes-of-death (accessed on 9 December 2020).
2. Collet, J.-P.; Thiele, H.; Barbato, E.; Barthélémy, O.; Bauersachs, J.; Bhatt, D.L.; Dendale, P.; Dorobantu, M.; Edvardsen, T.; Folliguet, T.; et al. 2020 ESC Guidelines for the management of acute coronary syndromes in patients presenting without persistent ST-segment elevation. *Eur. Heart J.* **2021**, *42*, 1289–1367. [PubMed]
3. Lawton, J.S.; Tamis-Holland, J.E.; Bangalore, S.; Bates, E.R.; Beckie, T.M.; Bischoff, J.M.; Bittl, J.A.; Cohen, M.G.; DiMaio, J.M.; Don, C.W.; et al. 2021 ACC/AHA/SCAI Guideline for Coronary Artery Revascularization: A Report of the American College of Cardiology/American Heart Association Joint Committee on Clinical Practice Guidelines. *Circulation* **2022**, *145*, e18–e114. [PubMed]
4. Knuuti, J.; Wijns, W.; Saraste, A.; Capodanno, D.; Barbato, E.; Funck-Brentano, C.; Prescott, E.; Storey, R.F.; Deaton, C.; Cuisset, T.; et al. 2019 ESC Guidelines for the diagnosis and management of chronic coronary syndromes. *Eur. Heart J.* **2020**, *41*, 407–477. [PubMed]
5. Zhang, D.; Liu, X.; Xia, J.; Gao, Z.; Zhang, H.; de Albuquerque, V.H.C. A Physics-guided Deep Learning Approach for Functional Assessment of Cardiovascular Disease in IoT-based Smart Health. *IEEE Internet Things J.* **2023**, 1. [CrossRef]
6. Menezes, M.N.; Silva, J.L.; Silva, B.; Rodrigues, T.; Guerreiro, C.; Guedes, J.P.; Santos, M.O.; Oliveira, A.L.; Pinto, F.J. Coronary X-ray angiography segmentation using Artificial Intelligence: A multicentric validation study of a deep learning model. *Int. J. Cardiovasc. Imaging* **2023**, *39*, 1385–1396. [CrossRef]
7. Zhang, H.; Gao, Z.; Zhang, D.; Hau, W.K.; Zhang, H. Progressive Perception Learning for Main Coronary Segmentation in X-Ray Angiography. *IEEE Trans. Med. Imaging* **2023**, *42*, 864–879.
8. Zhao, C.; Vij, A.; Malhotra, S.; Tang, J.; Tang, H.; Pienta, D.; Xu, Z.; Zhou, W. Automatic extraction and stenosis evaluation of coronary arteries in invasive coronary angiograms. *Comput. Biol. Med.* **2021**, *136*, 104667. [CrossRef]
9. Liu, X.; Wang, X.; Chen, D.; Zhang, H. Automatic Quantitative Coronary Analysis Based on Deep Learning. *Appl. Sci.* **2023**, *13*, 2975. [CrossRef]
10. Algarni, M.; Al-Rezqi, A.; Saeed, F.; Alsaeedi, A.; Ghabban, F. Multi-constraints based deep learning model for automated segmentation and diagnosis of coronary artery disease in X-ray angiographic images. *PeerJ Comput. Sci.* **2022**, *8*, e933. [CrossRef]
11. Cong, C.; Kato, Y.; De Vasconcellos, H.D.; Ostovaneh, M.R.; Lima, J.A.C.; Ambale-Venkatesh, B. Deep learning-based end-to-end automated stenosis classification and localization on catheter coronary angiography. *Front. Cardiovasc. Med.* **2023**, *10*, 944135. [CrossRef]
12. Szegedy, C.; Liu, W.; Jia, Y.; Sermanet, P.; Reed, S.; Anguelov, D.; Erhan, D.; Vanhoucke, V.; Rabinovich, A. Going deeper with convolutions. In Proceedings of the 2015 IEEE Conference on Computer Vision and Pattern Recognition (CVPR), Boston, MA, USA, 7–12 June 2015. pp. 1–9.
13. Moon, J.H.; Lee, D.Y.; Cha, W.C.; Chung, M.J.; Lee, K.-S.; Cho, B.H.; Choi, J.H. Automatic stenosis recognition from coronary angiography using convolutional neural networks. *Comput. Methods Programs Biomed.* **2020**, *198*, 105819. [CrossRef] [PubMed]
14. Woo, S.; Park, J.; Lee, J.-Y.; Kweom, I.S. CBAM: Convolutional block attention module. In Proceedings of the European Conference on Computer Vision (ECCV), Munich, Germany, 8–14 September 2018; Volume 11211, pp. 3–19.
15. Ling, H.; Chen, B.; Guan, R.; Xiao, Y.; Yan, H.; Chen, Q.; Bi, L.; Chen, J.; Feng, X.; Pang, H.; et al. Deep Learning Model for Coronary Angiography. *J. Cardiovasc. Transl. Res.* **2023**, *16*, 896–904. [CrossRef] [PubMed]
16. Du, T.; Liu, X.; Zhang, H.; Xu, B. Real-time Lesion Detection of Cardiac Coronary Artery Using Deep Neural Networks. In Proceedings of the 2018 International Conference on Network Infrastructure and Digital Content (IC-NIDC), Guiyang, China, 22–24 August 2018; pp. 150–154.
17. Ren, S.; He, K.; Girshick, R.; Sun, J. Faster R-CNN: Towards Real-Time Object Detection with Region Proposal Networks. *IEEE Trans. Pattern Anal. Mach. Intell.* **2017**, *39*, 1137–1149. [CrossRef] [PubMed]
18. Danilov, V.V.; Klyshnikov, K.Y.; Gerget, O.M.; Kutikhin, A.G.; Ganyukov, V.I.; Frangi, A.F.; Ovcharenko, E.A. Real-time coronary artery stenosis detection based on modern neural networks. *Sci. Rep.* **2021**, *11*, 7582. [CrossRef]
19. Antczak, K.; Liberadzki, A. Stenosis Detection with Deep Convolutional Neural Networks. *MATEC Web Conf.* **2018**, *210*, 04001. [CrossRef]
20. Ovalle-Magallanes, E.; Avina-Cervantes, J.G.; Cruz-Aceves, I.; Ruiz-Pinales, J. Transfer Learning for Stenosis Detection in X-ray Coronary Angiography. *Mathematics* **2020**, *8*, 1510. [CrossRef]
21. Du, T.; Xie, L.; Zhang, H.; Liu, X.; Wang, X.; Chen, D.; Xu, Y.; Sun, Z.; Zhou, W.; Song, L.; et al. Training and validation of a deep learning architecture for the automatic analysis of coronary angiography. *EuroIntervention* **2021**, *17*, 32–40. [CrossRef]
22. Pang, K.; Ai, D.; Fang, H.; Fan, J.; Song, H.; Yang, J. Stenosis-DetNet: Sequence consistency-based stenosis detection for X-ray coronary angiography. *Comput. Med. Imaging Graph.* **2021**, *89*, 101900. [CrossRef]
23. Dingli, P.; Gonzalo, N.; Escaned, J. Intravascular Ultrasound-guided Management of Diffuse Stenosis. *Radcl. Cardiol.* **2018**, *2018*, 1–18.
24. Levine, G.N.; Bates, E.R.; Blankenship, J.C.; Bailey, S.R.; Bittl, J.A.; Cercek, B.; Chambers, C.E.; Ellis, S.G.; Guyton, R.A.; Hollenberg, S.M.; et al. 2011 ACCF/AHA/SCAI Guideline for Percutaneous Coronary Intervention: A report of the American College of Cardiology Foundation/American Heart Association Task Force on Practice Guidelines and the Society for Cardiovascular Angiography and Interventions. *Circulation* **2011**, *124*, e574–e651.

25. Louvard, Y.; Thomas, M.; Dzavik, V.; Hildick-Smith, D.; Galassi, A.R.; Pan, M.; Burzotta, F.; Zelizko, M.; Dudek, D.; Ludman, P.; et al. Classification of coronary artery bifurcation lesions and treatments: Time for a consensus! *Catheter. Cardiovasc. Interv.* **2007**, *71*, 175–183. [CrossRef] [PubMed]
26. Ultralytics. GitHub-Ultralytics/Yolov5: YOLOv5 in PyTorch > ONNX > CoreML > TFLite. 2020. Available online: https://github.com/ultralytics/yolov5 (accessed on 26 June 2020).
27. Lin, T.Y.; Dollár, P.; Girshick, R.; He, K.; Hariharan, B.; Belongie, S. Feature Pyramid Networks for Object Detection. *arXiv* **2016**, arXiv:1612.03144.
28. Liu, S.; Qi, L.; Qin, H.; Shi, J.; Jia, J. Path Aggregation Network for Instance Segmentation. In Proceedings of the 2018 IEEE/CVF Conference on Computer Vision and Pattern Recognition, Salt Lake City, UT, USA, 18–23 June 2018; pp. 8759–8768.
29. Zheng, Z.; Wang, P.; Liu, W.; Li, J.; Ye, R.; Ren, D. Distance-IoU Loss: Faster and Better Learning for Bounding Box Regression. *arXiv* **2019**, arXiv:1911.08287. [CrossRef]
30. Rezatofighi, H.; Tsoi, N.; Gwak, J.; Sadeghian, A.; Reid, I.; Savarese, S. Generalized Intersection Over Union: A Metric and a Loss for Bounding Box Regression. In Proceedings of the 2019 IEEE/CVF Conference on Computer Vision and Pattern Recognition (CVPR), Long Beach, CA, USA, 15–20 June 2019; pp. 658–666.
31. Selvaraju, R.R.; Cogswell, M.; Das, A.; Vedantam, R.; Parikh, D.; Batra, D. Grad-CAM: Visual Explanations from Deep Networks via Gradient-based Localization. *arXiv* **2016**, arXiv:1610.02391.
32. Dinesh, M.G.; Bacanin, N.; Askar, S.S.; Abouhawwash, M. Diagnostic ability of deep learning in detection of pancreatic tumour. *Sci. Rep.* **2023**, *13*, 9725. [CrossRef]
33. Zahrawi, M.; Shaalan, K. Improving video surveillance systems in banks using deep learning techniques. *Sci. Rep.* **2023**, *13*, 7911. [CrossRef]
34. Chiriboga, M.; Green, C.M.; Hastman, D.A.; Mathur, D.; Wei, Q.; Díaz, S.A.; Medintz, I.L.; Veneziano, R. Rapid DNA origami nanostructure detection and classification using the YOLOv5 deep convolutional neural network. *Sci. Rep.* **2022**, *12*, 3871. [CrossRef]
35. Alyoubi, W.L.; Abulkhair, M.F.; Shalash, W.M. Diabetic Retinopathy Fundus Image Classification and Lesions Localization System Using Deep Learning. *Sensors* **2021**, *21*, 3704. [CrossRef]
36. Santos, C.; Aguiar, M.; Welfer, D.; Belloni, B. A New Approach for Detecting Fundus Lesions Using Image Processing and Deep Neural Network Architecture Based on YOLO Model. *Sensors* **2022**, *22*, 6441. [CrossRef]
37. Li, T.; Bo, W.; Hu, C.; Kang, H.; Liu, H.; Wang, K.; Fu, H. Applications of deep learning in fundus images: A review. *Med. Image Anal.* **2021**, *69*, 101971. [CrossRef]

Disclaimer/Publisher's Note: The statements, opinions and data contained in all publications are solely those of the individual author(s) and contributor(s) and not of MDPI and/or the editor(s). MDPI and/or the editor(s) disclaim responsibility for any injury to people or property resulting from any ideas, methods, instructions or products referred to in the content.

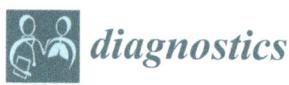

Article

Evaluation of Augmentation Methods in Classifying Autism Spectrum Disorders from fMRI Data with 3D Convolutional Neural Networks

Johan Jönemo [1,2], David Abramian [1,2] and Anders Eklund [1,2,3,*]

1. Division of Medical Informatics, Department of Biomedical Engineering, Linköping University, 581 83 Linköping, Sweden
2. Center for Medical Image Science and Visualization (CMIV), Linköping University, 581 83 Linköping, Sweden
3. Division of Statistics and Machine Learning, Department of Computer and Information Science, Linköping University, 581 83 Linköping, Sweden
* Correspondence: anders.eklund@liu.se

Abstract: Classifying subjects as healthy or diseased using neuroimaging data has gained a lot of attention during the last 10 years, and recently, different deep learning approaches have been used. Despite this fact, there has not been any investigation regarding how 3D augmentation can help to create larger datasets, required to train deep networks with millions of parameters. In this study, deep learning was applied to derivatives from resting state functional MRI data, to investigate how different 3D augmentation techniques affect the test accuracy. Specifically, resting state derivatives from 1112 subjects in ABIDE (Autism Brain Imaging Data Exchange) preprocessed were used to train a 3D convolutional neural network (CNN) to classify each subject according to presence or absence of autism spectrum disorder. The results show that augmentation only provide minor improvements to the test accuracy.

Keywords: functional MRI; resting state; deep learning; augmentation; autism

Citation: Jönemo, J.; Abramian, D.; Eklund, A. Evaluation of Augmentation Methods in Classifying Autism Spectrum Disorders from fMRI Data with 3D Convolutional Neural Networks. *Diagnostics* **2023**, *13*, 2773. https://doi.org/10.3390/diagnostics13172773

Academic Editor: Daniele Giansanti

Received: 9 August 2023
Revised: 24 August 2023
Accepted: 25 August 2023
Published: 27 August 2023

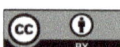

Copyright: © 2023 by the authors. Licensee MDPI, Basel, Switzerland. This article is an open access article distributed under the terms and conditions of the Creative Commons Attribution (CC BY) license (https://creativecommons.org/licenses/by/4.0/).

1. Introduction

Ever since the emergence of magnetic resonance imaging (MRI) in the 1980s, the absence of ionizing radiation and the flexibility of the acquisition procedure have made this an increasingly important imaging modality in the clinical sciences. The lack of contrast between different tissues in the brain and the interference of the mineralized tissue around it when using X-ray techniques make MRI especially useful in neuroimaging.

While a wide variety of neurological conditions can be diagnosed with MRI, psychiatric anomalies have proven illusive to detect. Presumably, this is because these affect many systems distributed throughout the brain and their manifestations are likely subtle as well as time variant. Furthermore, psychiatric anomalies can vary a lot between subjects. Functional MRI (fMRI) is a technique that seems particularly suited to capture this information, as it generates rich 4D data which can be used for studying brain activity as well as brain connectivity. In this work, it is investigated if deep-learning-based diagnosis of autism from resting state fMRI data can be further improved using 3D augmentation.

1.1. Resting State fMRI

Resting state fMRI has since 1995 been used to study brain connectivity [1,2]. A major advantage compared to task fMRI is that subjects can simply rest during the whole experiment, which normally takes 5–10 min (resulting in some 150–600 brain volumes, or put differently some 50,000 time series), instead of performing different tasks such as finger tapping or mental calculations. This makes it possible to include subjects which for some reason cannot perform certain tasks. A simple measure of the connectivity between two locations in the brain, called functional connectivity, is the correlation between the two corresponding time series, but several more advanced methods also exist. To limit the size of the 2D correlation matrix, the correlations are normally calculated between the mean time series of some 100–200 brain parcels (instead of some 50,000 voxels). The brain can be divided according to different (resting state) networks, such as the default mode network and the auditory network, and different diseases often affect specific networks.

1.2. Autism

Autism spectrum disorder (ASD) is a disorder characterized by certain features in social communication, and restricted, repetitive, or unusual sensory–motor behaviours [3]. The prevalence of ASD is 1–5% in developed countries [4]. The subject of autism has been studied extensively in recent years, and technology has already contributed to the development of treatments for autism, in terms of rehabilitation and communication.

Due to the lack of reliable biomarkers, the diagnosis is usually based on behaviour, which is very time consuming. Recent work has demonstrated that motor abnormalities can be very informative for detection of ASD [5,6], and that machine learning can be used to shorten the behavioral diagnosis [7]. As ASD results from early altered brain development and neural reorganisation [8,9], it should be possible to derive objective biomarkers from neuroimaging data to aid professionals (paediatricians, psychiatrists, or psychologists) in diagnosising ASD. Here, machine learning can be used to learn informative traits from the high-dimensional fMRI data.

1.3. Machine Learning for Diagnosis of ASD

Several large collaborative efforts have been made to collect and share neuroimaging data of healthy controls as well as diseased [10,11]. ABIDE (Autism Brain Imaging Data Exchange) [12] is one such effort that make available data for 539 subjects diagnosed with ASD as well as 573 typical controls. The ABIDE data originate from 17 sites, and the subjects were aged 7–64 years (median 14.7 years across groups). Using machine learning in an endeavour to classify (resting state) fMRI data according to the presence or absence of ASD has become increasingly popular recently. This classification can be performed in several ways, either using estimated functional connectivity network matrices (2D) or using derivatives (3D volumes), such as weighted and binarized degree centrality, as different approaches to compress the 4D fMRI data. In this work, 3D volumes are used, as it is not obvious how to augment network matrices.

The ASD classification problem seems hard in that accuracies seldom rise to more than 70% when the model classifies unseen data [13–18]. While 1112 subjects is a very large fMRI dataset, it is still small from a deep learning perspective (for example, the popular ImageNet database [19] contains several million images). To further increase the size of the training dataset, and to make convolutional neural networks (CNNs) robust to transformations such as rotation, data augmentation is often used [20,21]. In previous work, it was demonstrated that 3D augmentation for brain tumor segmentation significantly improves the segmentation accuracy [22]. In this work, the purpose is instead to see if 3D augmentation can help train a better ASD classifier, as well as what kind of augmentation techniques work the best.

1.4. Related Work

Several other researchers have used the same ABIDE dataset to train deep learning models for classification [16–18,23,24], but do not mention anything about augmentation. In a recent review on deep learning for autism by Khodatars et al. [25], only advanced augmentation techniques, such as generative adversarial methods (GANs), are briefly mentioned, but training a GAN requires a very large dataset to start from and there is very little work published on 3D GANs. Some researchers have employed resampling techniques wherein shorter time series have been cropped out of longer ones [13,14], typically for the double purpose of getting an augmented data set while also eliminating the extra complication of variable length sequences. Ji et al. [26] instead applied augmentation to the estimated network matrices. In our study, by contrast, different preprocessing pipelines are used to extract all relevant information from the time dimension, and manipulate data only in the spatial domain.

2. Materials and Methods

2.1. Data

Preprocessing of 4D resting state fMRI data is a complex process involving many different steps, and there is no consensus regarding what the optimal pipeline or toolbox is [27]. Head motion is a major problem in resting state fMRI, as it can, for example, result in erroneous group differences if two cohorts differ in the mean amount of head motion [28,29]. All processing pipelines therefore perform head motion correction, and use additional steps to further suppress motion related signal. ABIDE preprocessed [30] (http://preprocessed-connectomes-project.org/abide/, accessed on 10 February 2023) shares preprocessed ABIDE [12] data from structural MRI and resting state fMRI in various forms. As all the preprocessing has been completed, the focus in this work is on the machine-learning-based diagnosis, and other researchers can use the same preprocessed data to reproduce the presented findings. Resting state derivatives (3D volumes where the time dimension has been collapsed into different forms of statistics) resulting from two pipelines were downloaded from ABIDE preprocessed, for 1112 subjects.

One pipeline was the connectome computation system (CCS) [31], which performs slice timing correction, motion realignment, and global intensity normalisation. The data were cleaned from confounders by performing regression with the estimated head movement parameters, the time-dependent global mean intensity, as well as regressors for linear and quadratic drift. Each time series was also band pass filtered (0.01–0.1 Hz). This preprocessing corresponds to the strategy called global_filt. Each subject was, furthermore, registered to the MNI152 brain template using boundary based rigid body registration [32] for functional to anatomical registration, and FLIRT and FNIRT for anatomical to template registration [33].

Another such pipeline was "data processing assistant for resting-state fMRI" (DPARSF) [34]. It also performs slice timing correction and motion realignment, but does not perform any intensity normalisation. The same confounders are corrected for and the same band pass filtering is performed, whereupon functional to anatomical registration was performed with ordinary rigid body methods and anatomical to MNI152 brain template registration completed using DARTEL [35].

After preliminary testing of the 10 available derivatives available in ABIDE preprocessed (amplitude of low frequency fluctuations (ALFF), weighted and binarized degree centrality, dual regression, weighted and binarized eigenvector centrality, fractional ALFF, local functional connectivity density (LFCD), regional homogeneity (REHO), voxel-mirrored homotopic connectivity (VMHC)), the REHO derivative was chosen for comparing different augmentation strategies. Regional homogeneity is a measure of correlation between a voxel's time series and those of its neighbours [36], based on the non-parametric rank correlation statistic known as Kendall's Coefficient of Concordance (KCC) [37]. Each derivative volume from the resting state fMRI data has a size of $61 \times 73 \times 61$ voxels (each $3 \times 3 \times 3$ mm^3), which is fed into the 3D CNN described below. See Figure 1 for a preprocessed fMRI volume and the REHO derivative from the CCS pipeline, downloaded from ABIDE (https://s3.amazonaws.com/fcp-indi/data/Projects/ABIDE_Initiative/Outputs/ccs/filt_global/func_preproc/OHSU_0050147_func_preproc.nii.gz, accessed on 1 August 2023; https://s3.amazonaws.com/fcp-indi/data/Projects/ABIDE_Initiative/Outputs/ccs/filt_global/reho/OHSU_0050147_reho.nii.gz, accessed on 1 August 2023). The 539 subjects with ASD and the 573 controls were split 70/15/15 into training, validation, and test sets.

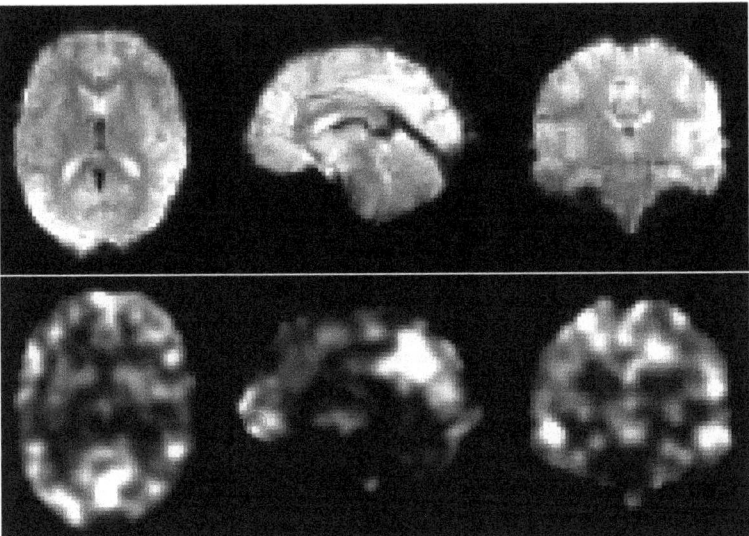

Figure 1. (**Top**): an fMRI volume obtained after preprocessing with the CCS pipeline. (**Bottom**): the REHO derivative obtained from the preprocessed 4D fMRI dataset, used by the 3D CNN to classify each subject as control or ASD. Different types of 3D augmentation were applied to each REHO volume, in an attempt to improve the test accuracy. Several other derivatives are available in ABIDE preprocessed, but were not used in this study due to time-consuming training.

2.2. Deep Learning

CNNs are often used for deep-learning-based classification and segmentation of image data, as learning a number of small filters is much more efficient compared to training a dense network (which models the relationship between all pixels in an image, instead of only looking at local correlations). While 2D CNNs are much more common, they are easily extended to 3D as convolution can be performed in any number of dimensions. Unfortunately, existing deep learning frameworks do not support 4D convolutions, which would be required to directly classify 4D fMRI data. The 3D CNN used in this work was implemented using Keras and consists of three convolutional layers (with ReLU activation), max-pooling layers, a dense layer with 16 nodes, and a final one-node layer with sigmoid activation. The first and second convolutional layers contain 8 filters each (size $3 \times 3 \times 3$), and the last convolutional layer uses 16 filters. The total number of trainable parameters in the 3D CNN is approximately 450 k. The CNN was trained with the Adam optimizer with a learning rate of 10^{-5} and a batch size of 16. To prevent overfitting, early stopping was used with a patience of 50 epochs. The training was run until validation accuracy did not improve, and the model was then restored to the state when the last improvement was seen. As an alternative, the models were also trained for 150 epochs with no conditional stopping. To obtain more robust estimates of the test accuracy, 10-fold cross validation was used and the mean test accuracy was calculated.

2.3. Augmentation

There are many types of augmentation that can be useful in 3D. Rotation, flipping, and scaling (zooming in or out) are common for training 2D CNNs, and can also easily be applied in 3D. Elastic (non-linear) deformations are common when training segmentation networks, but perhaps not as common for classification. Brightness augmentation can for example help if the data have been collected at several different MR scanners, as they normally generate data with different brightness [22].

While 2D augmentation functions are included in many deep learning frameworks such as Keras and Pytorch, the support for 3D augmentation is normally lacking. As mentioned by Chlap et al. [21], many researchers use 2D augmentation even if the data are 3D. The 3D augmentation used here is adapted from that of Cirillo et al. [22] and is written in Python/NumPy [38], without facilities for running on a GPU. The 3D augmentation techniques tested in this study are:

- *Flipping*: flipping of the x-axis or not.
- *Rotation*: rotation applied to each axis with angles randomly chosen from a uniform distribution with range between −7.5 and 7.5 degrees, −15 and 15 degrees, −30 and 30 degrees, or −45 and 45 degrees.
- *Scale*: scaling applied to each axis by a factor randomly chosen from a uniform distribution with range ±10% or ±20%.
- *Brightness*: power-law γ intensity transformation with its parameters gain (g) and γ chosen randomly between 0.8 and 1.2 from a uniform distribution. The intensity (I) is randomly changed according to the formula: $I_{new} = g \cdot I^{\gamma}$.
- *Elastic deformation*: elastic (non-linear) deformation with square deformation grid with displacements sampled from from a normal distribution with standard deviation $\sigma = 2, 4, 6,$ or 8 voxels [39], where the smoothing is done by a spline filter with order 3 in each dimension.

To investigate the effect of combining different types of augmentation, the CNNs were also trained with the two best-performing augmentation approaches according to the CCS pipeline.

The average training time for a single fold were between five minutes and 2.5 h—depending on the type of on-the-fly augmentation employed, the combination of elastic deformation, and an affine transformation being the slowest–using one Nvidia Tesla V100 graphics card for the early stopping models. For the training with a fixed number of epochs, the average single fold training time was at least 10 min but otherwise in the previously mentioned span. In the longer training runs, it is unlikely that the computation speed was bounded by the speed of the graphics card, as the on-the-fly augmentations were performed on the CPU and could be further optimized. In total, some 600 3D CNNs were trained in order to compare all settings.

3. Results

The results from all the different augmentation techniques, as well as baseline results obtained without augmentation, are presented in Figures 2 and 3 (CCS pipeline) and Figures 4 and 5 (DPARSF pipeline). As the dataset is balanced (similar number of ASD and control subjects), only classification accuracy is reported (instead of more advanced metrics, such as area under the curve and Matthew's correlation coefficient). In general, the 3D augmentation does not have a large effect on the test accuracy. For early stopping with the CCS pipeline, random scaling seems to be the best single augmentation approach, but the mean improvement over 10 cross-validation folds is only about 0.5 percentage units. Small elastic deformations also have a small positive effect, while large deformations give worse results.

With the DPARSF pipeline brightness changes appear to be the best augmentation with an increase of 1.9 percentage units, but with high variance over folds, the improvement is negligible. For a fixed number of training epochs, elastic deformations and rotations or combinations thereof seem to work best, with the best improvement of accuracy being 2.2 percentage units in the CCS pipeline and 2.9 percentage units in the DPARSF pipeline. No statistical test was performed to test if this improvement is significant.

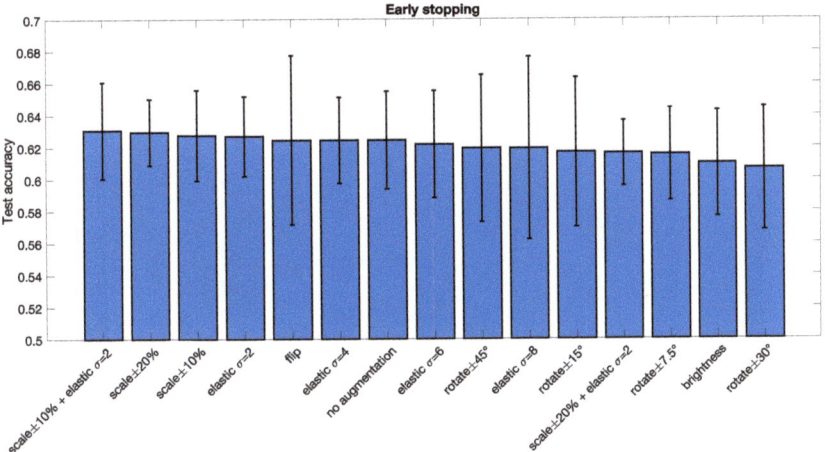

Figure 2. Test accuracy for classifying subjects as healthy or diseased for the ABIDE dataset processed with the CCS pipeline, for different data augmentation approaches. The error bar represents the standard deviation over the 10 cross-validation folds. Note that half of the augmentation approaches result in a test accuracy that is lower compared to the baseline model trained without augmentation, but overall, the differences are small. These results were obtained when using early stopping. Compared to no augmentation, the best augmentation approach increases the test accuracy by 0.6 percentage units.

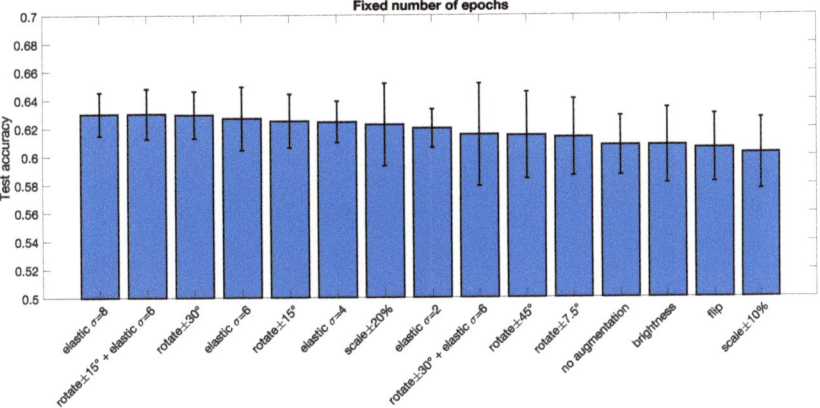

Figure 3. Test accuracy for classifying subjects as healthy or diseased for the ABIDE dataset processed with the CCS pipeline, for different data augmentation approaches. The error bar represents the standard deviation over the 10 cross-validation folds. These results were obtained when using a fixed number of epochs for each training. Compared to no augmentation, the best augmentation approach increases the test accuracy by 2.2 percentage units.

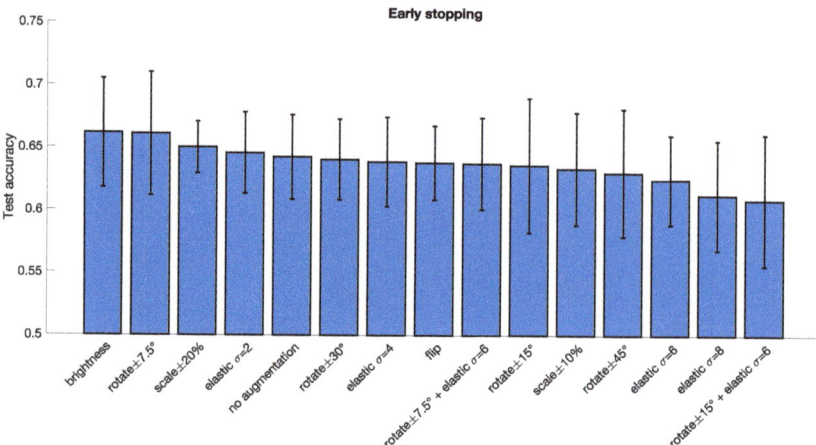

Figure 4. Test accuracy for classifying subjects as healthy or diseased for the ABIDE dataset processed with the DPARSF pipeline, for different data augmentation approaches. The error bar represents the standard deviation over the 10 cross-validation folds. Note that half of the augmentation approaches result in a test accuracy that is lower compared to the baseline model trained without augmentation, but overall, the differences are small. These results were obtained when using early stopping. Compared to no augmentation, the best augmentation approach increases the test accuracy by 1.9 percentage units.

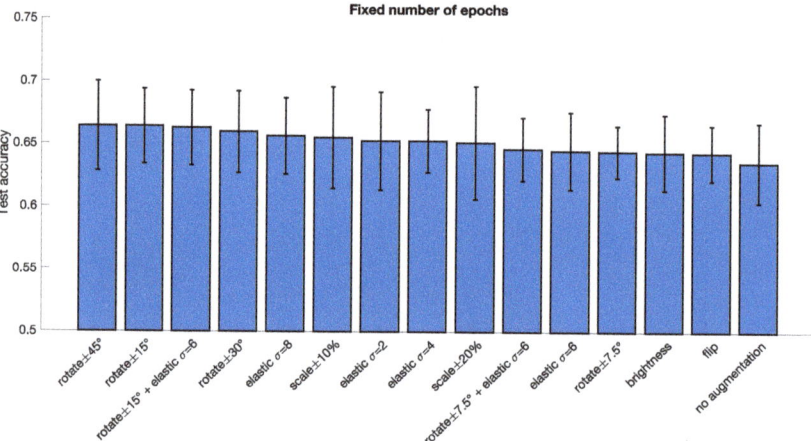

Figure 5. Test accuracy for classifying subjects as healthy or diseased for the ABIDE dataset processed with the DPARSF pipeline, for different data augmentation approaches. The error bar represents the standard deviation over the 10 cross-validation folds. These results were obtained when using a fixed number of epochs for each training. Compared to no augmentation, the best augmentation approach increases the test accuracy by 2.9 percentage units.

4. Discussion

Compared to previous work on 3D augmentation for brain tumor segmentation [22], where several 3D augmentation techniques were shown to significantly improve the segmentation accuracy on the test set, only minor improvements of the test accuracy were found in this study (even though the training accuracy is well above 90%, indicating overfitting). Volume classification is in general a problem which requires more training data compared to volume segmentation, as each volume only represents a single training example, which may partly explain the results.

In this study, brightness augmentation only helps for the DPARSF pipeline with early stopping, while it provided a major improvement for brain tumor segmentation for MR images collected at some 20 different sites [22]. A possible explanation is that the data in this study are not raw MR images, since many preprocessing steps have been used to normalize the intensities to a certain range, and to calculate different derivatives. On the contrary, as the ranges of values in the derivative volumes are not, in general, arbitrary in the same way, brightness augmentation can impair the performance. In DPARSF, no intensity normalization is performed, which may explain why the brightness augmentation results are different compared to the CCS pipeline.

Since all the subjects have been registered to MNI space, it was hypothesized that the results may be different if random transformations are applied to the test volumes, but test time augmentation did not change the findings (results not shown). The presented results are for a single preprocessing strategy (global signal regression and bandpass filtering), and a single derivative, and the preprocessing choice can at least in theory affect how much the augmentation helps.

The focus here has been on classifying ASD and controls, with a binary classifier. ASD criteria are based on DSM-5 criteria, and there are currently three levels of severity. It is possible that using 3D augmentation when training a classifier to distinguish the three severity levels could lead to different results.

The conclusion is that 3D augmentation only provides minor improvements in accuracy (0.6–2.9 percentage units) when training 3D CNNs for classification of ASD versus controls, but the results may be different for an easier task where the baseline test accuracy is for example 80%. The results may also differ for other derivatives in ABIDE preprocessed, and when using several derivatives at the same time using a multi-channel 3D CNN. However, to perform the trainings for many combinations of preprocessing, and for different derivatives, would be very time consuming.

Author Contributions: J.J. and D.A. implemented the 3D CNN and performed the experiments. J.J. and A.E. wrote the paper. A.E. supervised the work. All authors have read and agreed to the published version of the manuscript.

Funding: This work was supported by the Swedish research council grant 2017-04889, and by the ITEA/VINNOVA funded project Automation, Surgery Support and Intuitive 3D visualization to optimize workflow in IGT SysTems (ASSIST) (grant 2021-01954), and by the Åke Wiberg foundation (grant M22-0088).

Institutional Review Board Statement: This research study was conducted retrospectively using anonymized human subject data made available in open access by ABIDE preprocessed. Ethical approval was not required as confirmed by the ethics committee of Linköping.

Informed Consent Statement: Informed consent was obtained from all subjects involved in the study; see ABIDE for details.

Data Availability Statement: The datasets analyzed for this study can be found at http://preprocessed-connectomes-project.org/abide/, accessed on 10 February 2023.

Acknowledgments: Primary support for the work by Adriana Di Martino was provided by the (NIMH K23MH087770) and the Leon Levy Foundation. Primary support for the work by Michael P. Milham and the INDI team was provided by gifts from Joseph P. Healy and the Stavros Niarchos Foundation to the Child Mind Institute, as well as by an NIMH award to MPM (NIMH R03MH096321).

Conflicts of Interest: A.E. has previously received hardware from Nvidia. Otherwise, the authors declare that the research was conducted in the absence of any commercial or financial relationships that could be construed as a potential conflict of interest. The funders had no role in the design of the study; in the collection, analyses, or interpretation of data; in the writing of the manuscript; or in the decision to publish the results.

References

1. Biswal, B.; Zerrin Yetkin, F.; Haughton, V.M.; Hyde, J.S. Functional connectivity in the motor cortex of resting human brain using echo-planar MRI. *Magn. Reson. Med.* **1995**, *34*, 537–541. [CrossRef] [PubMed]
2. Van Den Heuvel, M.P.; Pol, H.E.H. Exploring the brain network: A review on resting-state fMRI functional connectivity. *Eur. Neuropsychopharmacol.* **2010**, *20*, 519–534. [CrossRef] [PubMed]
3. Lord, C.; Elsabbagh, M.; Baird, G.; Veenstra-Vanderweele, J. Autism spectrum disorder. *Lancet* **2018**, *392*, 508–520. [CrossRef] [PubMed]
4. Lyall, K.; Croen, L.; Daniels, J.; Fallin, M.D.; Ladd-Acosta, C.; Lee, B.K.; Park, B.Y.; Snyder, N.W.; Schendel, D.; Volk, H.; et al. The changing epidemiology of autism spectrum disorders. *Annu. Rev. Public Health* **2017**, *38*, 81–102. [CrossRef] [PubMed]
5. Simeoli, R.; Milano, N.; Rega, A.; Marocco, D. Using technology to identify children with autism through motor abnormalities. *Front. Psychol.* **2021**, *12*, 635696. [CrossRef] [PubMed]
6. Milano, N.; Simeoli, R.; Rega, A.; Marocco, D. A deep learning latent variable model to identify children with autism through motor abnormalities. *Front. Psychol.* **2023**, *14*, 1194760. [CrossRef] [PubMed]
7. Wall, D.P.; Dally, R.; Luyster, R.; Jung, J.Y.; DeLuca, T.F. Use of artificial intelligence to shorten the behavioral diagnosis of autism. *PLoS ONE* **2012**, *7*, e43855. [CrossRef] [PubMed]
8. Bauman, M.L.; Kemper, T.L. Neuroanatomic observations of the brain in autism: A review and future directions. *Int. J. Dev. Neurosci.* **2005**, *23*, 183–187. [CrossRef]
9. O'Reilly, C.; Lewis, J.D.; Elsabbagh, M. Is functional brain connectivity atypical in autism? A systematic review of EEG and MEG studies. *PLoS ONE* **2017**, *12*, e0175870. [CrossRef]
10. Mennes, M.; Biswal, B.B.; Castellanos, F.X.; Milham, M.P. Making data sharing work: The FCP/INDI experience. *Neuroimage* **2013**, *82*, 683–691. [CrossRef]
11. Poldrack, R.A.; Gorgolewski, K.J. Making big data open: Data sharing in neuroimaging. *Nat. Neurosci.* **2014**, *17*, 1510–1517. [CrossRef] [PubMed]
12. Di Martino, A.; Yan, C.G.; Li, Q.; Denio, E.; Castellanos, F.X.; Alaerts, K.; Anderson, J.S.; Assaf, M.; Bookheimer, S.Y.; Dapretto, M.; et al. The autism brain imaging data exchange: Towards a large-scale evaluation of the intrinsic brain architecture in autism. *Mol. Psychiatry* **2014**, *19*, 659. [CrossRef] [PubMed]
13. Dvornek, N.C.; Ventola, P.; Pelphrey, K.A.; Duncan, J.S. Identifying autism from resting-state fMRI using long short-term memory networks. In *Machine Learning in Medical Imaging: 8th International Workshop, MLMI 2017, Held in Conjunction with MICCAI 2017, Quebec City, QC, Canada, 10 September 2017*; Springer: Berlin/Heidelberg, Germany, 2017; pp. 362–370.
14. Huang, Z.A.; Zhu, Z.; Yau, C.H.; Tan, K.C. Identifying autism spectrum disorder from resting-state fMRI using deep belief network. *IEEE Trans. Neural Netw. Learn. Syst.* **2020**, *32*, 2847–2861. [CrossRef] [PubMed]
15. Arbabshirani, M.R.; Plis, S.; Sui, J.; Calhoun, V.D. Single subject prediction of brain disorders in neuroimaging: Promises and pitfalls. *Neuroimage* **2017**, *145*, 137–165. [CrossRef] [PubMed]
16. Heinsfeld, A.S.; Franco, A.R.; Craddock, R.C.; Buchweitz, A.; Meneguzzi, F. Identification of autism spectrum disorder using deep learning and the ABIDE dataset. *Neuroimage Clin.* **2018**, *17*, 16–23. [CrossRef] [PubMed]
17. Yang, X.; Schrader, P.T.; Zhang, N. A deep neural network study of the ABIDE repository on autism spectrum classification. *Int. J. Adv. Comput. Sci. Appl.* **2020**, *11*, 1–6. [CrossRef]
18. Thomas, R.M.; Gallo, S.; Cerliani, L.; Zhutovsky, P.; El-Gazzar, A.; van Wingen, G. Classifying autism spectrum disorder using the temporal statistics of resting-state functional MRI data with 3D convolutional neural networks. *Front. Psychiatry* **2020**, *11*, 440. [CrossRef]
19. Deng, J.; Dong, W.; Socher, R.; Li, L.J.; Li, K.; Fei-Fei, L. Imagenet: A large-scale hierarchical image database. In Proceedings of the 2009 IEEE Conference on Computer Vision and Pattern Recognition, Miami, FL, USA, 20–25 June 2009; pp. 248–255.
20. Shorten, C.; Khoshgoftaar, T.M. A survey on image data augmentation for deep learning. *J. Big Data* **2019**, *6*, 60. [CrossRef]
21. Chlap, P.; Min, H.; Vandenberg, N.; Dowling, J.; Holloway, L.; Haworth, A. A review of medical image data augmentation techniques for deep learning applications. *J. Med. Imaging Radiat. Oncol.* **2021**, *65*, 545–563. [CrossRef]
22. Cirillo, M.D.; Abramian, D.; Eklund, A. What is the best data augmentation approach for brain tumor segmentation using 3D U-Net? In Proceedings of the IEEE International Conference on Image Processing (ICIP), Anchorage, AK, USA, 19–22 September 2021.
23. Guo, X.; Dominick, K.C.; Minai, A.A.; Li, H.; Erickson, C.A.; Lu, L.J. Diagnosing autism spectrum disorder from brain resting-state functional connectivity patterns using a deep neural network with a novel feature selection method. *Front. Neurosci.* **2017**, *11*, 460. [CrossRef]
24. El-Gazzar, A.; Quaak, M.; Cerliani, L.; Bloem, P.; van Wingen, G.; Mani Thomas, R. A hybrid 3DCNN and 3DC-LSTM based model for 4D spatio-temporal fMRI data: An ABIDE autism classification study. In *OR 2.0 Context-Aware Operating Theaters and Machine Learning in Clinical Neuroimaging: Second International Workshop, OR 2.0 2019, and Second International Workshop, MLCN 2019, Held in Conjunction with MICCAI 2019, Shenzhen, China, 13–17 October 2019*; Springer: Cham, Switzerland, 2019; pp. 95–102.
25. Khodatars, M.; Shoeibi, A.; Sadeghi, D.; Ghaasemi, N.; Jafari, M.; Moridian, P.; Khadem, A.; Alizadehsani, R.; Zare, A.; Kong, Y.; et al. Deep learning for neuroimaging-based diagnosis and rehabilitation of autism spectrum disorder: A review. *Comput. Biol. Med.* **2021**, *139*, 104949. [CrossRef]
26. Ji, J.; Wang, Z.; Zhang, X.; Li, J. Sparse data augmentation based on encoderforest for brain network classification. *Appl. Intell.* **2022**, *52*, 4317–4329. [CrossRef]

27. Waheed, S.H.; Mirbagheri, S.; Agarwal, S.; Kamali, A.; Yahyavi-Firouz-Abadi, N.; Chaudhry, A.; DiGianvittorio, M.; Gujar, S.K.; Pillai, J.J.; Sair, H.I. Reporting of resting-state functional magnetic resonance imaging preprocessing methodologies. *Brain Connect.* **2016**, *6*, 663–668. [CrossRef] [PubMed]
28. Power, J.D.; Barnes, K.A.; Snyder, A.Z.; Schlaggar, B.L.; Petersen, S.E. Spurious but systematic correlations in functional connectivity MRI networks arise from subject motion. *Neuroimage* **2012**, *59*, 2142–2154. [CrossRef]
29. Eklund, A.; Nichols, T.E.; Afyouni, S.; Craddock, C. How does group differences in motion scrubbing affect false positives in functional connectivity studies? *BioRxiv* **2020**. [CrossRef]
30. Craddock, C.; Benhajali, Y.; Chu, C.; Chouinard, F.; Evans, A.; Jakab, A.; Khundrakpam, B.S.; Lewis, J.D.; Li, Q.; Milham, M.; et al. The Neuro Bureau Preprocessing Initiative: Open sharing of preprocessed neuroimaging data and derivatives. *Front. Neuroinform.* **2013**, *7*, 5.
31. Xu, T.; Yang, Z.; Jiang, L.; Xing, X.X.; Zuo, X.N. A connectome computation system for discovery science of brain. *Sci. Bull.* **2015**, *60*, 86–95. [CrossRef]
32. Greve, D.N.; Fischl, B. Accurate and robust brain image alignment using boundary-based registration. *Neuroimage* **2009**, *48*, 63–72. [CrossRef]
33. Jenkinson, M.; Beckmann, C.F.; Behrens, T.E.; Woolrich, M.W.; Smith, S.M. FSL. *Neuroimage* **2012**, *62*, 782–790. [CrossRef]
34. Yan, C.; Zang, Y. DPARSF: A MATLAB toolbox for "pipeline" data analysis of resting-state fMRI. *Front. Syst. Neurosci.* **2010**, *4*, 1377. [CrossRef]
35. Ashburner, J. A fast diffeomorphic image registration algorithm. *Neuroimage* **2007**, *38*, 95–113. [CrossRef] [PubMed]
36. Zang, Y.; Jiang, T.; Lu, Y.; He, Y.; Tian, L. Regional homogeneity approach to fMRI data analysis. *NeuroImage* **2004**, *22*, 394–400. [CrossRef] [PubMed]
37. Kendall, M.; Gibbons, J.D. *Rank Correlation Methods*; Oxford University Press: New York, NY, USA, 1990.
38. Harris, C.R.; Millman, K.J.; van der Walt, S.J.; Gommers, R.; Virtanen, P.; Cournapeau, D.; Wieser, E.; Taylor, J.; Berg, S.; Smith, N.J.; et al. Array programming with NumPy. *Nature* **2020**, *585*, 357–362. [CrossRef] [PubMed]
39. Ronneberger, O.; Fischer, P.; Brox, T. U-net: Convolutional networks for biomedical image segmentation. In Proceedings of the International Conference on Medical Image Computing and Computer-Assisted Intervention, Munich, Germany, 5–9 October 2015; Springer: Berlin/Heidelberg, Germany, 2015; pp. 234–241.

Disclaimer/Publisher's Note: The statements, opinions and data contained in all publications are solely those of the individual author(s) and contributor(s) and not of MDPI and/or the editor(s). MDPI and/or the editor(s) disclaim responsibility for any injury to people or property resulting from any ideas, methods, instructions or products referred to in the content.

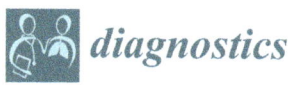

Article

Automatic Detection and Classification of Diabetic Retinopathy Using the Improved Pooling Function in the Convolution Neural Network

Usharani Bhimavarapu [1], Nalini Chintalapudi [2] and Gopi Battineni [2,3,*]

[1] Department of Computer Science and Engineering, Koneru Lakshmaiah Education Foundation, Vaddeswaram 522302, India
[2] Clinical Research Centre, School of Medicinal and Health Products Sciences, University of Camerino, 62032 Camerino, Italy
[3] The Research Centre of the ECE Department, V. R. Siddhartha Engineering College, Vijayawada 520007, India
* Correspondence: gopi.battineni@unicam.it

Abstract: Diabetic retinopathy (DR) is an eye disease associated with diabetes that can lead to blindness. Early diagnosis is critical to ensure that patients with diabetes are not affected by blindness. Deep learning plays an important role in diagnosing diabetes, reducing the human effort to diagnose and classify diabetic and non-diabetic patients. The main objective of this study was to provide an improved convolution neural network (CNN) model for automatic DR diagnosis from fundus images. The pooling function increases the receptive field of convolution kernels over layers. It reduces computational complexity and memory requirements because it reduces the resolution of feature maps while preserving the essential characteristics required for subsequent layer processing. In this study, an improved pooling function combined with an activation function in the ResNet-50 model was applied to the retina images in autonomous lesion detection with reduced loss and processing time. The improved ResNet-50 model was trained and tested over the two datasets (i.e., APTOS and Kaggle). The proposed model achieved an accuracy of 98.32% for APTOS and 98.71% for Kaggle datasets. It is proven that the proposed model has produced greater accuracy when compared to their state-of-the-art work in diagnosing DR with retinal fundus images.

Keywords: CNN; diabetic retinopathy; fundus image; pooling function

Citation: Bhimavarapu, U.; Chintalapudi, N.; Battineni, G. Automatic Detection and Classification of Diabetic Retinopathy Using the Improved Pooling Function in the Convolution Neural Network. Diagnostics 2023, 13, 2606. https://doi.org/10.3390/diagnostics13152606

Academic Editor: Daniele Giansanti

Received: 7 July 2023
Revised: 30 July 2023
Accepted: 2 August 2023
Published: 5 August 2023

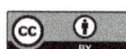

Copyright: © 2023 by the authors. Licensee MDPI, Basel, Switzerland. This article is an open access article distributed under the terms and conditions of the Creative Commons Attribution (CC BY) license (https://creativecommons.org/licenses/by/4.0/).

1. Introduction

Glucose in the body is converted into energy, which helps with everyday tasks. Diabetes is caused by obesity, poor nutrition, and limited physical activity. However, elevated blood glucose can build up in the blood vessels of several human organs, including the eye. People who have had diabetes for over a decade have the chance of getting diabetic retinopathy (DR) [1]. Globally, the population suffering from diabetes is expected to reach 552 million by 2030 [2]. Preventing visual loss is possible with early detection and sufficient treatment [3]. DR consists of five classes—no DR, mild, moderate, severe, and proliferative.

DR can affect blood vessels, in severe cases damaging, enlarging, or blocking them, or causing leaks; the abnormal growth of blood vessels can cause total blindness. Microaneurysms, haemorrhages, and exudates are the major signs of retinal DR. The level of the disease can be identified based on the shape, size, and overall appearance of the lesions. The main benefits of DR screening are its high effectiveness, low cost and minimal reliance on clinicians (i.e., ophthalmologists). The global eye screening tool for DR is the fundus photograph [4]. To prevent diabetes-related blindness, automated screening allows for clinically convenient and cost-effective detection [5].

From the field of computer science, deep learning can be a practical approach to automatic DR detection [6]. A deep learning system automatically identifies the DR with an accuracy that is equal to or better than that of ophthalmologists. The core deep learning model for medical image diagnosis prediction, and classification is the convolution neural network (CNN). However, there is the possibility to improve the performance of the model by tuning the hyperparameters in these deep learning-based models.

CNN models AlexNet and VGGNet-16 have been implemented for this purpose and the results suggest that VGG-19 performs best; however, the DR stages have not been explicitly ranked [7]. A hybrid technique incorporating image processing and deep learning was proposed for the detection and classification of DR in the publicly available dataset MESSIDOR, and Histogram Equalization (HE) and Contrast Limited Adaptive Histogram Equalization (CLAHE) were implemented to improve the contrast of the image [8]. Other CNN models, like Inception V3, Dense 121, Xception, Dense 169, and ResNet 50, have been explored for the enhanced classification of different DR phases [9].

In another study, the authors proposed a framework with a new loss function by implementing mid-level representations to improve DR detection performance [10]. Another report proved that VGGNet produced higher accuracy compared with other CNN models such as AlexNet, GoogleNet, and ResNet for DR classification [11]. A CNN model implementation with data augmentation for DR image classification was presented in [12].

Other frameworks for the early diagnosis and classification of DR were presented for Grampian [13], MESSIDOR [14], and EYEPACS datasets [15]. In [16], the authors mentioned that 90% of accuracy was achieved in diagnosing microaneurysms and extracting and classifying the candidate lesions. All of these existing studies have implemented built-in hyperparameters. However, model performance can be improved by adjusting hyperparameters within deep learning models. To counter the self-strengthening trend and ensure that as many candidate component models as possible have been properly trained, we have added balance loss to our model. The proposed approach could extract key features from the fundus images that can help make an accurate DR diagnosis.

2. Materials and Methods

The objective of the current study was to accurately categorize DR fundus images into different severities. We discussed an automated system for assessing the seriousness of diabetic retinopathy. The classification accuracy for diabetic retinopathy was improved in the current research using a modified CNN architecture. Figure 1 illustrates the proposed framework.

2.1. Dataset Collection

We collected the dataset from two publicly available fundus image datasets, i.e., APTOS [17] and Kaggle [18]. Table 1 tabulates the count for five categories in APTOS and Kaggle datasets. Figure 2 shows the sample fundus images from the two datasets. The first-row fundus images are from APTOS and the second-row fundus images are from the Kaggle dataset.

Table 1. Dataset distribution.

Dataset	NODR	Mild DR	Moderate DR	Severe DR	PDR	Count
APTOS	1805	370	999	193	295	3662
Kaggle	25,810	2443	5292	873	708	35,126

We employed data augmentation to increase the number of images throughout the training sample. Once provided with more DR to learn from, DL approaches generally improve their performance. Overfitting is avoided and the imbalance in the dataset is corrected by the application of data augmentation. Horizontal shift augmentation was one of the transformations considered for this study; it involves horizontally shifting an image's pixels while maintaining the original image's perspective. The dimension of this transition is specified by a number ranging from 0 to 1 and the viewing angle of the original image is preserved. The image can also be rotated with an additional type of transformation by a random amount between 0 and 180 degrees. By employing data augmentation methods, we were able to fix the problem of varying sample sizes and convoluted categorizations. After augmentation, the APTOS dataset classes were evenly distributed for the training set—1805 for NODR, 1850 for Mid, 1988 for Moderate, 1737 for Severe, and 1770 for PDR. After augmentation, the Kaggle dataset classes were evenly distributed for the training set—25,810 for NODR, 24,430 for Mid, 26,460 for Moderate, 25,317 for Severe, and 25,488 for PDR. Figure 3 shows some of the augmentation operations followed in this study. Table 2 tabulates the statistics of the data augmentation operations and the final augmented fundus images of each dataset.

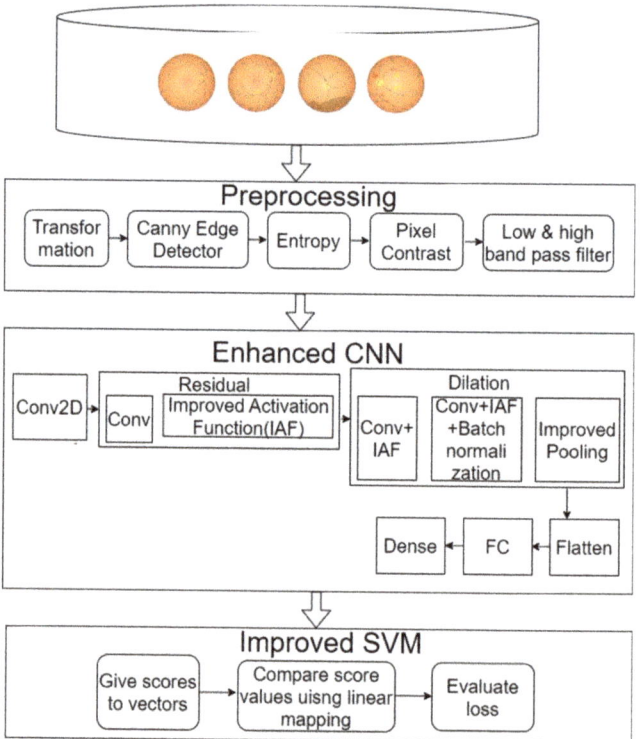

Figure 1. Experimental framework.

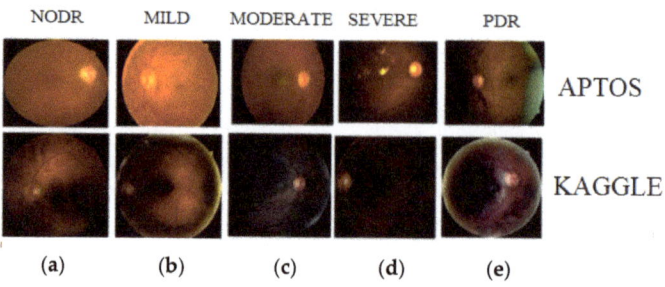

Figure 2. Multiclass of DR (a) NODR, (b) Mild DR, (c) Moderate DR, (d) Severe DR, and (e) PDR. (First row—APTOS dataset, second row—Kaggle dataset).

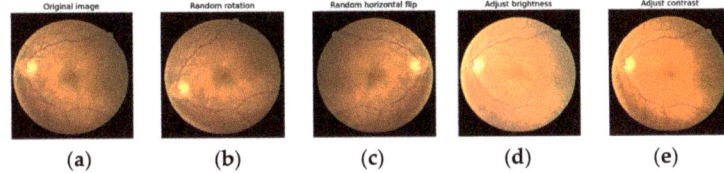

Figure 3. Augmentation (**a**) Original image, (**b**) rotation, (**c**) horizontal flip, (**d**) brightness, (**e**) contrast.

Table 2. Dataset augmentation operations.

Class	APTOS			Kaggle		
	Original	Operations	Augmented	Original	Operations	Augmented
NoDR	1805	0	1805	25,810	0	25,810
MildDR	370	5	1850	2443	10	24,430
Moderate DR	999	2	1998	5292	5	26,460
Severe DR	193	9	1737	873	29	25,317
PDR	295	6	1770	708	36	25,488
Total	3662		9160	35,126		127,505

2.2. Pre-Processing

In this study, we implemented the enhanced artificial bee colony (ABC) algorithm to improve the lesions' visual contents. Consider $\xi(i,j) \epsilon D$ with dimensions PXQ, where the values of P, Q are taken as 512 for every image in the database D.

The mathematical representation of the transformation function,

$$\Xi_f = \frac{1}{\int_0^1 x^{(c-1)}(1-x)^{d-1} dx} X \int_0^v x^{(c-1)}(1-x)^{d-1} dx, \quad (1)$$

where x is an integration variable and c and d are adjustable parameters of a given function where the maximum value of c is compared with d.

We evaluated the fitness function to adjust the values of c and d and also to measure the complete lesion image.

$$F(\xi_H(i,j)) = \log(\log(\sum_{j=1}(\Psi))) M_\Psi E(\xi_H) Y(\xi_H), \quad (2)$$

where $\sum_{j=1}(\Psi)$ represents the total edge intensities of an image evaluated through a canny edge detector. $Y(\xi_H)$ represents the contrast of the image $\xi_H(i,j)$, M_Ψ represents the total edge pixels of the processed image, and $E(\xi_H)$ represents the image entropy $\xi_H(i,j)$, represented as:

$$E(\xi_H) = \sum_{j=0}^m q_i \log_2(q_i), \quad (3)$$

where q_i represents the ith pixel intensity probability; the max value is 255.

The contrast of the image is represented as:

$$Y(\xi_H) = \sum_{j=0}^{mI} Y(\xi_H)(I_i), \quad (4)$$

where I_i represents the image blocks and mI represents the mth image block.

The contrasted local band of each block is represented as:

$$\begin{aligned}\xi_{Hy}(I_i) &= \sum_{(p,q)\epsilon I} Y(\xi_H)(p,q) \\ &= \sum_{(p,q)\in I} \frac{\xi_H(p,q) \otimes \phi_b}{\xi_H(p,q) \otimes \phi_c},\end{aligned} \quad (5)$$

where p, q represents the pixels of the rows and columns of each block, ϕ_b represents the bandpass filter, and ϕ_c represents the low pass filter.

2.3. Enhanced ResNet-50

The proposed model consists of convolution blocks and includes the improved pooling function, a drop-out layer, dense layers, and a SoftMax classification layer; Figure 4 presents the improved ResNet-50 model.

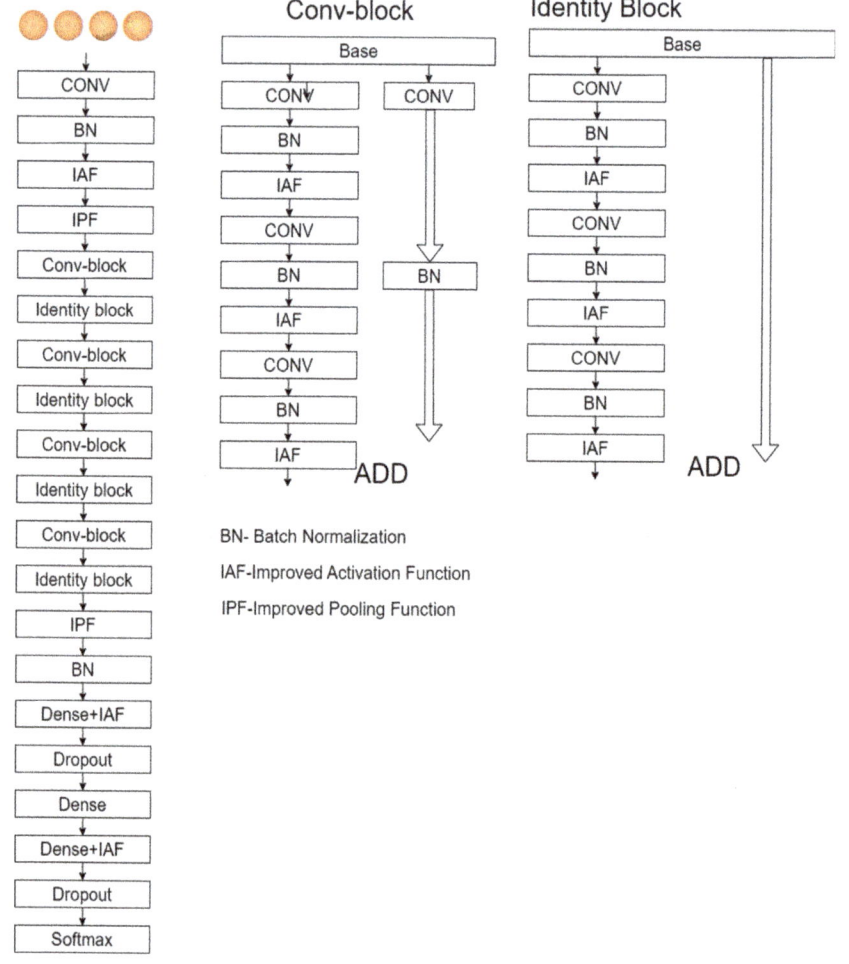

Figure 4. Improved ResNet-50 model.

Convolution Layer: The convolutional block is the fundamental building component, and each convolution block contains a convolution 2D, an improved activation function, and improved pooling with the average value. The vanishing gradient issue is solved using the improved activation function, simplifying the process so the network can understand and carry out its tasks promptly.

Kernel: The model's initial layer is the convolution layer. This layer initiates the process by applying the filters, also known as the kernel. The kernel size depends on two values—the width and height of the filter. In this study, we set the size of the filter as 3.

This filter enables and identifies the features that help understand low-level visual aspects like edges and curves.

Flattened layer: The flattened layer is located among the convolution and the dense layers. Tensor datatypes are used as inputs for the convolution layers, whereas dense layers demand a one-dimensional layout. The flattened layer was applied to translate the two-dimensional image representation into a one-dimensional input.

Dropout Layer: A dropout value of 0.2 was used in this study, which helps to avoid overfitting. This layer's function was to turn various components on and off to reduce the model's complexity and training time. The model thus acquires all the features that are required.

Dense Layer: A single matrix is accepted as input by the dense layer, which produces output based on the characteristics of the matrix. The identification and class labelling of fundus images occurs in these layers. The model's output is produced by a dense layer with five neurons and an improved activation function, and it assigns the image to one of five categories of diabetes: NoDR, Mild, Moderate, Severe, or Proliferative. After a few layers, the proposed activation is applied; this probability-based activation function measures the number of neurons by the entire number of classes.

Pooling function: The pooling function in the CNN is primarily used to downsample the feature maps and learn deeper image features that are resilient to subtle local alterations. The features from each spatial region are aggregated in this process. Pooling not only expands the receptive field of convolutional kernels across layers but also reduces memory needs and computational complexity by lowering the resolution of the feature maps while keeping critical features required for processing by the following layers. Pooling can be used in medical image analysis to manage variations in lesion sizes and positions [19,20]. Fundus images frequently have many lesions or parts, which causes their distributions of convolutional activations to be exceedingly complex since unimodal distributions cannot adequately capture statistics of convolutional activations, which limits the CNN performance.

We first pass Y throughout a group of prediction layers with parameters θ_p, i.e., $c(\theta_p; Y)$. The weights are outputted throughout by using a fully connected layer with additional noise.

The improved pooling function is presented as:

$$F_k(c(\theta_p; Y)) = T_k^h C(\theta_p; Y) + \sqrt{\delta . \log(1 + \exp(T_k^m C(\theta_p; Y)))}, \qquad (6)$$

where T_k^h and T_k^m are the fully connected layers, the kth parameter and additional noise, δ is the random variable, $C(\theta_p; Y)$ are the learned weights, and the weight function can be represented as:

$$w_k(Y) = \sqrt{\frac{\exp(TOP - Q(F_k(c(\theta_p; Y))))}{\sum_{k=1}^{m} \exp(TOP - Q(F_k(c(\theta_p; Y))))}}, \qquad (7)$$

where TOP-Q are the Q largest weights.

To make learned weights sparse, we maintained the TOP-Q weights and set the remaining ones as negative infinity and we used the improved activation function to normalize all the weights.

We added extra loss using the learned weights:

$$L_s = 3\sqrt{\beta\left(\frac{S\left(\sum_{s=1}^{N} w_k(Y_s)\right)}{M\left(\sum_{s=1}^{N} w_k(Y_s)\right)}\right)}, \qquad (8)$$

where Y_s is the mini-batch training sample, S and M are the standard deviation and the mean, and β is the parameter.

The improved activation function, which was recommended as a replacement for the activation function ReLU, is represented as:

$$f(x) = \begin{cases} x/2; if -2 \leq x < 2 \\ -1; if\ x < -2 \\ 1; if\ x > 2 \end{cases} \quad (9)$$

2.4. Classification

We applied the improved SVM in this study to improve classification accuracy. Initially, the SVM calculates the score for all the extracted features by using linear mapping on feature vectors and uses this to evaluate the loss. The improved SVM uses the linear mapping on extracted features to calculate the feature score for the parts of the region of interest used to differentiate the lesion types, which helps in the evaluation of loss function, which helps to obtain the classification results. Algorithm 1 for the improved SVM is presented below.

Algorithm 1 Improved SVM

- Initialize the values in the training set.
- Repeat for j = 1 to M.

Calculate the loss using the enhanced optimization for all values of j.
Compare the extracted regions in the liver images.
end

- Repeat for every score vector j − 1 to M.

Compute the SVM
argmax((w × p j) + b)
end

- Compute for all weights and finally evaluate the output.

---

3. Results

All experiments were implemented on Keras. The data split was performed based on an 80:20 ratio, where 80% of the data were used for training and 20% for testing. We implemented the proposed pooling function and activation function in the base models VGG-16, DenseNet, ResNet-50, Xception, and AlexNet for the fundus images. Table 3 tabulates the splitting of training and testing sets of fundus images for two augmented datasets.

Table 3. Augmented dataset image distribution.

Class	APTOS		Kaggle	
	Training	Testing	Training	Testing
NoDR	1444	361	20,648	5162
MildDR	1480	370	19,544	4886
Moderate DR	1598	400	21,166	5292
Severe DR	1390	347	20,254	5063
PDR	1416	354	20,390	5098
Total	7328	1832	102,004	25,501

3.1. Image Enhancement Evaluation

Image enhancement is a vital concept that changes the intensities of the original image to improve the image's perceptual quality. Figure 5 shows the contrast enhancement results for the APTOS dataset fundus image. Figure 5 compares the proposed model with some other existing enhancement models. Contrast-limited adaptive histogram equalization (CLAHE) models show insufficient image enhancement. The histogram modification framework (HMF) model enhances the image well; however, the hazy look is not adequately removed. The heuristic adaptive histogram equalization (HAHE) model produces an enhanced image with unwanted artefacts visible in the fundus image. The artificial bee colony algorithm (ABC) yields better results than the other existing models; still, it has some viewable artifacts in the fundus image. The proposed model generates an outstanding result compared to all other existing models and successfully improves every minor detail present in the fundus image.

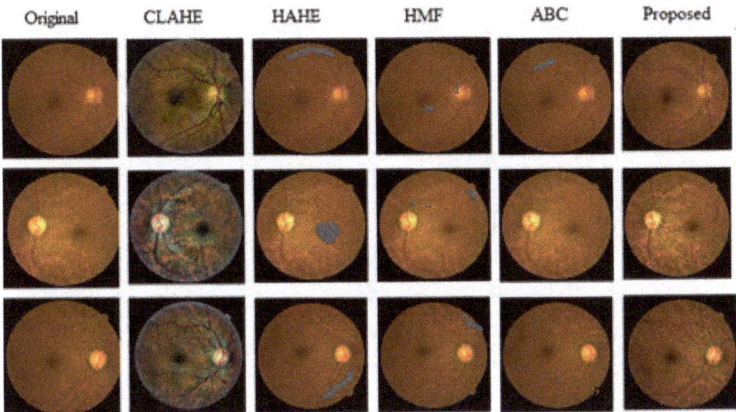

Figure 5. Comparison of the image enhancement of the proposed model with the existing models.

Evaluation and assessment are important for analysing the proposed model performance quantitatively. The proposed image enhancement model is accessed with performance measures such as entropy, peak signal-to-noise ratio (PSNR), the structural similarity index measure (SSIM), gradient magnitude similarity deviation (GMSD), and the patch-based contrast quality index (PCQI) [21–23].

Entropy defines the amount of information contained in the processed image.

$$\text{Entropy} = \sum_{y=0}^{255} P(n) \log_2(P(n)); \qquad (10)$$

where $P(n)$ represents the probability of the nth level of the image.

PSNR computes the amount of noise content in the processed image.

$$\text{PSNR} = 20 \log_{10} \frac{2}{\frac{1}{AB} \sum_{x=0}^{A-1} \sum_{y=0}^{B-1} |I_0(x,y) - I_i(x-y)|^2}, \qquad (11)$$

where A, B denotes the image size.

$$\text{SSIM} = \frac{(2\mu_{I_i}\mu_{I_o} + A_1)(2\sigma_{I_i}\sigma_{I_o} + A_2)}{(\mu_{I_i}^2 + \mu_{I_o}^2 + A_1)(\sigma_{I_i}^2 + \sigma_{I_o}^2 + A_2)}, \qquad (12)$$

where μ_{I_i}, μ_{I_o} represents the input and the output intensity values, σ_{I_i}, σ_{I_o} represent the input and the output standard deviation values, and A_1, A_2 represent the constant to limit the instability problem.

Table 4 tabulates the average scores for the augmented APTOS dataset. The performance of the proposed model was demonstrated by comparing six state-of-the-art existing models such as Clahe [24], exposure-based sub-image histogram equalization (ESIHE) [25], HAHE [26], BIMEF [27], HMF [28], and ABC. From Table 4, it is clear that the proposed model achieves a higher SSIM value, and its similarity level is up to the mark when compared with the original fundus image. The proposed enhanced model attains a lesser GMSD value for the images and holds more excellent visual quality compared to the other methods. The proposed model gains a higher PSNR value and the noise suppression level is very good compared with that of the other models. The proposed model holds a higher entropy value to the original image and the amount of information preserved is high compared with the state-of-the-art models. The proposed model obtains a more significant PCQI value compared with the other models, and generates a good quality image with minimum structural distortions. The proposed enhanced model offers less running time when compared to the state-of-the-art contrast enhancement models. The running time of the CLAHE and ESIHE models is approximately equal to that of the proposed model. But these models suffer from noise and distortion. From Table 4, we can recognise that the proposed enhanced model is superior in enriching content, maintaining similarity, and suppressing the noise and distortion. The proposed enhanced image enhancement model generated a crisp and clear output.

Table 4. Average scores for the augmented APTOS dataset.

Model	PSNR	GMSD	Entropy	SSIM	PCQI	Processing Time (s)
Clahe [24]	30.83	0.163	7.263	0.634	1.139	0.155
ESIHE [25]	31.93	0.074	7.316	0.635	1.282	0.153
HAHE [26]	32.82	0.125	7.226	0.693	1.001	0.373
BIMEF [27]	31.68	0.199	7.269	0.736	1.007	0.364
HMF [28]	32.63	0.085	7.283	0.636	1.103	0.218
ABC	34.83	0.048	7.834	0.877	1.378	0.173
Proposed	35.56	0.037	7.935	0.983	1.484	0.151

3.2. Segmentation Comparison

The proposed model obtains more accurate and robust segmentation results. From Figure 6 it can be noticed that the proposed model obtains more accurate results.

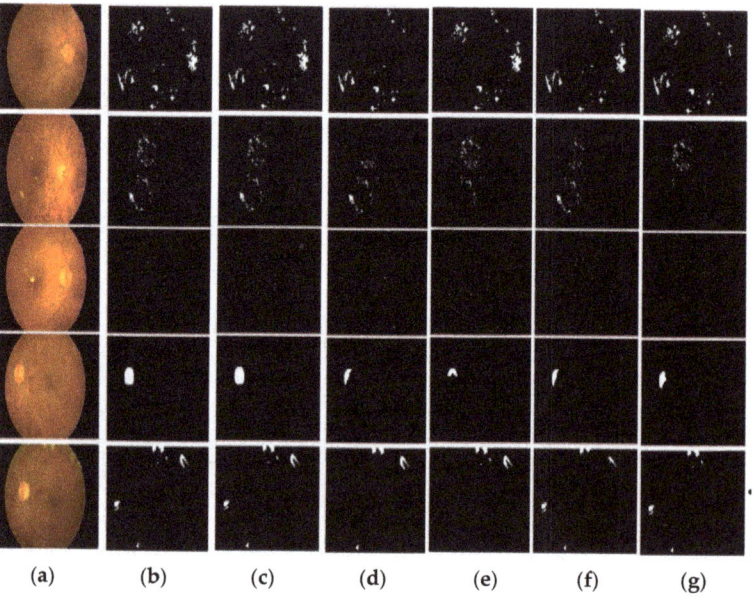

Figure 6. Segmentation results. (a) original image, (b) ground truth, (c) proposed model, (d) DenseNet, (e) Inception, (f) VGG-19, (g) AlexNet.

Table 5 tabulates the performance of the proposed enhanced ResNet-50 compared to the state-of-the-art models. The proposed system performed very accurately compared with the other lesion segmentation methods in the state-of-the-art models. It saves the obtained accuracy of abnormal fundus images. It achieves accurate, detailed segmentation results with small lesions, so it is the perfect choice for automatic computer-aided diagnosis (CAD) systems that depend on lesion segmentation results as it exceeds the estimations of the alternative models in terms of overall accuracy.

Table 5. Comparison of segmentation results for the APTOS dataset with the state-of-the-art models.

Model	Pool + Act	Accuracy	Precision	Recall
DenseNet [29]	Max + Relu	0.9484	0.8364	0.9584
Inception [12]	Max + Relu	0.9847	0.8578	0.9848
VGG-19 [30]	Max + Relu	0.9795	0.8479	0.9483
AlexNet [31]	Max + Relu	0.9858	0.9378	0.9847
ResNet-50	Proposed	0.9986	1.0000	1.0000
AlexNet	Proposed	0.9986	1.0000	0.9864
DenseNet	Proposed	0.9959	1.0000	0.9916
Inception	Proposed	0.9972	0.9864	0.9864
VGG-19	Proposed	0.9986	0.9866	1.0000

3.3. Evaluation of the APTOS Dataset

Figure 7 illustrates the confusion matrix for the APTOS dataset. We implemented five baseline models—VGG-16, DenseNet, ResNet-50, Xception, and AlexNet—and compared their performances on the APTOS dataset. From these five models, ResNet-50 showed the highest performance.

According to the 5-class confusion matrix mentioned above, the performance of each model was evaluated based on accuracy, recall, precision, and F1-score. Table 6 tabulates the APTOS fundus classification test set results. The improved SVM model achieved the highest accuracy of the remaining classification models. The results show that the augmented APTOS fundus classification for the ResNet-50 model achieves the highest accuracy for the improved SVM model.

Table 6. Performance metrics for APTOS augmented dataset.

CNN Model	Classifier	Accuracy	Precision	Recall	F1-Score	Class
DenseNet	ISVM	0.99781659	0.99445983	0.99445983	0.99445983	Normal
		0.99672489	0.98924731	0.99459459	0.99191375	Mild
		0.99617904	0.99002494	0.99250000	0.99126092	Moderate
		0.99727074	0.99137931	0.99423631	0.99280576	Severe
		0.99781659	1.0000000	0.98870056	0.99431818	PDR
	SVM	0.99617904	0.98895028	0.99168975	0.99031812	Normal
		0.99617904	0.98921833	0.99189189	0.99055331	Mild
		0.99508734	0.98753117	0.99000000	0.98876404	Moderate
		0.99617904	0.98850575	0.99135447	0.98992806	Severe
		0.99563319	0.99428571	0.98305085	0.98863636	PDR
	RF	0.99563319	0.98891967	0.98891967	0.98891967	Normal
		0.99290393	0.98113208	0.98378378	0.98245614	Mild
		0.99344978	0.98258706	0.98750000	0.98503741	Moderate
		0.99508734	0.98563218	0.98847262	0.98705036	Severe
		0.99344978	0.98857143	0.97740113	0.98295455	PDR
	NB	0.99454148	0.98347107	0.98891967	0.98618785	Normal
		0.99072052	0.97319035	0.98108108	0.97711978	Mild
		0.99399563	0.98503741	0.98750000	0.98626717	Moderate
		0.99290393	0.98265896	0.97982709	0.98124098	Severe
		0.99290393	0.98853868	0.97457627	0.98150782	PDR

Table 6. Cont.

CNN Model	Classifier	Accuracy	Precision	Recall	F1-Score	Class
ResNet-50	ISVM	0.99781659	0.99173554	0.99722992	0.99447514	Normal
		0.99836245	0.99460916	0.9972973	0.99595142	Mild
		0.99836245	0.99749373	0.9950000	0.99624531	Moderate
		0.99945415	1.00000000	0.99711816	0.99855700	Severe
		0.99945415	1.00000000	0.99717514	0.99858557	PDR
	SVM	0.99727074	0.99171271	0.99445983	0.99308437	Normal
		0.99727074	0.99191375	0.99459459	0.99325236	Mild
		0.99563319	0.98756219	0.9925000	0.99002494	Moderate
		0.99727074	0.99421965	0.99135447	0.99278499	Severe
		0.99836245	1.00000000	0.99152542	0.99574468	PDR
	RF	0.99617904	0.98895028	0.99168975	0.99031812	Normal
		0.99563319	0.98655914	0.99189189	0.98921833	Mild
		0.99563319	0.99000000	0.99000000	0.99000000	Moderate
		0.99617904	0.99132948	0.98847262	0.98989899	Severe
		0.99672489	0.99431818	0.98870056	0.99150142	PDR
	NB	0.99508734	0.98351648	0.99168975	0.98758621	Normal
		0.99399563	0.98123324	0.98918919	0.98519515	Mild
		0.99508734	0.98997494	0.98750000	0.98873592	Moderate
		0.99344978	0.98550725	0.97982709	0.98265896	Severe
		0.99508734	0.99145299	0.98305085	0.98723404	PDR
AlexNet	ISVM	0.99617904	0.98895028	0.99168975	0.99031812	Normal
		0.99454148	0.98648649	0.98648649	0.98648649	Mild
		0.99235808	0.98250000	0.98250000	0.98250000	Moderate
		0.99672489	0.99135447	0.99135447	0.99135447	Severe
		0.99727074	0.99433428	0.99152542	0.99292786	PDR
	SVM	0.99454148	0.98347107	0.98891967	0.98618785	Normal
		0.99454148	0.98913043	0.98378378	0.98644986	Mild
		0.99290393	0.98740554	0.98000000	0.98368883	Moderate
		0.99454148	0.98280802	0.98847262	0.98563218	Severe
		0.99508734	0.98591549	0.98870056	0.98730606	PDR
	RF	0.99344978	0.98071625	0.98614958	0.98342541	Normal
		0.99126638	0.97580645	0.98108108	0.97843666	Mild
		0.99126638	0.98484848	0.97500000	0.97989950	Moderate
		0.99235808	0.97982709	0.97982709	0.97982709	Severe
		0.99454148	0.98587571	0.98587571	0.98587571	PDR
	NB	0.99290393	0.97802198	0.98614958	0.98206897	Normal
		0.98962882	0.97050938	0.97837838	0.97442799	Mild
		0.99017467	0.98232323	0.97250000	0.97738693	Moderate
		0.99235808	0.9826087	0.97694524	0.97976879	Severe
		0.99235808	0.98022599	0.98022599	0.98022599	PDR
Inception	ISVM	0.99399563	0.97814208	0.99168975	0.98486933	Normal
		0.99126638	0.97326203	0.98378378	0.97849462	Mild
		0.99290393	0.99236641	0.97500000	0.98360656	Moderate
		0.99399563	0.98275862	0.98559078	0.98417266	Severe
		0.99508734	0.99145299	0.98305085	0.98723404	PDR
	SVM	0.99344978	0.97808219	0.98891967	0.98347107	Normal
		0.99181223	0.98102981	0.97837838	0.97970230	Mild
		0.98962882	0.97984887	0.97250000	0.97616060	Moderate
		0.99181223	0.97701149	0.97982709	0.97841727	Severe
		0.99290393	0.98300283	0.98022599	0.98161245	PDR
	RF	0.99181223	0.97527473	0.98337950	0.97931034	Normal
		0.98908297	0.97297297	0.97297297	0.97297297	Mild
		0.98744541	0.97243108	0.9700000	0.97121402	Moderate
		0.99126638	0.97971014	0.9740634	0.97687861	Severe
		0.99126638	0.97740113	0.97740113	0.97740113	PDR
	NB	0.99072052	0.96994536	0.98337950	0.97661623	Normal
		0.98962882	0.97820163	0.97027027	0.97421981	Mild
		0.98635371	0.97229219	0.96500000	0.96863237	Moderate
		0.98744541	0.96285714	0.97118156	0.96700143	Severe
		0.99126638	0.98011364	0.97457627	0.97733711	PDR

Table 6. *Cont.*

CNN Model	Classifier	Accuracy	Precision	Recall	F1-Score	Class
VGG-19	ISVM	0.99290393	0.97540984	0.98891967	0.98211829	Normal
		0.98908297	0.96791444	0.97837838	0.97311828	Mild
		0.99017467	0.98477157	0.97000000	0.97732997	Moderate
		0.99454148	0.98840580	0.98270893	0.98554913	Severe
		0.99290393	0.98300283	0.98022599	0.98161245	PDR
	SVM	0.99181223	0.97267760	0.98614958	0.97936726	Normal
		0.99072052	0.98092643	0.97297297	0.97693351	Mild
		0.98744541	0.97721519	0.96500000	0.97106918	Moderate
		0.99126638	0.97421203	0.97982709	0.97701149	Severe
		0.98962882	0.97183099	0.97457627	0.97320169	PDR
	RF	0.99126638	0.97260274	0.98337950	0.97796143	Normal
		0.98853712	0.97289973	0.97027027	0.97158322	Mild
		0.98689956	0.97474747	0.96500000	0.96984925	Moderate
		0.98962882	0.97126437	0.97406340	0.97266187	Severe
		0.98799127	0.96892655	0.96892655	0.96892655	PDR
	NB	0.98853712	0.96195652	0.98060942	0.97119342	Normal
		0.98635371	0.96495957	0.96756757	0.96626181	Mild
		0.98580786	0.97222222	0.96250000	0.96733668	Moderate
		0.98799127	0.96829971	0.96829971	0.96829971	Severe
		0.98689956	0.97142857	0.96045198	0.96590909	PDR

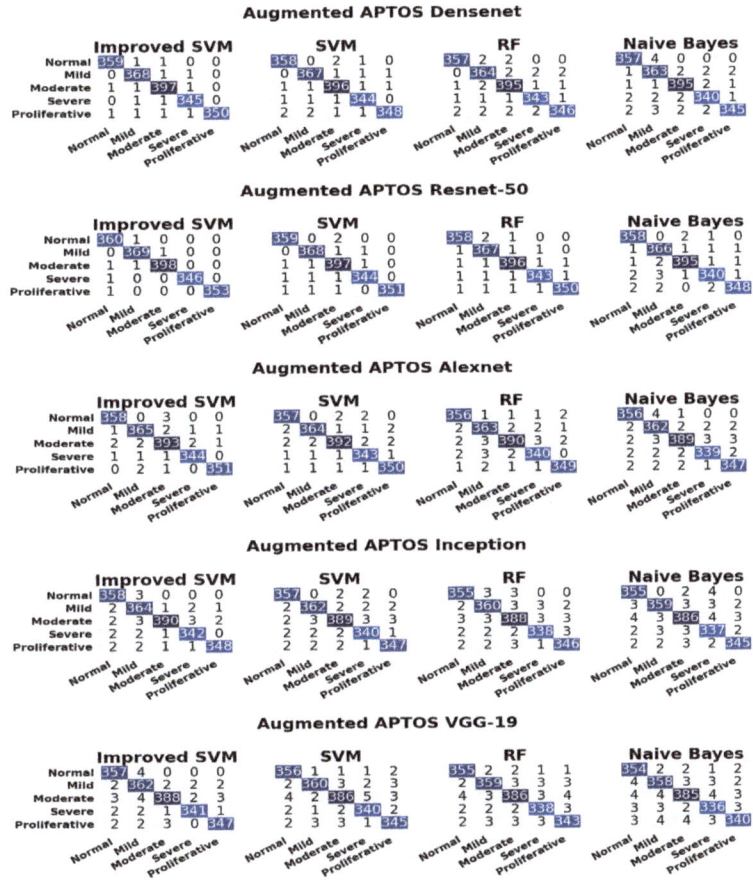

Figure 7. Confusion matrix for APTOS augmented dataset on different CNN models.

3.4. Evaluation of the Kaggle Dataset

Figure 8 illustrates the confusion matrix for the Kaggle dataset. We implemented five baseline models-VGG-16, DenseNet, ResNet-50, Xception, and AlexNet-and compared their performances on the Kaggle dataset. From these five models, ResNet-50 showed the highest performance. In 203 NODR fundus images, the proposed ISVM classifier accurately classified 202 fundus images for the ResNet-50 model. In 54 Mild images, the ISVM classifier accurately classified 54. Out of 69 moderate fundus images, ISVM accurately identified 68. Out of 15 images, ISVM accurately identified 14 for severe, and out of 7 images, ISVM accurately identified 6 for PDR for the ResNet-152 model. For the ResNet-50 model, the SVM classifier accurately identified 201 NODR images, 53 mild and 67 moderate, 14 severe, and 5 for PDR. For the ResNet-152 model, the RF classifier accurately identified 201 NODR images, 53 mild and 66 moderate, 13 severe, and 5 for PDR. For the ResNet-50 model, the NB classifier accurately identified 201 NODR images, 52 mild and 65 for moderate, 12 for severe, and 5 for PDR. Table 6 tabulated the Kaggle classification test set results.

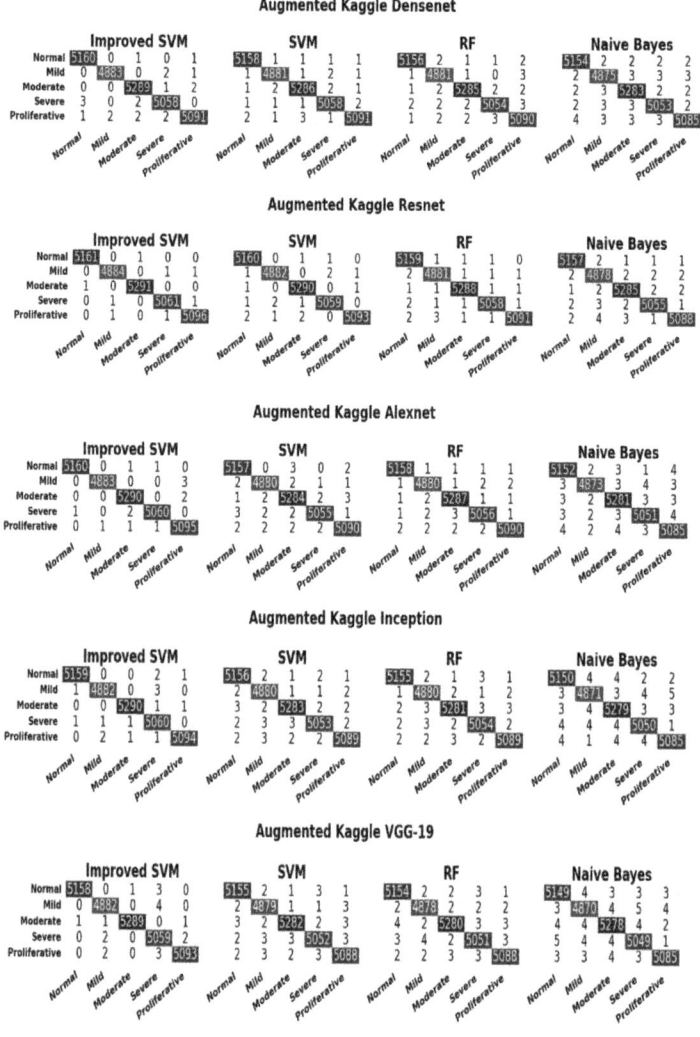

Figure 8. Confusion matrix for Kaggle augmented dataset on different CNN models.

From Table 7, we can see that the improved SVM model achieved the highest accuracy compared to the remaining classification models. The achieved results revealed that the overall testing accuracy and the performance metrics for the improved ResNet-50 with the improved SVM are the most appropriate for diabetic retinopathy detection, with a testing accuracy of 99.9% for fundus images.

Table 7. Performance metrics for Kaggle augmented dataset.

CNN Model	Classifier	Accuracy	Precision	Recall	F1-Score	Class
DenseNet	ISVM	0.99976472	0.99922541	0.99961255	0.99941894	Normal
		0.99980393	0.99959058	0.99938600	0.99948828	Mild
		0.99968629	0.99905553	0.99943311	0.99924428	Moderate
		0.99960786	0.99901244	0.99901244	0.99901244	Severe
		0.99956864	0.99921492	0.99862691	0.99892083	PDR
	SVM	0.99964707	0.99903157	0.99922511	0.99912833	Normal
		0.99960786	0.99897667	0.99897667	0.99897667	Mild
		0.99952943	0.99886621	0.99886621	0.99886621	Moderate
		0.99956864	0.99881517	0.99901244	0.99891379	Severe
		0.99952943	0.99901884	0.99862691	0.99882284	PDR
	RF	0.99956864	0.99903120	0.99883766	0.99893442	Normal
		0.99949022	0.99836367	0.99897667	0.99867008	Mild
		0.99949022	0.99886600	0.99867725	0.99877161	Moderate
		0.99941179	0.99881423	0.9982224	0.99851823	Severe
		0.99929415	0.99803922	0.99843076	0.99823495	PDR
	NB	0.99929415	0.99806352	0.99845021	0.99825683	Normal
		0.99913729	0.99774867	0.99774867	0.99774867	Mild
		0.99921572	0.99792218	0.99829932	0.99811071	Moderate
		0.99921572	0.99802489	0.99802489	0.99802489	Severe
		0.99913729	0.99823322	0.99744998	0.99784144	PDR
ResNet-50	ISVM	0.99992157	0.99980628	0.99980628	0.99980628	Normal
		0.99984314	0.99959067	0.99959067	0.99959067	Mild
		0.99992157	0.99981104	0.99981104	0.99981104	Moderate
		0.99984314	0.99960498	0.99960498	0.99960498	Severe
		0.99984314	0.99960769	0.99960769	0.99960769	PDR
	SVM	0.99972550	0.99903195	0.99961255	0.99932217	Normal
		0.99972550	0.99938588	0.99918133	0.99928359	Mild
		0.99976472	0.99924443	0.99962207	0.99943321	Moderate
		0.99972550	0.99940735	0.99920995	0.99930864	Severe
		0.99972550	0.99960746	0.99901922	0.99931325	PDR
	RF	0.99960786	0.99864499	0.99941883	0.99903176	Normal
		0.99956864	0.99877225	0.99897667	0.99887445	Mild
		0.99968629	0.99924414	0.99924414	0.99924414	Moderate
		0.99964707	0.99920980	0.99901244	0.99911111	Severe
		0.99960786	0.99941107	0.99862691	0.99901884	PDR
	NB	0.99952943	0.99864446	0.99903138	0.99883788	Normal
		0.99925493	0.99775005	0.99836267	0.99805627	Mild
		0.99941179	0.99848857	0.99867725	0.99858290	Moderate
		0.99945100	0.99881446	0.99841991	0.99861715	Severe
		0.99937257	0.99882214	0.99803845	0.99843014	PDR
AlexNet	ISVM	0.99988236	0.99980624	0.99961255	0.99970939	Normal
		0.99984314	0.99979525	0.99938600	0.99959058	Mild
		0.99976472	0.99924443	0.99962207	0.99943321	Moderate
		0.99980393	0.99960490	0.99940747	0.99950617	Severe
		0.99968629	0.99901961	0.99941153	0.99921553	PDR
	SVM	0.99949022	0.99845111	0.99903138	0.99874116	Normal
		0.99952943	0.99877200	0.99877200	0.99877200	Mild
		0.99933336	0.99829964	0.99848828	0.99839395	Moderate
		0.99949022	0.99901186	0.99841991	0.99871580	Severe
		0.99941179	0.99862664	0.99843076	0.99852869	PDR
	RF	0.99964707	0.99903157	0.99922511	0.99912833	Normal
		0.99949022	0.99856763	0.99877200	0.99866980	Mild
		0.99952943	0.99867775	0.99905518	0.99886643	Moderate
		0.99949022	0.99881470	0.99861742	0.99871605	Severe
		0.99949022	0.99901865	0.99843076	0.99872461	PDR
	NB	0.99909807	0.99748306	0.99806277	0.99777283	Normal
		0.99917650	0.99836099	0.99733934	0.99784990	Mild
		0.99905886	0.99754439	0.99792139	0.99773285	Moderate
		0.99909807	0.99782695	0.99762986	0.99772840	Severe
		0.99894122	0.99725436	0.99744998	0.99735216	PDR

Table 7. Cont.

CNN Model	Classifier	Accuracy	Precision	Recall	F1-Score	Class
Inception	ISVM	0.99980393	0.99961248	0.99941883	0.99951564	Normal
		0.99972550	0.99938588	0.99918133	0.99928359	Mild
		0.99984314	0.99962207	0.99962207	0.99962207	Moderate
		0.99960786	0.99861851	0.99940747	0.99901283	Severe
		0.99976472	0.99960754	0.99921538	0.99941142	PDR
	SVM	0.99941179	0.99825750	0.99883766	0.99854750	Normal
		0.99937257	0.99795501	0.99877200	0.99836334	Mild
		0.99937257	0.99867675	0.99829932	0.99848800	Moderate
		0.99933336	0.99861660	0.99802489	0.99832066	Severe
		0.99937257	0.99862637	0.99823460	0.99843045	PDR
	RF	0.99945100	0.99864394	0.99864394	0.99864394	Normal
		0.99937257	0.99795501	0.99877200	0.99836334	Mild
		0.99925493	0.99848743	0.99792139	0.99820433	Moderate
		0.99929415	0.9982224	0.9982224	0.9982224	Severe
		0.99933336	0.99843045	0.9982346	0.99833252	PDR
	NB	0.99898043	0.99728892	0.99767532	0.99748208	Normal
		0.99890200	0.99733825	0.99693000	0.99713408	Mild
		0.99890200	0.99716660	0.99754346	0.99735500	Moderate
		0.99898043	0.99743235	0.99743235	0.99743235	Severe
		0.99905886	0.99784144	0.99744998	0.99764567	PDR
VGG-19	ISVM	0.99980393	0.99980616	0.99922511	0.99951555	Normal
		0.99964707	0.99897688	0.99918133	0.99907910	Mild
		0.99984314	0.99981096	0.99943311	0.99962200	Moderate
		0.99945100	0.99802722	0.99920995	0.99861824	Severe
		0.99968629	0.99941130	0.99901922	0.99921522	PDR
	SVM	0.99937257	0.99825716	0.99864394	0.99845051	Normal
		0.99933336	0.99795459	0.99856734	0.99826087	Mild
		0.99933336	0.99867650	0.99811036	0.99839335	Moderate
		0.99921572	0.99822170	0.99782738	0.99802450	Severe
		0.99921572	0.99803845	0.99803845	0.99803845	PDR
	RF	0.99925493	0.99787028	0.99845021	0.99816016	Normal
		0.99929415	0.99795417	0.99836267	0.99815838	Mild
		0.99917650	0.99829836	0.99773243	0.99801531	Moderate
		0.99909807	0.99782695	0.99762986	0.99772840	Severe
		0.99925493	0.99823426	0.99803845	0.99813634	PDR
	NB	0.99890200	0.99709527	0.99748160	0.99728840	Normal
		0.99878436	0.99692938	0.99672534	0.99682735	Mild
		0.99886279	0.99716607	0.99735450	0.99726027	Moderate
		0.99886279	0.99703791	0.99723484	0.99713637	Severe
		0.99909807	0.99803729	0.99744998	0.99774355	PDR

Figure 9 presents the evaluation of the performance metrics for the different models. According to the achieved results, overall testing accuracy, and performance metrics, the proposed model is appropriate for detecting and classifying DR with a testing accuracy of 98.32% on the APTOS dataset.

Table 8 tabulates the varying sizes of the training and testing sets and the corresponding mean and standard deviation.

Table 8. Varying training and test size.

Dataset	Training	Testing	Accuracy	Mean	Standard Deviation
APTOS	70	30	0.981225	0.982543	0.0011409
	75	25	0.983202		
	80	20	0.983202		
Kaggle	70	30	0.971344	0.980237	0.0080882
	75	25	0.982213		
	80	20	0.987154		

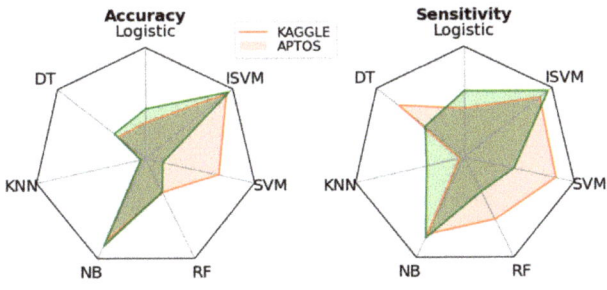

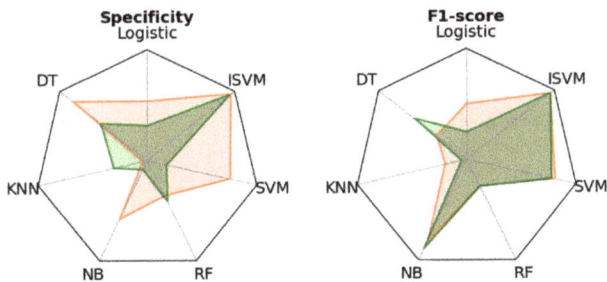

Figure 9. DR classification comparison of various classifiers of different datasets. It displays the performance results of the two datasets. Pink color represents the messidor and the green represents the APTOS.

4. Discussion

This study aimed to identify and classify DR based on fundus images from two different datasets. Initially, all the images in the dataset were of different sizes; the images were resized to 225 × 225 using the RGB colour. The hyperparameters were tuned to optimize the proposed model. Model training can be accelerated, and the possibility of performance improved using the pooling function. There is no ideal batch size, and we implemented the experiments with various batch sizes. If we find the suitable batch size in addition to the suitable kernel and hidden layers, the model will yield a high performance. Batch size 64 produces better results than batch sizes 16 or 32. The batch size was 64 for the fundus images because this study's dataset was large. From previous studies, we observed that the batch sizes, in conjunction with a suitable kernel and hidden layer, will yield a high performance. The parameters (i.e., a batch size of 64, epochs of 1000, and a learning rate of 0.001) were adjusted to achieve a high performance.

After extracting the features, the improved SVM classifies the lesions. In [15], the authors implemented AdaBoost to extract the features and the Gaussian mixture model, KNN, and SVM to classify the lesions and analyse the retina fundus images with different illuminations and views. A new unsupervised approach based on PCA for detecting microaneurysms was presented in [16]. The manual identification and differentiation of diabetic retinopathy from fundus images is time-consuming. Table 9 presents the processing time analysis of the existing techniques for the Kaggle and APTOS datasets to calculate the computation overhead. The achieved results revealed that the overall processing time for the improved SVM classifier is the most appropriate for diabetic retinopathy classification, with a minimum of 14 ms for Kaggle and 15 ms for APTOS datasets.

Table 9. DR classification comparison of the processing time for the proposed model with different optimizations.

Classifier	Kaggle (s)	APTOS (s)
Logistic regression [32]	21	29
DT [33]	15	21
KNN [34]	23	30
NB [35]	20	25
RF [36]	20	23
SVM [37]	22	31
Improved SVM	14	15

A study based on feature extraction using the RF model produced 74% accuracy in DR image classification [38]. Another two proposed hybrid models are based on combining the Gaussian mixture model and SVM to diagnose microaneurysms [18] and using KNN for the detection and classification of DR [39]. All the above-discussed studies used the existing classifiers to classify the DR lesions.

Some studies implemented CNN models to perform the binary classification of DR datasets [40,41]. Dropout regularization, augmentation, and pre-processing were performed manually by using the image editing tools in [42]. A deep CNN was proposed by [43] to classify normal and NPDR with two neural networks (i.e., the global and the local) and model performance was evaluated by the kappa score. The main disadvantage of this work is that it classifies only normal and NPPR, but it only works to detect the PDR.

To overcome those issues, the diagnostic results of the proposed model proved that it can achieve a satisfactory diagnostic performance, which can significantly assist the medical professional in the decision-making process in the early stages of detecting the infection, and timely treatment can decrease risk. Automatic screening and differentiation of diabetic retinopathy from fundus images will significantly reduce the effort of the medical professional and accelerate the diagnosis process.

Five class classifications are realized in the model, providing feasibility for the diagnosis of DR and its severity levels. The proposed model for the feature extraction and classification of DR performs better than the state-of-the-art models with high accuracy and less complexity. We will further optimize the model to model the accuracy of DR diagnosis and try to develop a more powerful DR detection model to assist doctors in clinical examinations.

The limitation of this model is that it is trained with only fundus image-level supervision, making it very challenging to accurately locate some minute lesion regions. Next, we need to specify the coarse location of the lesion along with the DR grading, which will help from the perspective of clinical application.

5. Conclusions

High blood pressure leads to DR, which causes retinal damage. Retinal vascularization is damaged by DR and can lead to blindness and potentially death. Fundoscopy examinations, which are time-consuming and expensive, allow ophthalmologists to see retinal vascular swelling. There is a need to automatically identify diabetic retinopathy by examining retinal fundus images. This study proposed an enhanced pooling function technique to minimize the loss to detect retina lesions, and an improved SVM classifier to classify the lesions using linear mapping. Five pre-trained deep learning models were recognized during the selection of the implementation, namely VGG-16, DenseNet, ResNet-50, Inception, and AlexNet. The proposed pooling and activation function results outperformed all the existing models. This study's proposed model provided efficient accuracy results compared to the existing models.

Author Contributions: Methodology, U.B., N.C. and G.B.; Software, U.B.; Validation, G.B.; Investigation, U.B. and N.C. All authors have read and agreed to the published version of the manuscript.

Funding: This research received no external funding.

Informed Consent Statement: This study does not include any human subject or clinical trial information.

Data Availability Statement: Not applicable.

Conflicts of Interest: The authors declare no conflict of interest.

References

1. Wild, S.H.; Roglic, G.; Green, A.; Sicree, R.; King, H. Global Prevalence of Diabetes: Estimates for the Year 2000 and Projections for 2030. *Diabetes Care* **2004**, *27*, 2569. [CrossRef]
2. Scully, T. Diabetes in numbers. *Nature* **2012**, *485*, S2–S3. [CrossRef]
3. Wu, L.; Fernandez-Loaiza, P.; Sauma, J.; Hernandez-Bogantes, E.; Masis, M. Classification of diabetic retinopathy and diabetic macula+r edema. *World J. Diabetes* **2013**, *4*, 290. [CrossRef]
4. Khansari, M.M.; O'neill, W.D.; Penn, R.D.; Blair, N.P.; Shahidi, M. Detection of Subclinical Diabetic Retinopathy by Fine Structure Analysis of Retinal Images. *J. Ophthalmol.* **2019**, *2019*, 5171965. [CrossRef]
5. Tufail, A.; Rudisill, C.; Egan, C.; Kapetanakis, V.V.; Salas-Vega, S.; Owen, C.G.; Rudnicka, A.R. Automated diabetic retinopathy image assessment software: Diagnostic accuracy and cost-effectiveness compared with human graders. *Ophthalmology* **2017**, *124*, 343–351. [CrossRef]
6. Gulshan, V.; Rajan, R.; Widner, K.; Wu, D.; Wubbels, P.; Rhodes, T.; Whitehouse, K.; Coram, M.; Corrado, G.; Ramasamy, K.; et al. Performance of a Deep-Learning Algorithm vs Manual Grading for Detecting Diabetic Retinopathy in India. *JAMA Ophthalmol.* **2019**, *137*, 987–993. [CrossRef]
7. García, G.; Gallardo, J.; Mauricio, A.; López, J.; Del Carpio, C. Detection of diabetic retinopathy based on a convolutional neural network using retinal fundus images. In *Artificial Neural Networks and Machine Learning–ICANN 2017, Proceedings of the 26th International Conference on Artificial Neural Networks, Alghero, Italy, 11–14 September 2017*; Springer International Publishing: Cham, Switzerland, 2017; pp. 635–642, Proceedings, Part II 26.
8. Hemanth, D.J.; Deperlioglu, O.; Kose, U. An enhanced diabetic retinopathy detection and classification approach using deep convolutional neural network. *Neural Comput. Appl.* **2019**, *32*, 707–721. [CrossRef]
9. Qummar, S.; Khan, F.G.; Shah, S.; Khan, A.; Shamshirband, S.; Rehman, Z.U.; Khan, I.A.; Jadoon, W. A Deep Learning Ensemble Approach for Diabetic Retinopathy Detection. *IEEE Access* **2019**, *7*, 150530–150539. [CrossRef]
10. Costa, P.; Galdran, A.; Smailagic, A.; Campilho, A. A Weakly-Supervised Framework for Interpretable Diabetic Retinopathy Detection on Retinal Images. *IEEE Access* **2018**, *6*, 18747–18758. [CrossRef]
11. Wan, S.; Liang, Y.; Zhang, Y. Deep convolutional neural networks for diabetic retinopathy detection by image classification. *Comput. Electr. Eng.* **2018**, *72*, 274–282. [CrossRef]
12. Bhatkar, A.P.; Kharat, G.U. Detection of diabetic retinopathy in retinal images using MLP classifier. In Proceedings of the 2015 IEEE International Symposium on Nanoelectronic and Information Systems, Indore, India, 21–23 December 2015; IEEE: New York, NY, USA, 2015; pp. 331–335.
13. Xu, J.; Zhang, X.; Chen, H.; Li, J.; Zhang, J.; Shao, L.; Wang, G. Automatic Analysis of Microaneurysms Turnover to Diagnose the Progression of Diabetic Retinopathy. *IEEE Access* **2018**, *6*, 9632–9642. [CrossRef]
14. Antal, B.; Hajdu, A. An Ensemble-Based System for Microaneurysm Detection and Diabetic Retinopathy Grading. *IEEE Trans. Biomed. Eng.* **2012**, *59*, 1720–1726. [CrossRef]
15. Dutta, S.; Manideep, B.C.; Basha, S.M.; Caytiles, R.D.; Iyengar, N.C.S.N. Classification of Diabetic Retinopathy Images by Using Deep Learning Models. *Int. J. Grid Distrib. Comput.* **2018**, *11*, 99–106. [CrossRef]
16. Lunscher, N.; Chen, M.L.; Jiang, N.; Zelek, J. Automated Screening for Diabetic Retinopathy Using Compact Deep Networks. *J. Comput. Vis. Imaging Syst.* **2017**, *3*, 1–3. [CrossRef]
17. Available online: https://www.kaggle.com/competitions/aptos2019-blindness-detection/data (accessed on 2 October 2022).
18. Available online: https://www.kaggle.com/competitions/diabetic-retinopathy-detection/discussion/234309 (accessed on 2 October 2022).
19. Nirthika, R.; Manivannan, S.; Ramanan, A.; Wang, R. Pooling in convolutional neural networks for medical image analysis: A survey and an empirical study. *Neural Comput. Appl.* **2022**, *34*, 5321–5347. [CrossRef]
20. Yamashita, R.; Nishio, M.; Do, R.K.G.; Togashi, K. Convolutional neural networks: An overview and application in radiology. *Insights Imaging* **2018**, *9*, 611–629. [CrossRef]
21. Kumar, M.; Bhandari, A.K. Contrast Enhancement Using Novel White Balancing Parameter Optimization for Perceptually Invisible Images. *IEEE Trans. Image Process.* **2020**, *29*, 7525–7536. [CrossRef]
22. Niu, Y.; Wu, X.; Shi, G. Image Enhancement by Entropy Maximization and Quantization Resolution Upconversion. *IEEE Trans. Image Process.* **2016**, *25*, 4815–4828. [CrossRef]
23. Veluchamy, M.; Bhandari, A.K.; Subramani, B. Optimized Bezier Curve Based Intensity Mapping Scheme for Low Light Image Enhancement. *IEEE Trans. Emerg. Top. Comput. Intell.* **2021**, *6*, 602–612. [CrossRef]

24. Pizer, S.M. Contrast-limited adaptive histogram equalization: Speed and effectiveness stephen m. pizer, r. eugene johnston, james p. ericksen, bonnie c. yankaskas, keith e. muller medical image display research group. In Proceedings of the First Conference on Visualization in Biomedical Computing, Atlanta, GA, USA, 22–25 May 1990; Volume 337, p. 2.
25. Singh, K.; Kapoor, R. Image enhancement using Exposure based Sub Image Histogram Equalization. *Pattern Recognit. Lett.* **2014**, *36*, 10–14. [CrossRef]
26. Kansal, S.; Tripathi, R.K. New adaptive histogram equalisation heuristic approach for contrast enhancement. *IET Image Process.* **2020**, *14*, 1110–1119. [CrossRef]
27. Yang, K.-F.; Zhang, X.-S.; Li, Y.-J. A Biological Vision Inspired Framework for Image Enhancement in Poor Visibility Conditions. *IEEE Trans. Image Process.* **2019**, *29*, 1493–1506. [CrossRef]
28. Arici, T.; Dikbas, S.; Altunbasak, Y. A Histogram Modification Framework and Its Application for Image Contrast Enhance-ment. *IEEE Trans. Image Process.* **2009**, *18*, 1921–1935. [CrossRef]
29. Mishra, M.; Menon, H.; Mukherjee, A. Characterization of S1 and S2 Heart Sounds Using Stacked Autoencoder and Convo-lutional Neural Network. *IEEE Trans. Instrum. Meas.* **2018**, *68*, 3211–3220. [CrossRef]
30. Simonyan, K.; Zisserman, A. Very deep convolutional networks for large-scale image recognition. *arXiv* **2014**, arXiv:1409.1556.
31. Li, H.-Y.; Dong, L.; Zhou, W.-D.; Wu, H.-T.; Zhang, R.-H.; Li, Y.-T.; Yu, C.-Y.; Wei, W.-B. Development and validation of medical record-based logistic regression and machine learning models to diagnose diabetic retinopathy. *Graefe's Arch. Clin. Exp. Ophthalmol.* **2022**, *261*, 681–689. [CrossRef]
32. Tsao, H.Y.; Chan, P.Y.; Su, E.C.Y. Predicting diabetic retinopathy and identifying interpretable biomedical features using machine learning algorithms. *BMC Bioinform.* **2018**, *19*, 111–121. [CrossRef]
33. Bhatia, K.; Arora, S.; Tomar, R. Diagnosis of diabetic retinopathy using machine learning classification algorithm. In Proceedings of the 2016 2nd International Conference on Next Generation Computing Technologies (NGCT), Dehradun, India, 14–16 October 2016; IEEE: New York, NY, USA, 2016; pp. 347–351.
34. Chen, Y.; Hu, X.; Fan, W.; Shen, L.; Zhang, Z.; Liu, X.; Du, J.; Li, H.; Chen, Y.; Li, H. Fast density peak clustering for large scale data based on kNN. *Knowl.-Based Syst.* **2019**, *187*, 104824. [CrossRef]
35. Cao, K.; Xu, J.; Zhao, W.Q. Artificial intelligence on diabetic retinopathy diagnosis: An automatic classification method based on grey level co-occurrence matrix and naive Bayesian model. *Int. J. Ophthalmol.* **2019**, *12*, 1158. [CrossRef]
36. Alzami, F.; Megantara, R.A.; Fanani, A.Z. Diabetic retinopathy grade classification based on fractal analysis and random forest. In Proceedings of the 2019 International Seminar on Application for Technology of Information and Communication (iSemantic), Se-marang, Indonesia, 21–22 September 2019; IEEE: New York, NY, USA, 2019; pp. 272–276.
37. Yu, S.; Tan, K.K.; Sng, B.L.; Li, S.; Sia, A.T.H. Lumbar Ultrasound Image Feature Extraction and Classification with Support Vector Machine. *Ultrasound Med. Biol.* **2015**, *41*, 2677–2689. [CrossRef]
38. Seoud, L.; Chelbi, J.; Cheriet, F. Automatic grading of diabetic retinopathy on a public database. In Proceedings of the Ophthalmic Medical Image Analysis International Workshop, Munich, Germany, 8 October 2015; University of Iowa: Iowa City, IA, USA, 2015; Volume 2. No. 2015.
39. Savarkar, S.P.; Kalkar, N.; Tade, S.L. Diabetic retinopathy using image processing detection, classification and analysis. *Int. J. Adv. Comput. Res.* **2013**, *3*, 285.
40. Gondal, W.M.; Kohler, J.M.; Grzeszick, R.; Fink, G.A.; Hirsch, M. Weakly-supervised localization of diabetic retinopathy lesions in retinal fundus images. In Proceedings of the 2017 IEEE International Conference on Image Processing (ICIP), Beijing, China, 17–20 September 2017; pp. 2069–2073. [CrossRef]
41. Wang, Z.; Yin, Y.; Shi, J.; Fang, W.; Li, H.; Wang, X. Zoom-in-net: Deep mining lesions for diabetic retinopathy detection. In *Medical Image Computing and Computer Assisted Intervention—MICCAI 2017, Proceedings of the 20th International Conference, Quebec City, QC, Canada, 11–13 September 2017*; Springer International Publishing: Cham, Switzerland, 2017; pp. 267–275, Proceedings, Part III 20.
42. Chandrakumar, T.; Kathirvel, R.J.I.J.E.R.T. Classifying diabetic retinopathy using deep learning architecture. *Int. J. Eng. Res. Technol.* **2016**, *5*, 19–24.
43. Yang, Y.; Li, T.; Li, W.; Wu, H.; Fan, W.; Zhang, W. Lesion detection and grading of diabetic retinopathy via two-stages deep convolutional neural networks. In *Medical Image Computing and Computer Assisted Intervention—MICCAI 2017, Proceedings of the 20th International Conference, Quebec City, QC, Canada, 11–13 September 2017*; Springer International Publishing: Cham, Swit-zerland, 2017; pp. 533–540, Proceedings, Part III 20.

Disclaimer/Publisher's Note: The statements, opinions and data contained in all publications are solely those of the individual author(s) and contributor(s) and not of MDPI and/or the editor(s). MDPI and/or the editor(s) disclaim responsibility for any injury to people or property resulting from any ideas, methods, instructions or products referred to in the content.

MDPI
St. Alban-Anlage 66
4052 Basel
Switzerland
www.mdpi.com

Diagnostics Editorial Office
E-mail: diagnostics@mdpi.com
www.mdpi.com/journal/diagnostics

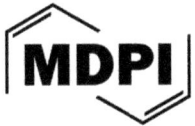

Disclaimer/Publisher's Note: The statements, opinions and data contained in all publications are solely those of the individual author(s) and contributor(s) and not of MDPI and/or the editor(s). MDPI and/or the editor(s) disclaim responsibility for any injury to people or property resulting from any ideas, methods, instructions or products referred to in the content.

www.ingramcontent.com/pod-product-compliance
Lightning Source LLC
LaVergne TN
LVHW070736100526
838202LV00013B/1248